FOOTFALLS

ON THE

BOUNDARY OF ANOTHER WORLD.

WITH NARRATIVE ILLUSTRATIONS.

BY

ROBERT DALE OWEN.

FORMERLY MEMBER OF CONGRESS, AND AMERICAN MINISTER TO NAPLES.

"As it is the peculiar method of the Academy to interpose no personal judgment, but to admit those opinions which appear most probable, to compare arguments, and to set forth all that may be reasonably stated in favor of each proposition, and so, without obtruding any authority of its own, to leave the judgment of the hearers free and unprejudiced, we will retain this custom which has been handed down from Socrates; and this method, dear brother Quintus, if you please, we will adopt, as often as possible, in all our dialogues together."—CICERO *de Divin. Lib.* ii. §72.

PHILADELPHIA:

J. B. LIPPINCOTT & CO.

1868.

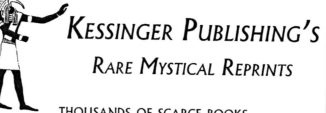
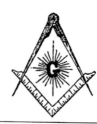

PREFACE.

It may interest the reader, before perusing this volume, to know some of the circumstances which preceded and produced it.

The subjects of which it treats came originally under my notice in a land where, except to the privileged foreigner, such subjects are interdicted,—at Naples, in the autumn of 1855. Up to that period I had regarded the whole as a delusion which no prejudice, indeed, would have prevented my examining with care, but in which, lacking such examination, I had no faith whatever.

To an excellent friend and former colleague, the Viscount de St. Amaro, Brazilian Minister at Naples, I shall ever remain debtor for having first won my serious attention to phenomena of a magneto-psychological character and to the study of analogous subjects. It was in his apartments, on the 4th of March, 1856, and in presence of himself and his lady, together with a member of the royal family of Naples, that I witnessed for the first time, with mingled feelings of surprise and incredulity, certain physical movements apparently without material agency. Three weeks later, during an evening at the Russian Minister's, an incident occurred, as we say, fortuitously, which, after the strictest scrutiny, I found myself unable to explain without referring it to some intelligent agency foreign to the spectators present,—not one of whom, it may be added, knew or had practiced any thing connected with what is called Spiritualism or mediumship. From that day I determined to test the matter thoroughly. My public duties left me, in winter, few leisure hours, but many during the summer and autumn months; and that leisure, throughout more than two years, I devoted to an investigation (conducted partly by personal ob-

3

servations made in domestic privacy, partly by means of books) of the great question whether agencies from another phase of existence ever intervene here, and operate, for good or evil, on mankind.

For a time the observations I made were similar to those which during the last ten years so many thousands have instituted in our country and in Europe, and my reading was restricted to works for and against Animal Magnetism and for and against the modern Spiritual theory. But, as the field opened before me, I found it expedient to enlarge my sphere of research,—to consult the best professional works on Physiology, especially in its connection with mental phenomena, on Psychology in general, on Sleep, on Hallucination, on Insanity, on the great Mental Epidemics of Europe and America, together with treatises on the Imponderables,—including Reichenbach's curious observations, and the records of interesting researches recently made in Prussia, in Italy, in England and elsewhere, on the subject of Human Electricity in connection with its influence on the nervous system and the muscular tissues.

I collected, too, the most noted old works containing narrative collections of apparitions, hauntings, presentiments, and the like, accompanied by dissertations on the Invisible World, and toiled through formidable piles of chaff to reach a few gleanings of sound grain.

Gradually I became convinced that what by many have been regarded as new and unexampled phenomena are but modern phases of what has ever existed. And I ultimately reached the conclusion that, in order to a proper understanding of much that has excited and perplexed the public mind under the name of Spiritual Manifestations, historical research should precede every other inquiry,—that we ought to look throughout the past for classes of phenomena, and seek to arrange these, each in its proper niche.

I was finally satisfied, also, that it behooved the student in this field (in the first instance, at least) to devote his attention to spontaneous phenomena, rather than to those that are evoked,—to appearances and disturbances that present themselves occasionally only, it is true, but neither sought nor looked for; like the rainbow, or the Aurora Porealis, or the wind that bloweth where it listeth, uncontrolled by the wishes or the agency of man. By restricting the inquiry to these, all suspicion of being misled by epidemic excitement or expectant attention is completely set aside.

A record of such phenomena, carefully selected and authenticated, constitutes the staple of the present volume. In putting it forth, I am not to be held, any more than is the naturalist or the astronomer, to the imputation of tampering with holy things. As regards the special purpose of this work, no charge of necromantic efforts or unlawful seeking need be met, since it cannot possibly apply. The accusation, if any be brought, will be of a different character. If suspicion I incur, it will be not of sorcery, but of superstition,—of an endeavor, perhaps, to revive popular delusions which the lights of modern science have long since dispelled, or of stooping to put forth as grave relations of fact what are no better than idle nursery-tales.

Accepting this issue, I am content to put myself on the country. I demand a fair trial before a jury who have not prejudged the cause. I ask for my witnesses a patient hearing, well assured that the final verdict, be it as it may, will be in accordance with reason and justice.

I aspire not to build up a theory. I doubt, as to this subject, whether any man living is yet prepared to do so. My less ambitious endeavor is to collect together solid, reliable building-stones which may serve some future architect. Already beyond middle age, it is not likely that I shall continue here long enough to see the edifice erected. But others may. The race endures, though the individual pass to another stage of existence.

If I did not esteem my subject one of vast importance, I should be unworthy to approach its treatment. Had I found other writers bestowing upon it the attention which that importance merits, I should have remained silent. As it is, I have felt, with a modern author, that "the withholding of large truths from the world may be a betrayal of the greatest trust."*

I am conscious, on the other hand, that one is ever apt to

---

* "*Friends in Council,*" Art. Truth.

1*

overestimate the importance of one's own labors. Yet even an effort such as this may suffice to give public opinion a true or a false direction. Great results are sometimes determined by humble agencies. "A ridge-tile of a cottage in Derbyshire," says Gisborne, "decides whether the rain which falls from heaven shall be directed to the German Ocean or the Atlantic."

Let the reader, before he enters on the inquiry whether ultramundane interference be a great reality or a portentous delusion, permit me one additional remark. He will find that, in treating that hypothesis, I have left many things obscure and uninterpreted. Where no theory was clearly indicated, I preferred to state the facts and waive all explanation, having reached that period of life when, if good use has been made of past years, one is not ashamed to say, "I do not know," in any case in which that is the simple truth. We do well, however, to bear in mind that a difficulty unsolved does not amount to an argument in opposition.*

To the many friends whose kindness has aided my undertaking, these pages owe their chief value. To some therein named I am enabled here to tender my grateful acknowledgments. To others who have assisted in private I am not less deeply indebted.

I doubt not that if I were to delay the publication of this book for some years I should find much to modify, something to retract. But if, in this world, we postpone our work till we deem it perfect, death comes upon us in our hesitation, and we effect nothing, from bootless anxiety to effect too much.

R. D. O.

₊ On page 511 will be found "Addenda to the Tenth Thousand."

---

* "Where we cannot answer all objections, we are bound, in reason and in candor, to adopt the hypothesis which labors under the least."—"*Elements of Logic*," by Archbishop Whately.

"That is accounted probable which has better argument producible for it than can be brought against it."—South.

TABLE OF CONTENTS.

BOOK I.

PRELIMINARY.

CHAPTER I.

Is ultramundane interference reality, or delusion?—The inquiry practical, but hitherto discouraged—Time an essential element—Isaac Taylor—Jung Stilling—Swedenborg—Animal Magnetism—Arago's opinion—Dr. Carpenter's admissions—The American epidemic—Phenomena independent of opinions—Sentiment linked to action—The home on the other side—Hades—Johnson's, Byron's, Addison's, and Steele's opinions—Truth in every rank—The Ghost-Club—Contempt corrects not—Spiritualism an influential element—Dangers of over-credulity—Demoniac manifestations—Reason the appointed pilot—Duty of research—How dispose of spontaneous phenomena?—Martin Korky—Courage and impartiality demanded—A besetting temptation—Feeble belief—Skepticism—Georget's conversion—Evidence of sense—Some truths appeal to consciousness—Severe test applied to the subject selected.

CHAPTER II.

Columbus in Barcelona—The marvel of marvels—Presumption—There may be laws not yet in operation—Modern study of the imponderables—Arago's and Cuvier's admissions—What may be.

CHAPTER III.

Modern miracles rejected—Hume—The Indian prince—Definition of a miracle—Change-bearing laws—Illustration from

BOOK III.

DISTURBANCES POPULARLY TERMED HAUNTINGS.

CHAPTER I.

No proof of gaudy supernaturalism—A startling element presents itself—Poltergeister—What we find, not what we may expect to find—Ancient haunted houses.

CHAPTER II.

Disturbances at Tedworth—First example of responding of the sounds—Glanvil's observations—Mr. Mompesson's attestation—The Wesley disturbances—John Wesley's narrative—Emily Wesley's narrative, and her experience thirty-four years later—Opinions of Dr. Clarke, Dr. Priestley, Southey, and Coleridge—The New Havensack case—Mrs. Golding and her maid—The Castle of Slawensik—Disturbances in Silesia—Dr. Kerner's inquiries—Councilor Hahn's attestation—Twenty-five years after—Disturbances in the dwelling of the Seeress of Prevorst—Displacement of house-rafters—The law-suit—Disturbances legally attested—The farm-house of Baldarroch—An alleged discovery—The cre-

CHAPTER II.

How Senator Linn's life was saved—Was it clairvoyance, or prescience?—Help amid the snow-drifts—Unexpected consolation—Gaspar—The rejected suitor—Is spiritual guardianship an unholy or incredible hypothesis?

BOOK VI.

THE SUGGESTED RESULTS.

CHAPTER I.

A theory must not involve absurd results—Whence can the dead return?—Character but slightly changed at death—Spiritual theory involves two postulates—Hades swept out along with purgatory—How the matter stands historically—The Grecian Hades—The Jewish Sheol—What becomes of the soul immediately after death?—An abrupt metamorphosis?—A final doom, or a state of progress?—How human character is formed here—The postulates rational—What has resulted from discarding Hades—Enfeebling effect of distance—The loss of identity—The conception of two lives—Man cannot sympathize with that for which he is not prepared—The virtuous reasonably desire and expect another stage of action—Human instincts too little studied—Man's nature and his situation—The Ideal—The utterings of the presaging voice—Man remains, after death, a human creature—Footfalls—A master-influence in another world—We are journeying toward a land of love and truth—What death is—What obtains the rites of sepulture.

CHAPTER II.

Admissions demanded by reason—The invisible and inaudible world—We may expect outlines rather than filling up—Man's choice becomes his judge—Pneumatology of the Bible—More light hereafter.

LIST OF AUTHORS CITED.

Abercrombie. Intellectual Powers.

Abrantès, Mémoires de Madame la Duchesse de, écrits par elle-même, Paris, 1835.

Account of the French Prophets and their Pretended Inspirations, London, 1708.

Alexander ab Alexandro; about 1450.

Arago. Biographie de Jean-Sylvain Bailly, Paris, 1853.

Aristotle. De Divinatione et Somniis.

Aubrey's Miscellanies.

Babbage. Ninth Bridgewater Treatise, London, 1838.

Bacon's Essays, London, 1597.

Baillarger. Des Hallucinations.

Bailly. Report on Mesmerism, made to the King of France, August 11, 1784.

Baxter. The Certainty of the World of Spirits, London, 1691.

Beaumont. An Historical, Physiological, and Theological Treatise of Spirits, London, 1705.

Beecher, Rev. Charles. Review of Spiritual Manifestations.

Bennett, Professor. The Mesmeric Mania, Edinburgh, 1851.

Bertrand. Traité du Somnambulisme, Paris, 1823.

Bichât. Récherches Physiologiques sur la Vie et la Mort, Paris, 1805.

Binns, Edward, M.D. The Anatomy of Sleep, 2d ed., London, 1845.

Blackstone's Commentaries.

Boismont, De. Des Hallucinations, Paris, 1852.

Bovet. The Devil's Cloyster, 1684.

Braid, James. Neurypnology, or the Rationale of Sleep, London, 1843.

Brewster, Sir David. The Martyrs of Science, London, 1856.

Brodie, Sir B. Psychological Inquiries, 3d ed., London, 1856.

Browne, Sir Thomas. Works.

Burdach. Traité de Physiologie, Paris, 1839.

Bushnell, Horace. Nature and the Supernatural, New York, 1858.

Butler's Analogy of Religion to the Constitution and Course of Nature.

Calmeil. De la Folie, Paris, 1845.

Capron. Modern Spiritualism, Boston, 1853.

Carlyon, Clement, M.D. Early Years and Late Reflections.

Carpenter, William B., M.D. Principles of Human Physiology, 5th ed., 1855.

Causes Célèbres.

Chalmers's Evidences of the Christian Religion.

Chaucer's Tale of the Chanon Yeman.

Christmas, Rev. Henry. Cradle of the Twin Giants, Science and History, London, 1849.

Cicero de Divinatione.
      de Naturâ Deorum.

Clairon, Mémoires de Mademoiselle, Actrice du Théatre Français, écrits par elle-même, Paris, 1822.

Clarke, Dr. Memoirs of the Wesley Family, 2d ed., London, 1843.

Coleridge's Lay Sermons.

Court, M. Histoire des Troubles des Cevennes, Alais, 1819.

Crowe, Catherine. Night Side of Nature, 1848. Ghosts and Family Legends, 1859.

Cuvier. Leçons d'Anatomie comparée.

Dechambre. Analyse de l'Ouvrage du Docteur Szafkowski sur les Hallucinations, 1850.

De Foe, Daniel. Universal History of Apparitions, London, 1727.

Dendy, W. C. Philosophy of Mystery.

Du Bois-Reymond. Untersuchungen über thierische Elektricität, Berlin, 1848–49.

Eclipse of Faith.

Edwards, Henry, D.D. The Doctrine of the Supernatural Established, London, 1845.

Ennemoser. Geschichte der Magie, Leipzig, 1844.

Essays written during the Intervals of Business, London, 1853.

Faraday. Experimental Researches in Chemistry and Physics, London, 1859.

Ferriar, John, M.D. Essay towards a Theory of Apparitions.

Foissac. Rapports et Discussions de l'Academie Royale de Médecine sur le Magnetisme Animal, Paris, 1833.

Friends in Council, London.

Garinet. Histoire de la Magie en France.

Gasparin, Comte de. Des Tables tournantes, du Surnaturel en Général, et des Esprits, Paris, 1855.

Georget. De la Physiologie du Système nerveux, Paris, 1821.

Glanvil. Sadducismus Triumphatus, 3d ed., London, 1689.

Goethe. Aus meinem Leben.

Grose, Francis, F.A.S. Provincial Glossary and Popular Superstition, London, 1790.

Hare, Robert, M.D. Experimental Examination of the Spirit-Manifestations, 4th ed., New York, 1856.

Hazlitt's Round Table.

Herschel, Sir John. Preliminary Discourse on the Study of Natural History, 2d ed., London, 1851.

Histoire des Diables de Loudun, Amsterdam, 1693.

Holland. Chapters on Mental Physiology, London, 1852.

Huidekoper, Frederick. The Belief of the First Three Centuries concerning Christ's Mission to the Underworld.

Humboldt, Baron. Cosmos.

Versuche über die gereizte Muskel- und Nervenfaser.

Hume's Essays.

Insulanus, Theophilus. Treatise on Second-Sight, Dreams, and Apparitions, Edinburgh, 1763.

Johnson's Rasselas.

Jones, Bence, M.D. On Animal Electricity: being an Abstract of the Discoveries of Émil Du Bois-Reymond, London, 1852.

Kepleri Epistolæ.

Kerner, Justinus. Die Seherin von Prevorst, 4th ed., Stuttgart, 1846.

Kerr, Robert. Memoirs of the Life of William Smellie, Edinburgh, 1811.

La Flèche. La Démonomanie de Loudun, 1634.

La Place. Théorie analytique des Probabilités, Paris, 1847.

Locke on the Human Understanding.

Macario. Du Sommeil, des Rêves, et du Somnambulisme, Lyons, 1857.

Mackay's Popular Delusions.

Macnish. Philosophy of Sleep.

Martin. Description of the Western Islands of Scotland, London, 1706.

Matteucci, Carlo. Traite des Phénomènes électro-physiologiques des Animaux, 1844.

Mayo, Herbert. On the Truths contained in Popular Superstitions, Edinburgh and London, 1851.

Ménardaye, M. de la. Examen et Discussions critiques de l'Histoire des Diables de Loudun, Paris, 1747.

Mirville, Marquis de. Des Esprits, et de leurs Manifestations fluidiques, 3d ed., Paris, 1854.

Misson. Théatre sacré des Cevennes, London, 1707.

Montgéron, Carré de. La Vérité des Miracles opérés par l'Intercession de M. de Pâris, 2d ed., Cologne, 1745.

Müller's Manuel de Physiologie, Paris, 1845.

Neander's Church History.

Plautus' Mostellaria, a Comedy.

Priestley, Dr. Original Letters by the Rev. John Wesley and his Friends, London, 1791.

Racine. Abrégé de l'Histoire de Port-Royal, Paris, 1693.

Raikes, Thomas. A Portion of the Journal kept by, London, 1856.

Reichenbach. Untersuchungen über die Dynamide.

Sensitive Mensch.

Reid's Essays on the Mind.

Réponse à l'Examen de la Possession des Religieuses de Louviers, Rouen, 1643.

Report of the Mysterious Noises at Hydesville, Canandaigua, April, 1848.

Ricard. Traité du Magnetisme Animal.

Rogers' Table-Talk.

Rogers, E. C. Philosophy of Mysterious Agents, Human and Mundane, Boston, 1853.

Roman Ritual.

Roscoe, William. The Life of Lorenzo de' Medici.

Rutter. Animal Electricity.

Scheffer. Histoire de Laponie, Paris, 1778.

Scott, Sir Walter. Letters on Demonology and Witchcraft, 2d ed., 1857.

Sears, Edmund H. Foregleams of Immortality, 4th ed., Boston, 1858.

Siljeström. Minnesfest öfver Berzelius, Stockholm, 1849.

Sinclair. Satan's Invisible World Discovered, Edinburgh, 1789.

Spectator for July 6, 1711.

Spicer. Facts and Fantasies, London, 1853.

Stilling, Jung. Theorie der Geisterkunde, 1809.

Stöber. Vie de J. F. Oberlin.

Strahan, Rev. George, D.D. Prayers and Meditations of Dr. Samuel Johnson, London, 1785.

Strauss. Life of Jesus.

Taylor, Isaac. Physical Theory of Another Life, London, 1839.

Taylor, Joseph. Danger of Premature Interment.

Theologia Mystica, ad usum Directorum Animarum, Paris, 1848.

Tillotson's Sermons.

Tissot, le Père. Histoire Abrégée de la Possession des Ursulines de Loudun, Paris, 1828.

Torquemada. Flores Curiosas, Salamanca, 1570.

Walton, Isaac. The Lives of Dr. John Donne, Sir Henry Wotton, &c., Oxford edition, 1824.

Warton's History of English Poetry.

Welby, Horace. Signs before Death, London, 1825.

Whately, Archbishop. Historic Doubts relative to Napoleon Buonaparte 12th ed., London, 1853.

Whately, Archbishop. Elements of Logic.

Wigan. Duality of the Mind, London, 1844.

Wraxall, Sir N. William. Historical Memoirs of my Own Time.

FOOTFALLS

ON THE

BOUNDARY OF ANOTHER WORLD.

BOOK I.

PRELIMINARY.

CHAPTER I.

STATEMENT OF THE SUBJECT.

"As I did ever hold, there mought be as great a vanitie in retiring and withdrawing men's conceites (except they bee of some nature) from the world as in obtruding them; so, in these particulars, I have played myself the Inquisitor, and find nothing to my understanding in them contrarie or infectious to the state of Religion or manners, but rather, as I suppose, medecinable."—BACON: *Dedication to Essays*, 1597.

IN an age so essentially utilitarian as the present, no inquiry is likely to engage the permanent attention of the public, unless it be practical in its bearings.

Even then, if the course of such inquiry lead to the examination of extraordinary phenomena, it will be found that evidence the most direct, apparently sufficing to prove the reality of these, will usually leave the minds of men incredulous, or in doubt, if the appearances be of isolated character, devoid of authentic precedent in the past, and incapable of classification, in the proper niche, among analogous results; much more, in case they involve a suspension of the laws of nature.

If I entertain a hope of winning the public ear, while
I broach, broadly and frankly, the question whether
occasional interferences from another world in this be
reality or delusion, it is, first, because I feel confident
in being able to show that the inquiry is of a practical
nature; and, secondly, because the phenomena which I
purpose to examine in connection with it are not of isolated, still less of miraculous, character. In the etymo-
logical sense of the term, they are not *unlikely*, there
being many of their like to be found adequately attested
throughout history. They appear in groups, and lend
themselves, like all other natural phenomena, to classification.

Extraordinary, even astounding, they will usually be
considered; and that, not so much because they are
really uncommon, as because they have been, in a measure, kept out of sight. And this again arises, in part,
because few dispassionate observers have patiently
examined them; in part, because prejudice, which discredits them, has prevented thousands to whom they
have presented themselves from bearing public or even
private testimony to what they have witnessed; in part,
again, because, although these phenomena are by no
means of modern origin, or determined by laws but
recently operative, they appear to have much increased
in frequency and variety, and to have reached a new
stage of development, in the last few years; and finally,
because they are such as readily stir up in weak minds
blind credulity or superstitious terror, the prolific
sources of extravagance and exaggeration. Thus the
intelligent conceal and the ignorant misstate them.

This condition of things complicates the subject, and
much increases the difficulty of treating it.

Again: though no article of human faith is better
founded than the belief in the ultimate prevalence of
truth, yet, in every thing relating to earthly progress,

time enters as an essential element. The fruit drops not till it has ripened: if nipped by early blight or plucked by premature hand it is imperfect and worthless. And the world of mind, like that of physical nature, has its seasons: its spring, when the sap rises and the buds swell; its summer, of opened flower and blossom; its autumn, of yellow grain. We must not expect to reap, in any field, until harvest-time.

Yet, how gradual soever time's innovations and the corresponding progress of the human mind, there are certain epochs at which, by what our short sight calls chance, particular subjects spring forth into notice, as it were, by a sudden impulse, attracting general attention, and thus predisposing men's minds to engage in their investigation. At such epochs, words that at other times would fall unheeded may sink deep and bear good fruit.

It seldom happens, however, at the first outbreak of any great excitement, when some strange novelty seems bursting on the world, that the minds of men, whether of supporters or of opponents, maintain due moderation, either in assent or in denial. The hasty ardor of new-born zeal, and the sense, quick to offense when first impinged upon, of prejudice long dominant, alike indispose to calm inquiry, are alike unfavorable to critical judgment.

And thus, at the present day, perhaps, (when the din of the earliest onset has subsided and the still small voice can be heard,) rather than at any period of the last ten years, during which our country has witnessed the rise and progress of what may be called a revival of Pneumatology, may the subject be discussed with less of passion and received with diminished prejudice. And if a writer, in treating of it at this juncture, escape some of those shoals upon which earlier inquirers have stranded, it may be due as much to a happy selection of time, as to any especial merit or superior discernment.

Then, too, as to the great question of which I purpose to examine the probabilities, recent events have not only enlisted the attention of the audience : they have also, in a measure, opened way for the speaker. The strictness of the taboo is relaxed. And this was greatly to be desired. For the inquiry touching the probability of ultramundane intervention—though it cannot be said to have been lost sight of at any moment since the dawn of civilization, though Scripture affirm it as to former ages, and though, throughout later times, often in various superstitious shapes, it has challenged the terrors of the ignorant—had seemed, for a century past, to be gradually losing credit and reputable standing, and to be doomed to exclusion from respectable society or philosophical circles. Able men cared not to jeopard a reputation for common sense by meddling with it at all.

With honorable exceptions, however. Of these I have met with none so original in thought, so philosophic in spirit, as Isaac Taylor. Yet he has treated, with a master's hand, one branch only of the subject,—the analogical.*

Another portion of this field of research has been partially occupied, from time to time, by a class of writers, often German, usually set down as superstitious dreamers; of which Jung Stilling, perhaps, is one of the fairest examples.† Pious, earnest, able, of a pro-

---

* *"Physical Theory of Another Life,"* by the Author of the "Natural History of Enthusiasm," (Isaac Taylor,) 1 vol. 12mo, pp. 336. London, 1839.

† *"Theorie der Geisterkunde,"* ("Theory of Spiritualism," or, literally, of Spirit-Knowledge,) by Jung Stilling, originally published in 1809. Johann Heinrich Jung, better known by his adjunct name of Stilling, born in the Duchy of Nassau in 1740, rose from poverty and the humblest position to ne, first, Professor of Political Economy at Heidelberg, and afterward a member of the Aulic Council of the Grand Duke of Baden.

bity beyond suspicion, but somewhat mystical withal, the Aulic Councilor of Baden sought proofs of his speculations in alleged actual occurrences, (as apparitions, house-hauntings, and the like,) the records of which he adopted, and thereupon erected his spirit-theory with a facility of belief for which the apparent evidence seems, in many of the examples cited, to be insufficient warrant. In our day others have pursued a similar line of argument; in one instance, at least, if sixteen editions in six years may vouch for the fact, attracting the sympathy of the public.*

Jacob Böhme is by some exalted to the highest rank among pneumatologists; but I confess to inability to discover much that is practical, or even intelligible, in the mystical effusions of the worthy shoemaker of Görlitz. The fault, however, may be in myself; for, as some one has said, "He is ever the mystic who lives in the world farthest removed from our own."

Swedenborg, the great spiritualist of the eighteenth century, is a writer as to whose voluminous works it would be presumptuous to offer an opinion without a careful study of them; and that I have not yet been able to give. This, however, one may safely assert,—that whatever judgment we may pass on what the Swedish seer calls his spiritual experience, and how little soever we may be prepared to subscribe to the exclusive claims unwisely set up for him by some of his disciples, an eminent spirit and power speak from his writings, which, even at a superficial glance, must arrest the attention of the right-minded. His idea of Degrees and Progression, reaching from earth to heaven; his doctrine of Uses, equally removed from ascetical dreamery and from Utilitarianism in its hard, modern sense; his allegation of Influx, or, in other words, of constant influence exerted from the spiritual world on the material; even his strange theory of Correspondences; but, last and chief, his glowing appreciation of that principle of Love which is the fulfilling of the Law; these and other kindred characteristics of the Swedenborgian system are of too deep and genuine import to be lightly passed by. To claim for them nothing more, they are at least marvelously suggestive, and therefore highly valuable.

For the rest, one may appreciate Swedenborg outside of Swedenborgianism. "For ourselves," said Margaret Fuller, "it is not as a seer of Ghosts, but as a seer of Truths, that Swedenborg interests us."

* "*Night Side of Nature,*" by Catherine Crowe, London, 1 vol. 12mo, pp. 502. The work, originally published in 1848, reached its sixteenth thousand in 1854. In common with the older narrative collections of Glanvil, Mather, Baxter, Beaumont, Sinclair, De Foe, and others of similar stamp,

It may be conceded, however, that these narratives
have commonly been read rather to amuse an idle hour
than for graver purpose. They have often excited
wonder, seldom produced conviction. But this, as I
think, is due, not to actual insufficiency in this field,
but rather, first, to an unphilosophical manner of presenting the subject,—a talking of wonders and miracles,
when there was question only of natural, even if ultramundane, phenomena; and, secondly, to an indiscri-
minate mixing-up of the reliable with the apocryphal,
to lack of judgment in selection and of industry in verification. I have not scrupled freely to cull from this
department; seeking, however, to separate the wheat
from the chaff, and content, in so doing, even if the available material that remains shall have shrunk to somewhat petty dimensions.

Essentially connected with this inquiry, and to be
studied by all who engage therein, are the phenomena
embraced in what is usually called Animal Magnetism.
First showing itself in France, three-quarters of a century
ago, its progress arrested at the outset, when its claims
were vague and its chief phenomena as yet unobserved,
by the celebrated report of Bailly,* often falling into

---

it is obnoxious to the same criticism as that of Stilling; yet any one who
feels disposed to cast the volume aside as a mere idle trumping-up of ghost-
stories might do well first to read its Introduction, and its Tenth Chapter on
"the future that awaits us."

A recent volume by the same author ("Ghosts and Family Legends,"
1859) makes no pretension to authenticity, nor to any higher purpose
than to help while away a winter evening.

* Made to the King of France, on the 11th of August, 1784. It was
signed, among other members of the commission, by Franklin and Lavoisier.

It should especially be borne in mind that, while the commissioners, in
that report, speak in strong terms against the magnetism of 1784, with its
baquets, its *crises*, and its convulsions,—against Mesmer's theory, too, of
a universal fluid with flux and reflux, the medium of influence by the celestial
bodies on the human system, and a universal curative agent,—they express
no opinion whatever, favorable or unfavorable, in regard to somnambulism

the hands of untrained and superficial observers, sometimes of arrant charlatans, its pretensions extravagantly
stated by some and arrogantly denied by others, Animal
Magnetism has won its way through the errors of its

---

properly so called. It is usually admitted that somnambulism, with its attendant phenomena, in the form now known to us, was observed, for the first time,
by the Marquis de Puységur, on his estate of Buzancy, near Soissons, on the 4th
of March, 1784; but Puységur made public his observations only at the close
of that year, four months after the commissioners' report was made. Bailly
and his associates, learned and candid as they were, must not be cited as
condemning that which they had never seen nor heard of. To this fact
Arago, a man who rose superior to the common prejudices of his associates,
honestly testifies. I translate from his notice of the life and career of the
unfortunate Bailly, published in the "Annuaire du Bureau des Longitudes"
for 1853. "The report of Bailly," says he, "upset from their foundations the
ideas, the system, the practice, of Mesmer and his disciples: let us add, in
all sincerity, that we have no right to evoke its authority against modern
somnambulism. Most of the phenomena now grouped around that name
were neither known nor announced in 1783. A magnetizer undoubtedly
says one of the least probable things in the world, when he tells us that
such an individual, in a state of somnambulism, can see every thing in perfect darkness, or read through a wall, or even without the aid of the eyes.
But the improbability of such assertions does not result from the celebrated
report. Bailly does not notice such marvels, either to assert or to deny
them. The naturalist, the physician, or the mere curious investigator, who
engages in somnambulic experiments, who thinks it his duty to inquire
whether, in certain states of nervous excitement, individuals are really
endowed with extraordinary faculties,—that, for instance, of reading through
the epigastrium or the heel,—who desires to ascertain positively up to what
point the phenomena announced with so much assurance by modern magnetizers belong only to the domain of the rogue or the conjurer,—all such
inquirers, we say, are not in this case running counter to a judgment rendered; they are not really opposing themselves to a Lavoisier, a Franklin, a
Bailly. They are entering upon a world entirely new, the very existence
of which these illustrious sages did not suspect."—(pp. 444–445.)

A little further on in the same article, Arago adds, "My object has been
to show that somnambulism ought not to be rejected a priori, especially by
those who have kept up with the progress of modern physical science."
And, in reproof of that presumption which so often denies without examining, he quotes these excellent lines, which, he says, the truly learned ought
to bear constantly in mind:—

" Croire tout découvert est une erreur profonde ;

C'est prendre l'horizon pour les bornes du monde."

friends and the denunciations of its enemies, and (what is harder yet to combat) through frequent mystifications by impostors and occasional gross abuse of its powers, to the notice and the researches of men of unquestioned talent and standing,—among them, eminent members of the medical profession,—and has at last obtained a modest place even in accredited and popular treatises on physiological science.*

The alleged proofs and analogical arguments above alluded to in favor of ultramundane intercourse, together with such corroboration as the phenomena of somnambulism afford, were all given to the world previous to the time when, in the obscure village of Hydesville, a young girl,† responding to the persistent knockings which for several nights had broken the rest of her mother and sisters, chanced upon the discovery that

---

* An example may be found in "Principles of Human Physiology," by William B. Carpenter, M.D., F.R.S. and F.G.S., 5th edition, London, 1855, ₴ 696, (at pages 647 et seq.,) under the head "Mesmerism." Dr. Carpenter discredits the higher phenomena of Clairvoyance, but admits, 1st. A state of complete insensibility, during which severe surgical operations may be performed without the consciousness of the patient. 2d. Artificial somnambulism, with manifestation of the ordinary power of mind, but no recollection, in the waking state, of what has passed. 3d. Exaltation of the senses during such somnambulism, so that the somnambule perceives what in his natural condition he could not. 4th. Action, during such somnambulism, on the muscular apparatus, so as to produce, for example, artificial catalepsy; and, 5th. Perhaps curative effects.

Dr. Carpenter says his mind is made up as to the reality of these phenomena, and that "he does not see why any discredit should attach to them." (Note at page 649.)

The character and standing of this gentleman's numerous works on physiology and medical science are too widely known to need indorsement.

† Kate, youngest daughter of Mr. and Mrs. John D. Fox, and then aged nine. It was on the night of the 31st of March, 1848. This was, however, as will be seen in the sequel, by no means the first time that the observation had been made that similar sounds showed appearance of intelligence.

For the particulars of the Hydesville story, see the last narrative in Book III.

these sounds seemed to exhibit characteristics of intelligence.

From that day a new and important phase has offered itself to the attention of the student in pneumatology, and with it a new duty; that of determining the true character of what is sometimes termed the American Epidemic, more wonderful in its manifestations, far wider spread in its range, than any of the mental epidemics, marvelous in their phenomena as some of them have been, recorded by physicians and psychologists of continental Europe.

From that day, too, there gradually emerged into notice a new department in the science of the soul,—the positive and experimental. Until now the greater number of accredited works on psychology or pneumatology have been made up exclusively of speculations drawn either from analogy or from history, sacred or profane,—eminent sources, yet not the only ones. No such work ought now to be regarded as complete without an examination of phenomena as well as a citation of authorities. And thus, though a portion of the present volume consists of historical recallings, since the wonders of the present can seldom be fitly judged without the aid of the past, another and larger portion embraces narratives of modern date, phenomena of comparatively recent occurrence, the evidence for which has been collected with the same care with which a member of the legal profession is wont to examine his witnesses and prepare his case for trial.

In perusing a work of this character, the reader will do well to bear in mind that phenomena exist independently of all opinions touching their nature or origin. A fact is not to be slighted or disbelieved because a false theory may have been put forth to explain it. It has its importance, if it be important at all, irrespective of all theories.

And if it should be alleged, as to this class of facts, that they *have* no intrinsic importance, the reply is, first, that although the present age, as at the outset I have admitted, be a utilitarian one,—though it seek the positive and hold to the practical,—yet the positive and the practical may be understood in a sense falsely restrictive. Man does not live by bread alone. He lives to develop and to improve, as much as to exist. And development and improvement are things as real as existence itself. That which brings home to our consciousness noble ideas, refined enjoyment, that which bears good fruit in the mind, even though we perceive it not with our eyes nor touch it with our hands, is something else than an idle dream. The poetry of life is more than a metaphor. Sentiment is linked to action. Nor is the world, with all its hard materialism, dead to these truths. There is a corner, even in our work-a-day souls, where the IDEAL lurks, and whence it may be called forth, to become, not a mere barren fancy, but the prolific parent of progress. And from time to time it *is* thus called forth, to ennoble and to elevate. It is not the enthusiast only who aspires. What is civilization but a realization of human aspirations?

Yet I rest not the case here, in generalities. When I am told that studies such as form the basis of this work are curious only, and speculative in their character, leading to nothing of solid value, and therefore unworthy to engage the serious attention of a business world, my further reply is, that such allegation is a virtual begging of the very question which in this volume I propose to discuss. It is an assuming of the negative in advance; it is a taking for granted that the phenomena in question cannot possibly establish the reality of ultramundane interference.

For, if they do, he must be a hardy or a reckless man who shall ask, "Where is the good?" This is not our abiding-place; and though, during our tenancy of sixty or seventy years, it behoove us to task our best energies in the cause of earthly improvement and happiness,—though it be our bounden duty, while here, to care, in a measure, for the worldly welfare of all, more especially for the wants and comforts of our own domestic hearth,—and though, as human workers, much the larger portion of our thoughts and time must be, or ought to be, thus employed,—yet, if our permanent dwelling-place is soon to be established elsewhere; if, as the years pass, our affections are stealing thither before us; if the home-circle, gradually dissolving here, is to be reconstituted, fresh and enduring, in other regions,* shall we hold it to be matter of mere idle curiosity, fantastic and indifferent, to ascertain, whether, in sober truth, an intimation from that future home is ever permitted to reach us, here on our pilgrimage, before we depart?

We cannot curtly settle this question, as some assume to do, by an *a priori* argument against the possibility of human intercourse with the denizens of another world. Especially is the Bible Christian barred from employing

---

* "We start in life an unbroken company: brothers and sisters, friends and lovers, neighbors and comrades, are with us: there is circle within circle, and each one of us is at the charmed center, where the heart's affections are aglow and whence they radiate outward on society. Youth is exuberant with joy and hope; the earth looks fair, for it sparkles with May-dews wet, and no shadow hath fallen upon it. We are all here, and we could live here forever. The home-center is on the hither side of the river; and why should we strain our eyes to look beyond? But this state of things does not continue long. Our circle grows less and less. It is broken and broken, and then closed up again; but every break and close make it narrower and smaller. Perhaps before the sun is at his meridian the majority are on the other side; the circle there is as large as the one here; and we are drawn contrariwise and vibrate between the two. A little longer, and almost all have crossed over; the balance settles down on the spiritual side, and the home-center is removed to the upper sphere. At length you see nothing but an aged pilgrim standing alone on the river's bank and looking earnestly toward the country on the other side."—"*Foregleams of Immortality,*" by Edmund H. Sears, 4th ed., Boston, 1858: chap. xvi., "Home," p. 136.

any such. That which has been may be.* The Scriptures teach that such intercourse did exist in earlier days; and they nowhere declare that it was thenceforth to cease forever.

And when, in advance of any careful examination of this question, we decide that, in our day at least, no such intervention is possible, it might be well that we consider whether our Sadducism go not further than we think for; whether, without our consciousness perhaps, it strike not deeper than mere disbelief in modern spiritual agencies. Let us look to it, that, in slightingly discarding what it is the fashion to regard as superstition, we may not be virtually disallowing also an essential of faith.† Does the present existence of another world come home to us as a living truth? Do we *verily believe* that beings of another sphere are around us, watching, caring, loving? Is it with our hearts, or

---

* "Why come not spirits from the realms of glory,
  To visit earth, as in the days of old,—
  The times of ancient writ and sacred story?
  Is heaven more distant? or has earth grown cold? . . .

"To Bethlehem's air was their last anthem given
  When other stars before the One grew dim?
  Was their last presence known in Peter's prison,
  Or where exulting martyrs raised the hymn?"

JULIA WALLICE.

† Whence do such able reasoners as Dr. Strauss derive their most efficient weapons in the assault upon existing faith? From the modern fashion of denying all ultramundane intrusion. That which we reject as incredible if alleged to have happened to-day, by what process does it become credible by being moved back two thousand years into the past?

"The totality of finite things," says Strauss, "forms a vast circle, which, except that it owes its existence and laws to a superior power, suffers no intrusion from without. This conviction is so much a habit of thought with the modern world, that in actual life the belief in a supernatural manifestation, an immediate divine agency, is at once attributed to ignorance or imposture."—*"Life of Jesus,"* vol. i. p. 71.

with our lips only, that we assent, if indeed we do assent,* to the doctrine contained in Milton's lines?—

> "Millions of spiritual creatures walk the earth,
> Unseen, both when we wake and when we sleep."

If all this be more to us than mere idle sound, with what show of reason can we take it for granted, as a point settled prior to all discussion of it, that intercourse with another world is no longer vouchsafed to us in this?

All reasoning *a priori*, if resorted to at all, tells in favor of such intervention. One of the strongest natural arguments in proof of the soul's immortality has ever been held to be the universality of man's belief in an after-life; a sentiment so common to all ages and nations that it may claim the character of an instinct.† But the belief in the occasional appearance,

---

* "Men have ever been familiar with the idea that the spirit does not rest with the body in the grave, but passes at once into new conditions of being. The opinion has gained adherence, and disputes the ground with the more material one, that it rests in sleep with the body to await one common day of awakening and judgment; and so confused are the common impressions on the subject that you may hear a clergyman, in his funeral sermon, deliberately giving expression to both in one discourse, and telling you, in the same breath, that my lady lately deceased is a patient inhabitant of the tomb, and a member of the angelic company. But the idea of uninterrupted life has so strong a hold on the affections, which cannot bear the idea of even the temporary extinction of that which they cling to, that it has the instinctive adherence of almost every one who has felt deeply and stood face to face with death."—(London) *National Review* for July, 1858, p. 32.

The question of a mediate state of existence commencing at the moment of death, the Hades alike of the ancients and of early Christianity, will be touched upon later in this volume.

There are those who admit the objective reality of apparitions, yet, denying the existence of any mediate state after death, adopt the theory that it is angels of an inferior rank created such, who, for good purpose, occasionally personate deceased persons, and that the departed never return. This is De Foe's hypothesis, and is ably advocated by him in his "*Universal History of Apparitions*," London, 1727.

The broad question is, whether "spiritual creatures," be they angels or departed souls, are present around us.

† The best analogical argument which I remember to have met with in

3*

or influence on human affairs, of disembodied spirits,* is scarcely less general or less instinctive; though it is to be admitted that in the Dark Ages it commonly degenerated into demonology.† The principle, however, may be true and the form erroneous; a contingency of constant recurrence throughout the history of the human mind, as when religion, for example, assumed and maintained for ages the pagan form.

The matter at issue, then, must be grappled with more closely. We have no right to regard it as a closed question, bluffly to reject it as involving incredible assumptions, or to dismiss it with foregone conclusions under terms of general denial.‡ It is neither

---

favor of the immortality of the soul is contained in Isaac Taylor's work already referred to, the "*Physical Theory of Another Life,*" at pp. 64 to 69. This argument from analogy must, I think, be regarded as much more forcible than the abstract logic by which the ancient philosophers sought to establish the truth in question. When Cicero, following Socrates and Plato, says of the soul, "*Nec discerpi, nec distrahi potest, nec igitur interire,*" the ingenuity of the reasoning is more apparent than its conclusiveness.

* *Disembodied,* disconnected from this natural body; not *unembodied;* for I by no means impugn the hypothesis of a spiritual body.—1 Cor. xv. 44.

† "To deny the possibility, nay, actual existence, of witchcraft and sorcery, is at once flatly to contradict the revealed word of God, in various passages both of the Old and New Testament; and the thing itself is a truth to which every nation in the world hath, in its turn, borne testimony, either by examples seemingly well attested, or by prohibitory laws, which at least suppose the possibility of commerce with evil spirits."—*Blackstone's Commentaries,* b. 4, c. 4, § 6.

I adduce the above from so distinguished a source on account of its bearings on the universality of man's belief in ultramundane intercourse, and to rebut a presumption against that intercourse, now in vogue; not as proof of the reality of such intercourse.

‡ It may not be amiss here to remind the reader that by such men as Johnson and Byron the universal belief of man in intercourse with the spirits of the departed was regarded as probable proof of its occasional reality. It will be remembered that the former, in his "Rasselas," puts into the mouth of the sage Imlac this sentiment:—"That the dead are seen no more I will not undertake to maintain against the concurrent testimony

logical nor becoming for men to decide, in advance of
investigation, that it is contrary to the divine economy
that there should be ultramundane interference. It is
our business to examine the Creator's works, and
thence, if needs we must, to derive conclusions as to His
intentions. It is our province to seek out and establish

---

of all ages and all nations. There is no people, rude or unlearned, among
whom apparitions of the dead are not related and believed. This opinion,
which prevails as far as human nature is diffused, could become universal
only by its truth: those that never heard of one another would not have
agreed in a tale which nothing but experience could make credible. That
it is doubted by single cavilers can very little weaken the general evidence; and some who deny it with their tongues confess it with their
fears."

To this passage Byron alludes in the following:—

"I merely mean to say what Johnson said,
      That, in the course of some six thousand years,
All nations have believed that from the dead
      A visitant at intervals appears.
And what is strangest upon this strange head,
      Is, that, whatever bar the reason rears
'Gainst such belief, there's something stronger still
In its behalf, let those deny who will."

Addison's opinion on the same subject is well known. It is contained
in one of the numbers of The Spectator ascertained to be from his pen,—
namely, No. 110, published Friday, July 6, 1711,—and is in these words:—

"I think a person who is thus terrified with the imagination of ghosts
and specters much more reasonable than one who, contrary to the reports
of all historians, sacred and profane, ancient and modern, and to the
traditions of all nations, thinks the appearance of spirits fabulous and
groundless. Could not I give myself up to this general testimony of mankind, I should to the relations of particular persons who are now living,
and whom I cannot distrust in other matters of fact."

Another distinguished contributor to The Spectator seems to have shared
the same opinion. The author of "A Treatise on Second-Sight, Dreams, and
Apparitions," a Highland clergyman, I believe, named Macleod, but writing
under the signature of Theophilus Insulanus, says,—

"What made me inquire more narrowly into the subject, was in consequence of a conversation I had with Sir Richard Steele, who engaged me
to search for instances of it well attested."—Treatise on Second-Sight, &c.,
Edinburgh, 1763, p. 97.

facts, and then to build upon them; not to erect on the sand of preconception hazarded theories of our own, which Science, in her onward march, may assault and overthrow, as did the system of Galileo the theology of the Roman inquisitors.*

As little defensible is it, in case we should happen in search of its proofs to come upon the testimony of the humble and the unlettered, that we refuse audience to any well-attested fact because we may not consider its origin sufficiently reputable. We may learn from all classes. We shall find truth in every rank. Things that escape the reputed wise and prudent may be perceived by those who in technical knowledge are but children in comparison. Mere learning does not

---

* Taylor has a passage on this subject well deserving our notice. Speaking of the belief in " occasional interferences of the dead with the living," which, he says, " ought not to be summarily dismissed as a mere folly of the vulgar," he adds :—

" In considering questions of this sort, we ought not to listen, for a moment, to those frequent but impertinent questions that are brought forward with a view of superseding the inquiry; such, for example, as these: —' What good is answered by the alleged extra-natural occurrences?' or, ' Is it worthy of the Supreme Wisdom to permit them?' and so forth. The question is a question, first, of *testimony*, to be judged of on the established principles of evidence, and then of *physiology;* but neither of theology nor of morals. Some few human beings are wont to walk in their sleep; and during the continuance of profound slumber they perform, with precision and safety, the offices of common life, and return to their beds, and yet are totally unconscious when they awake of what they have done. Now, in considering this or any such extraordinary class of facts, our business is, in the first place, to obtain a number of instances supported by the distinct and unimpeachable testimony of intelligent witnesses; and then, being thus in possession of the facts, to adjust them, as well as we can, to other parts of our philosophy of human nature. Shall we allow an objector to put a check to our scientific curiosity on the subject, for instance, of somnambulism, by saying, ' Scores of these accounts have turned out to be exaggerated or totally untrue,' or, ' This walking in the sleep ought not to be thought possible, or as likely to be permitted by the Benevolent Guardian of human welfare'?"—*Physical Theory of Another Life*, p. 27.

always enlighten: it may but distort and obscure.
That is a shrewd touch of satire, often applicable in
practical life, which Goethe puts in the mouth of him
of the Iron Hand, stout "Götz of Berlichingen."
When his little son, after repeating his well-conned
lesson in geography about the village and castle of Jaxt-
hausen,—the Berlichingen family-seat, on the banks of
the river Jaxt,—could not reply to his parent's question as to what castle he was talking about, the old
warrior exclaims, "Poor child! he knows not, for very
learning, his own father's house!"

The majority of educated men set aside, with little
thought or scruple, all stories of haunted houses, all narratives of apparitions, all allegations touching prophetic
or clear-sighted dreams, and similar pretensions, as the
ignoble offshoots of vulgar superstition. Yet there has
been of late a reaction in this matter. Here and there
we come upon indications of this. It is within my knowledge, that a few years since, at one of the chief English
universities, a society was formed out of some of its most
distinguished members, for the purpose of instituting,
as their printed circular expresses it, "a serious and
earnest inquiry into the nature of the phenomena
which are vaguely called supernatural." They subjected these to careful classification, and appealed to
their friends outside of the society to aid them in
forming an extensive collection of authenticated cases,
as well of remarkable dreams as of apparitions,
whether of persons living or of the deceased; the use
to be made of these to be a subject for future consideration.*

---

* The society referred to was formed in the latter part of the year 1851,
at Cambridge, by certain members of the University, some of them now
at the head of well-known institutions, most of them clergymen and fellows
of Trinity College, and almost all of them men who had graduated with
the highest honors. The names of the more active among them were kindly

C

It is to be conceded, however, that examples such as these, significant though they be, are but exceptions. The rule is to treat all alleged evidences for dream-revealings, or for the objective character of apparitions, or for the reality of those disturbances that go by the name of hauntings, as due either to accidental coincidence, to disease, to delusion, or to willful deception. One of the objects of the present volume is to inquire whether in so doing we are overlooking any actual phenomena.

Beyond this, upon a cognate subject, I do not propose to enter. I am not, in this work, about to investigate what goes by the name of spiritual manifestations,—such as table-moving, rapping, mediumship, and the like. As the geologist prefers first to inspect the rock *in situ*, so

---

furnished to me by the son of a British peer, himself one of the leading members. To him, also, I am indebted for a copy of the printed circular of the society, an able and temperate document, which will be found at length in the Appendix, (*Note A.*) The same gentleman informed me that the researches of the society had resulted in a conviction, shared, he believed, by all its members, that there *is* sufficient testimony for the appearance, about the time of death or after it, of the apparitions of deceased persons; while in regard to other classes of apparitions the evidence, so far as obtained, was deemed too slight to prove their reality.

To a gentleman who had been one of the more active members of the society, the Rev. Mr. W——, I wrote, giving him the title of the present work, and stating in general terms the spirit and manner in which I proposed to write it. In his reply he says, " I wish that I were able to make any contribution to your proposed work at all commensurate with the interest which I feel in the subject of it." . . . . " I rejoice extremely to learn that the subject is likely to receive a calm and philosophic treatment. This, at least, it demands; and, for my own part, I feel little doubt that great good will result from the publication of the work which you are preparing. My own experience has led me to form a conclusion similar to that which you express,—that the possibility of supramundane interference is a question which is gradually attracting more and more attention, especially with men of education. This circumstance makes me the more anxious that a selection of facts should be fairly laid before them."

The society, popularly known as the " Ghost Club," attracted a good deal of attention outside its own circle. Its nature and objects first came to my knowledge through the Bishop of ——, who took an interest in its proceedings and bestirred himself to obtain contributions to its records.

I think it best, at this time and in this connection, to examine the *spontaneous* phenomena, rather than those which are *evoked;* the phenomena which seem to come unsought, or, as we usually phrase it, by the visitation of God, rather than those which appear to be called up through the deliberate efforts of man. I have studied the former much more carefully than the latter; and space would fail me in a single volume to dispose of both.

But, if I had space, and felt competent to the task, it should not deter me that the subject is still in bad odor and sometimes in graceless hands. I well know it to be the fashion—and a very reprehensible fashion it is— to pass by with ridicule or contempt the extraordinary results which seem to present themselves in this connection. Be the facts as they may, such a course is impolitic and unwise. It is not by despising error that we correct it. No sensible man well informed as to the facts denies that, like every other subject professing to reach beyond the grave, this has its fanatics, misled by fantasies, dealing in vagaries of the imagination. But we are not justified in summarily setting aside, untested, any class of allegations because we may have detected among their supporters loose observation and false logic. Rational opinions may be irrationally defended. A creed may be true though some of its advocates can give no sufficient reason for the faith that is in them. Origanus, the astronomical instructor of Wallenstein's famous attendant, Seni, was one of the earliest defenders of the Copernican system; yet his arguments to prove the earth's motion are quite on a par, as to the absurdity of their character, with those advanced on the opposite side in favor of its immobility.

There is, then, nothing conclusive in it, that the investigator of such a subject is met with a thousand exaggerations. It does not settle the question, that at every step we detect errors and absurdities. The main problem lies deeper than these. "There are errors," says Coleridge, "which no wise man will treat with rudeness while there is a probability that they may be the refraction of some great truth as yet below the horizon."* And he must be a skeptic past saving who has critically examined the phenomena in question without reaching the conclusion that, how inaccurately soever they may have been interpreted until now, our best powers of reason are worthily taxed to determine their exact character.

Some wonders there are, in this connection, opening to human view. They may be purely scientific in their bearings, but, if so, none the less well deserving a place beside the marvels of electricity in its various phases. Nor, even if they finally prove to be phenomena exclusively physical, should those, meanwhile, be browbeat or discouraged who seek to detect therein ultramundane agencies. There are researches in which, if no pains and industry be spared, honestly to fail is as reputable as to succeed in others. And some of the most important discoveries have been made during a search after the impossible. Muschenbrœck stumbled upon the invention of the Leyden jar while endeavoring, it is said, to collect and confine Thales's electric effluvium.

Moralists and statesmen, too, should bear in mind that they have here to deal with an element which already seriously influences human opinion. The phenomena sometimes called spiritual, whether genuine or spurious, have attracted the attention, and won more or less of the belief, not of thousands only,—of millions, already.†

---

* In his first "*Lay Sermon.*"

† My friend William Howitt, the well-known author, who, with his amiable wife, has devoted much time and thought to this subject, says, in a recent reply to the Rev. Edward White's discourses, delivered in St. Paul's Chapel, Kentish Town, in October, November, and December, 1858,

And if these astounding novelties are permitted to spread
among us without chart or compass whereby to steer

"Spiritualism is said to have convinced three millions of people in America
alone. In Europe, I believe, there are not less than another million; and
the rapidity with which it is diffusing itself through all ranks and classes,
literally from the highest to the lowest, should set men thinking. It would
startle some people to discover in how many royal *palaces* in Europe it is
firmly seated, and with what vigor it is diffusing itself through all ranks
and professions of men, who do not care to make much noise about it; men
and women of literary, religious, and scientific fame."

I have not the means of judging as to the accuracy of Mr. Howitt's total
estimate. It must necessarily be an uncertain one. But as to the latter
portion of that gentleman's remarks, I can indorse it from personal knowledge. I found, in Europe, interested and earnest inquirers into this subject
in every rank, from royalty downward; princes, and other nobles, statesmen,
diplomatists, officers in the army and navy, learned professors, authors,
lawyers, merchants, private gentlemen, fashionable ladies, domestic mothers
of families. Most of these, it is true, prosecute their investigations in private, and disclose their opinions only to intimate or sympathizing friends.
But none the less does this class of opinions spread, and the circle daily
enlarge that receives them.

If further evidence of these allegations, so far as they relate to England,
be required, it is to be found in a late number of a well-known London
Quarterly, than which it would be difficult to name a periodical more opposed
to this movement. In the Westminster Review for January, 1858, in an
elaborate article devoted to the subject. the writer says, "We should be in
much error if we suppose that table-turning, or that group of asserted phenomena which in this country is embodied under that name, and which in
America assumes the loftier title of Spiritualism, in ceasing to occupy the
attention of the public generally, has also ceased to occupy the attention of
every part of it. The fact is very much otherwise. Our readers would be
astonished were we to lay before them the names of several of those who
are unflinching believers in it, or who are devoting themselves to the study
or reproduction of its marvels. Not only does it survive, but survives with
all the charm and all the stimulating attractiveness of a secret science.
Until the public mind in England shall be prepared to receive it, or until
the evidence shall be put in a shape to enforce general conviction, the present policy is to nurse it in quiet and enlarge the circle of its influence by
a system of noiseless extension. Whether this policy will be successful
remains to be seen; but there can be no doubt that, should ever the time
arrive for the revival of this movement, the persons at its head would be
men and women whose intellectual qualifications are known to the public
and who possess its confidence and esteem."—p. 32.

our course through an unexplored ocean of mystery, we
may find ourselves at the mercy of very sinister influences.

Among the communications heretofore commonly obtained, alleged to be ultramundane, are many which
seem to justify that old saying of Pythagoras: "It is
not out of every log of wood that a Mercury can be
made." Whether coming to us from another world or
from this, not a few of them contain a large mingling
of falsehood with truth, and a mass of puerilities alternating with reason. At times they disclose evil passions;
occasionally they are characterized by profanity; and
some of them, even where no fraud or conscious agency
is presumable, exhibit unmistakable evidence of a mundane origin or influence; as all candid, sensible advocates of the spiritual theory, after sufficient experience,
freely admit.*

---

* De Gasparin considers it a conclusive argument against the spiritual
theory, that "the particular opinions of each medium may be recognized in
the dogmas he promulgates in the name of the spirits." ("*Des Tables Tournantes, du Surnaturel en Général, et des Esprits*," par le Comte Agénor de
Gasparin, Paris, 1855, vol. ii. p. 497.) He is only partially accurate as to
the fact. It is the questioner as often perhaps as the medium who receives
back his own opinions. But this is only sometimes true of either. It is,
however, beyond all doubt, sometimes true; and the fact, however explained,
points, with many others, to the urgent necessity, on the part of those who
adopt the spiritual hypothesis, of receiving with the utmost care, and only
after the strictest scrutiny, any communications, no matter what their pretensions.

Until Spiritualists take such precautions,—until they sit in judgment on
what they receive, and separate the chaff from the wheat,—they cannot
reasonably complain if the majority of intelligent men reject all because a
part is clearly worthless. Nor, meanwhile, though a witty squib prove
nothing, can the point be denied of that which Saxe launches against some
alleged spirit communicators of our modern day :—

"If in your new estate you cannot rest,
    But must return, oh, grant us this request:
    Come with a noble and celestial air,
    And prove your titles to the names you bear;

Hence, under any hypothesis, great danger to the weak-minded and the over-credulous.

This danger is the greater, because men are wont to take it for granted that, when we shall have demonstrated (if we can demonstrate) the spiritual character of a communication, there needs no further demonstration as to the truth of the facts alleged and the opinions expressed therein.

This is a very illogical conclusion, though distinguished men have sometimes arrived at it.* It is one thing to determine the ultramundane origin of a communication, and quite another to prove its infallibility, even its authenticity. Indeed, there are more plausible reasons than many imagine for the opinion entertained by some able men, Protestants as well as Catholics,† that the

---

Give some clear token of your heavenly birth;
Write as good English as you wrote on earth:
And, what were once superfluous to advise,
Don't tell, I beg you, such egregious lies."

* See, for an example, *"Experimental Examination of the Spirit Manifestations,"* by Robert Hare, M.D., Emeritus Professor of Chemistry in the University of Pennsylvania, 4th ed., 1856, pp. 14, 15. When the venerable author obtained, as he expressed it, "the sanction of the spirits under test conditions," that is, by means most ingeniously contrived by him to prevent human deception, or (again to use his own words) "so that it was utterly out of the power of any mortal to pervert the result from being a pure emanation from the spirits whose names were given," he received as authentic, without further doubt or question, certain extraordinary credentials purporting to come from another world. Professor Hare is now himself a denizen of that world where honest errors find correction, and where to uprightness is meted out its reward.

† As by the Rev. Charles Beecher, in his *"Review of Spiritual Manifestations,"* chap. vii., where will be found the quotation given in the text.

De Mirville (*"Des Esprits et de leurs Manifestations fluidiques,"* par le Marquis de Mirville, Paris, 3d ed., 1854) is the ablest modern exponent of the Catholic doctrine of Demonology. The 4th edition of his work, so his publishers inform me, is (May, 1859) nearly exhausted. The Church of Rome, it is well known, recognizes the doctrine of possession by evil spirits as an article of faith:—"Quod dæmon corpora hominum *possidere* et *obsidere* possit, certum de fide est."—*Theologia Mystica, ad usum Directorum*

communications in question come from the Powers of Darkness, and that "we are entering on the first steps of a career of demoniac manifestation, the issues whereof man cannot conjecture." But I see no just cause whatever for such an opinion. The reasons for this revival of an antiquated belief seem to me plausible only. God has suffered evil to exist in this world; yet we do not, for that reason, conclude that hell reigns upon earth. We reflect that perhaps through this very antagonism may lie the path of progress. Or, at least, we weigh the good against the evil, and believe in the beneficence of the Creator. But His power is not limited to this side the grave. And if He *does* permit communication from the other side, is it in accordance with His attributes that such communication should resolve itself into mere demoniac obsession?

The reasons for a belief so gloomy and discouraging appear to me mainly to rest, among Protestants at least, upon an error of very mischievous influence, and to which, in a subsequent chapter, on the Change at Death, I shall have occasion to advert at large. I allude to the opinion, held by many, that the character of man undergoes, after death, a sudden transformation; and that the peculiarities and prejudices which distinguish the individual in this world do not pass with him into another. If they do, the motley character of communications thence obtained (if such communications there be) can excite no surprise. It is precisely what we may reasonably expect. God permits that from our many-charactered fellow-creatures of this world mingled truth and falsehood shall reach us: why not also

---

Animarum, Paris, 1848, vol. i. p. 376. The Roman Ritual (*Cap. De exorcizandis obsessis a dæmonio*) supplies, in detail, the rules for exorcising the Demon; and, in point of fact, exorcisms, at Rome and elsewhere throughout Catholic countries, are at this time of daily occurrence, though usually conducted in private, and little spoken of outside the pale of the Church.

from our fellow-creatures of another world, if the same variety of feeling and opinion prevail there? We are constantly called upon, by the exercise of our reason, to separate the genuine from the spurious in the one case. Where do we find warrant for the opinion that we are released from such a duty in the other? Lest we should imagine that, when we are commanded to prove *all* things, the injunction relates to mundane agencies only, an express text is added, declaring that spirits also must be tested.*

A world in which men should be exonerated from the duty, or forbidden the right, to bring the judgment into play,—to sift, by the strict dictates of conscience, good from evil, the right from the wrong,—would be a world disgraced and degraded. If such a principle were fully carried out, it would at last become a world lacking not only the exercise of reason, but reason itself. Use, to an extent which it is difficult to determine, is essential to continued existence. That which ceases to fulfill its purpose finally ceases to be. The eyes of fishes found far in the interior of the Mammoth Cave of Kentucky, shut out forever from the light of day, are rudimental only.†

But it is not conceivable that, under the Divine Economy, an order of things should ever be permitted, in which man should be shorn of his noblest attribute; that which, more than any other, stamps his superiority,

---

* 1 John iv. 1.

† This fact has been verified by dissection. The fish in question (the only known species of the genus *Amblyopsis Spelæus*) is, however, I believe, found only in similar localities. Nor is it certain that this fish is without the power to distinguish light from darkness; for the optic lobe remains. Drs. Telkampf, of New York, and Wyman, of Boston, have published papers on the subject.

It would be an interesting experiment to bring some of these fishes to the light, and ascertain whether, in the course of generations, their eyes would gradually become perfect.

4*

on this earth, over the lower animal races which share with him its occupation and its enjoyments. Human reason is the appointed pilot of human civilization; fallible, indeed, like any other steersman, but yet essential to progress and to safety. That pilot once dismissed from the helm, the bark will drift at random, abandoned to the vagrant influence of every chance current or passing breeze.

Let us conceive a case in illustration. Let us suppose that, from some undeniably spiritual source, as through speech of an apparition, or by a voice sounding from the upper air, there should come to us the injunction to adopt the principle of polygamy, either as that system is legally recognized in Turkey, or in its unavowed form, as it appears in the great cities of the civilized world. In such a case, what is to be done? The world is God's work. The experience of the world is God's voice. Are we to set aside that experience, proclaiming to us, as it does, that under the principle of monogamy alone have man's physical powers and moral attributes ever maintained their ascendency, while weakness and national decadence follow in the train of polygamy, whether openly carried out, as in Deseret and Constantinople, or secretly practiced, as in London and New York? Are we to give up the certain for the uncertain?—the teachings of God, through His works, for the biddings of we know not whom?

The folly and danger of so doing are apparent. Intimations from another world (supposing their reality) may be useful; they may be highly suggestive; they may supply invaluable materials for thought: just as the opinions of some wise man or the advice of some judicious friend, here upon earth, might do. But no opinion, no advice, from friend or stranger, ought to be received as infallible, or accepted as a rule of action, until Reason shall have sat in judgment upon it and decided, to the best of her ability, its truth and worth.

There exist not, nor can arise, any circumstances whatever that shall justify the reception by man, as infallible and mandatory, of any such communication. Let us suppose the extreme case. Let us imagine that, from some intelligence clearly ultramundane, there should come to us a certain communication which, fairly tested by reason, we decide to exceed, in depth and wisdom, any thing which that reason unaided could originate. Are we, because of the evident excellence of that communication, to receive with unquestioning acquiescence all its fellows coming apparently from the same source? In the chapter on Sleep cases will be adduced in proof that our intellectual powers during sleep *sometimes* surpass any waking effort. Yet what rational man would thence infer that we ought to be governed by our dreams?

If I have dwelt at length, and insisted with some iteration, on this matter, it is because of the wide spread mischief to which, in this connection, blindly assenting credulity has, in these later times especially, given rise; it is because of the urgent necessity for judgment to discriminate, for caution to scrutinize. But the necessity is as urgent to bear in mind, that judgment and caution are the very opposites of proscription and prejudice. On the supposition that spirits do actually communicate, if those who ought to give tone and direction to public opinion content themselves with arrogantly denouncing the whole as a portentous imposture, they lose all power or opportunity to regulate a reality of which they deny the existence.* And in

---

* Dining, in February, 1859, with a gentleman commercially well known in London, and sitting at table next to the lady of the house, she broached the subject of Spiritualism. I asked her if she had seen any of its alleged phenomena. She replied that she had not; that, from what she had heard,

the case here supposed, our moral and religious guides
risk the loss of influence and position by putting aside
an all-important inquiry,—a contingency which as a
body they appear to have overlooked.

The claims of the subject to the notice of the clergy
and of other public teachers are not founded alone upon
the fact that this heresy (if heresy it be) has penetrated
to every rank and class of society, and now influences,
more or less, the opinions and the conduct of millions
throughout the civilized world. These claims reach
further still. They derive from the necessity of the
case. The question as to investigation or no investigation is one of time only. Once mooted and seized upon
by popular sympathy, a matter like this *must* be probed

---

she was convinced there was some reality in it; but, being of a nervous
temperament, and not assured of her own self-control, she had refrained
from examining its manifestations. "Then I know," she added, "that it
has done so much harm. Has it not?" (appealing to a gentleman sitting
near us.) He assented in strong terms. I begged him to give me an example. "I could give you many," he replied, "in the circle of my acquaintance; but one in particular occurs to me. The daughter of a friend
of mine, in a family of the utmost respectability, and herself amiable and
intelligent, is, at this very time, quite carried away with its delusions. She
had raps from the table, and is in the habit of shutting herself up, day
after day, in the garret of her father's house, spelling out communications
which she imagines to come from departed spirits. She will not even take
the exercise necessary to her health; alleging that while she is gone she
may lose the chance of receiving some divine message. The remonstrances
of her parents, who are not at all affected with the mania, are unavailing;
and it causes them much grief."

Let us put what interpretation we may upon that which has been called
the spirit-rap and the communications thus obtained, it is evident that
such a case as the above savors of fanaticism and urgently demands regu-
lation. No condition of mind can be healthy—scarcely sane—which with-
draws all thoughts from the duties of earthly life, even from the care of
bodily health, and suffers them to be wholly engrossed by such communications; above all, when these are received, unquestioned, as divine and infallible revelation.

But to deny actual phenomena is not the proper mode to win over a misled or diseased mind.

to the bottom. There is nothing else for it. We can get rid of it on no other terms. We cannot hush it up if we would; we ought not if we could. Viewed in its scientific aspect, we might as reasonably interdict the study of electricity or the employment of the magnetic wires. And as regards its spiritual pretensions, either these are a perilous delusion, to be detected and exploded, as by carefully prosecuted researches every delusion can be, or else a reality important beyond any that crosses our daily path. If they be a delusion, leading astray the flock, on whom so strictly as on its pastor devolves the task of exposure?—but of exposure *after investigation;* since, in the words of a wise man of old, "He that answereth a matter before he heareth it, it is folly and shame unto him."* If, on the other hand, it should prove to be a reality, how grave their responsibility who blindly oppose it! In such a case, research on the part of public teachers rises to the rank of a sacred duty, lest haply, like the unbelievers of Gamaliel's day, they be found fighting against God.

And this duty is bounden the rather because of a great difficulty, suggested by the narratives forming the staple of this volume, which necessarily attends the policy of non-investigation. There is the question, how far we are to carry out that policy. Men, during the last ten years, and in our country especially, have, in this connection, had their attention mainly directed to what, in one sense, may be called the artificial phase of the subject. They have been chiefly occupied in examining phenomena which occur as the result of express intention and calculated method; which are elicited, not merely witnessed; such as the manifestations which come to light through what is called mediumship, in spiritual circles, through writing by impression, during artificial

---

* Proverbs xviii. 13.

somnambulism, and the like. These constitute but a small fraction of a great subject. They have for the most part been called forth during a few years only; while the vast mass of phenomena evidently allied to them, but purely spontaneous in their character, are spread over ages and come to us through all past history. These latter present themselves not merely unexpected, not unsought only, but often unwished for, deprecated, occasionally even in spite of entreaty and prayer. Often, indeed, they assume the character of ministration by spirits loving and gentle; but at other times they put on the semblance of persecution, retributive and terrible.* The former appear to bear out the doctrine of celestial guardianship, while the latter seem sent by God as he sends on the material world the hurricane and the earthquake. But both are independent of man's will or agency. They come as the rain falls or as the lightning flashes.

This complicates the case. We may condemn as Pythonism, or denounce as unlawful necromancy, the seeking after spiritual phenomena.† But in so doing we dispose of a small branch of the subject only. How are we to deal with ultramundane manifestations, in case it should prove that they do often occur not only without our agency but in spite of our adjuration? Grant that it were unwise, even sinful, to go in search of spiritual intervention: what are we to say of it if it overcome us sudden and unsolicited, and, whether for

---

* See, as an example of the former, the narrative entitled "*The rejected Suitor,*" and, as a specimen of the latter, that called "*What an English Officer suffered:*" both given in subsequent chapters of this work.

† In the records of the past we come, from time to time, upon proof that men have been disposed to regard that which they imperfectly understood as savoring of unhallowed mystery. In Chaucer's tale of the Chanon Yeman, chemistry is spoken of as an elfish art; that is, taught or conducted by spirits. This, Warton says, is an Arabian idea. See "*Warton's History of English Poetry,*" vol. i. p. 169.

good or for evil, a commissioned intruder on our earthly path? Under that phase also (if under such it be found really to present itself) are we to ignore its existence? Ought we, without any inquiry into the character of its influence, to prejudge and to repulse it? Let it assume what form it may, are we still, like the Princess Parizade of the Arabian tale, to stop our ears with cotton against the voices around us?

The abstract right to investigate the broad question as to the reality of ultramundane interference will not, in these United States, be seriously questioned. There never was a period in the world's history when human tyranny could close, except for a season, the avenue to any department of knowledge which the Creator has placed within the reach of man; least of all, one involving interests so vital as this. Nor is there any country in the civilized world where the attempt could be made with less chance of success than in ours.

Many, however, who concede the right deem its exercise to be fraught with danger to human welfare and happiness. Some danger, beyond question, there is. What thing in nature is one-sided? Which of our studies may not be injudiciously undertaken or imprudently pursued? Something, in all human endeavors, we must risk; and that risk is the greatest, usually, for the most important objects. Religious researches involve more risk than secular: they demand, therefore, greater caution and a more dispassionate spirit. Are we to avoid them for that reason? Would their interdiction subserve man's welfare and happiness?

That theory of the solar system which is now admitted by every astronomer and taught to every school-boy was once alleged to be fraught with danger to the welfare and happiness of mankind, and its author was compelled on his knees to pledge his oath that he would never more propagate it, by word or writing. Yet what

scientific hypothesis, do men at the present day scruple
to examine?   And, if scientific, why not spiritual also?
Are we prepared to trust our reason in the one case but
reject its conclusions in the other?—to declare of that
noble faculty, as a German caviler did of the telescope
which first revealed to human sight the satellites of
Jupiter, that "it does wonders on the earth, but falsely
represents celestial objects"?*

Let us take courage, and trust to the senses God has
given us.   There is no safety in cowardice, no expe-
diency, even if there were possibility, in evasion.   If to
the investigation of these matters we must come
sooner or later, it is the part of wisdom and manliness
to undertake it at once.

A large portion of the periodicals of the day have
hitherto either wholly ignored the subject of ultramundane interference, or else passed it by with superficial
and disparaging notice.   After a time there will be a
change in this.†   The subject is gradually attaining

---

* Martin Korky, in one of the *"Kepleri Epistolæ."*   He it was who declared to his master Kepler, "I will never concede his four planets to that
Italian from Padua, though I die for it," and of whom, when he afterward
begged to be forgiven for his presumptuous skepticism, Kepler wrote to
Galileo, "I have taken him again into favor upon this express condition,
to which he has agreed, that I am to show him Jupiter's satellites, and *he
is to see them* and own that they are there."

There are a good many Martin Korkys of the present day, with whom,
as to some of the phenomena to be noticed in this volume, the same agreement should be made.

† Respectable periodicals, untinctured by peculiarities of opinion, have
already begun to treat the general subject with more deference than formerly.   For example, in a long article, entitled "Ghosts of the Old and
New School," in one of the London Quarterlies, while the chief phenomena
called spiritual are discredited, there occur such admissions as the following:—"There are sets of facts that demand a more searching and perse-
vering investigation than they have yet received,—either that they may be
finally disposed of as false, or reduced to scientific order.   Such are the appearance of ghosts, the power of second-sight, of clairvoyance, and other

a breadth and importance and winning a degree of attention which will be felt by the better portion of the press as entitling it to that respectful notice which is the due of a reputable opponent. And surely this is as it should be. Let the facts be as they may, the duty of the press and of the pulpit is best fulfilled, and the dangers incident to the subject are best averted, by promoting, not discouraging, inquiry;* but inquiry, thorough, searching, sedulously accurate, and in the strictest sense of the term impartial.

The first requisite in him who undertakes such an investigation—more important, even, than scientific training to accurate research—is that he shall approach it unbiased and unpledged, bringing with him no favorite theory to be built up, no preconceived opinions to be gratified or offended, not a wish that the results should be found to be of this character or of that character, but a single, earnest desire to discover *of what character they are.*

To what extent I bring to the task such qualifications, they who may read these pages can best decide. No man is an impartial judge of his own impartiality. I distrust mine. I am conscious of a disturbing element; a leaning in my mind, aside from the simple wish to detect what really is. Not that on the strictest self-scrutiny I can accuse myself of a desire to foist into such an inquiry any preconceptions, scientific or theolo-

---

phenomena of magnetism and mesmerism; the nature of sleep and dreams, of spectral illusions, (in themselves a decisive proof that the sense of sight may be fully experienced independently of the eye;) the limits and working of mental delusion and enthusiastic excitement."—*National Review* for July, 1858, p. 13.

* "Éclairons-nous sur les vérités, quelles qu'elles soient, qui se présentent à notre observation; et loin de craindre de favoriser la superstition en admettant de nouveaux phénomènes, quand ils sont bien prouvés, soyons-persuadés que le seul moyen d'empêcher les abus qu'on peut en faire, c'est d'en répandre la connaissance."—BERTRAND.

gical, nor yet of the least unwillingness to accept or to surrender any opinions, orthodox or heterodox, which the progress of that inquiry might establish or disprove. Not that. But I *am* conscious of a feeling that has acquired strength within me as these researches progressed; a desire other than the mere readiness to inspect with dispassionate equanimity the phenomena as they appeared; an earnest hope, namely, that these might result in furnishing to the evidence of the soul's independent existence and immortality a contribution drawn from a source where such proof has seldom, until recently, been sought.

Against the leaning incident to that hope, interwoven with man's nature as it is, the explorer of such a field as this should be especially on his guard. It is one of the many difficulties with which the undertaking is beset. "It is easy," truly said Bonnet, the learned Genevese,—"it is easy and agreeable to believe; to doubt requires an unpleasant effort." And the proclivity to conclude on insufficient evidence is the greater when we are in search of what we strongly wish to find. Our longings overhurry our judgments. But what so earnestly to be desired as the assurance that death, the much dreaded, is a friend instead of an enemy, opening to us, when the dark curtain closes on earthly scenes, the portals of a better and happier existence?

It is a common opinion that the all-sufficient and only proper source whence to derive that conviction is sacred history.

But, how strongly soever we may affirm that the Scripture proofs of the soul's immortality ought to command the belief of all mankind, the fact remains that they do not.* Some rest unbelievers; many more carry

---

* The number of materialists throughout the educated portion of civilized

about with them, as to the soul's future destiny, a faith inanimate and barren; and, even among those who profess the most, the creed of the greater number may be summed up in the exclamation, "Lord, I believe: help Thou mine unbelief!"*

Since, then, no complaint is more common from the pulpit itself than of the world-wide discrepancy daily to be found, even among the most zealously pious, between faith and practice, may we not trace much of that discrepancy to the feeble grade of credence, so far below the living conviction which our senses bring home to us of earthly things, which often makes up this wavering faith?†

---

society, especially in Europe, is much greater than on the surface it would appear. If one broaches serious subjects, this fact betrays itself. I was conversing one day with a French lady of rank, intelligent and thoughtful beyond the average of her class, and happened to express the opinion that progression is probably a law of the next world, as of this. " You really believe, then, in another world?" she asked.

"Certainly, Madame la Comtesse."

"Ah! you are a fortunate man," she replied, with some emotion. "How many of us do not!"

* We shall often find, in the expressions employed by distinguished men (especially the leaders in science) to express their sense of the importance of a firm religious belief, rather a desire to obtain it, and envy of those who possess it, than an assertion that they themselves have found all they sought. Here is an eloquent example:—

" I envy no qualities of the mind and intellect in others,—nor genius, nor power, nor wit, nor fancy; but if I could choose what would be most delightful and, I believe, most useful to me, I should prefer a firm religious belief to every other blessing. For it makes life a discipline of goodness, creates new hopes when all earthly hopes vanish, and throws over the decay, the destruction, of existence, the most gorgeous of all lights; awakens life in death, and calls out from corruption and decay beauty and everlasting glory."—Sir Humphry Davy.

† One among a thousand illustrations of this discrepancy is to be found in the bitter anguish—the grief refusing to be comforted—with which survivors often bewail the dead; a grief infinitely more poignant than that with which they would see them embark for another hemisphere, if it were even without expectation of their return and with no certainty of their

It is important also to distinguish among those who go by the general name of unbelievers. Of these, a few deny that man has an immortal soul; others allege that they have as yet found no conclusive proof of the soul's ultramundane existence: and the latter are much more numerous than the former.

The difference between the two is great. The creed of the one may be taxed with presumption, of the other with insufficiency only. The one profess already to have reached the goal; the others declare that they are still on the road of inquiry.

But as to these latter, any additional class of proofs we can find touching the nature of the soul are especially important. Here we come upon the practical bearings of the question. For, while men are so diversely constituted and so variously trained as we find them, the same evidence will never convince all minds. And it is equally unchristian,* unphilosophical, and

happiness. If we do not forget, do we practically realize, that article of faith which teaches that it is only *to us* they die? The German idiomatic expression, in this connection, is as correct as it is beautiful :—

"Den Oberlin hatte zuweilen die Ahnung wie ein kalter Schauer durchdrungen, dass sein geliebtes Weib *ihm* sterben könne."—"*Das grosse Geheimniss der menschlichen Doppelnatur*," Dresden, 1855.

* Matthew vii. 1. It is quite contrary to the fact to assume as to skeptics in general that they are willfully blind. Many, it is true, especially in the heyday of youth, fall into unbelief, or an indifference much resembling it, from sheer heedlessness; while some deliberately avoid the thoughts of another world, lest these should abridge their pleasures in this; but the better and probably the more numerous portion belong to neither of these classes. They scruple because difficulties are thrust upon them. They doubt unwillingly and perforce. The author of the "*Eclipse of Faith*" (written in reply to Newman's "*Phases of Faith*") gives, as the confession of such a one, what is appropriate to hundreds of thousands :—

"I have been rudely driven out of my old beliefs; my early Christian faith has given way to doubt; the little hut on the mountain-side, in which I had thought to dwell with pastoral simplicity, has been shattered by the tempest, and I turned out to the blast without a shelter. I have wandered long and far, but have not found that rest which you tell me is to be ob-

unjust to condemn one's neighbor, because the species of testimony which convinces us leaves him in doubt or disbelief. Shall we imagine a just God joining in such a condemnation? Or may we not, far more rationally, believe it probable that, in the progressive course of His economy, He may be providing for each class of minds that species of evidence which is best fitted for its peculiar nature?

A Paris physician of the highest standing, Dr. Georget, the well-known author of a Treatise on the Physiology of the Nervous System,* made his will on the 1st of March, 1826, dying shortly after. To that document a clause is appended, in which, after alluding to the fact that in the treatise above referred to he had

---

tained. As I examine all other theories, they seem to me pressed by at least equal difficulties with that I have abandoned. I cannot make myself *contented*, as others do, with believing nothing; and yet I have nothing to believe. I have wrestled long and hard with my Titan foes, but not successfully. I have turned to every quarter of the universe in vain. I have interrogated my own soul, but it answers not. I have gazed upon nature, but its many voices speak no articulate language to *me ;* and, more especially, when I gaze upon the bright page of the midnight heavens, those orbs gleam upon me with so cold a light and amidst so portentous a silence that I am, with Pascal, terrified at the spectacle of the infinite solitude." —p. 70.

* *" De la Physiologie du Système Nerveux, et spécialement du Cerveau."* Par M. Georget, D. M. de la Faculté de Paris, ancien Interne de première classe de la division des Aliénées de l'Hospice de la Salpetrière: 2 vols., Paris, 1821.

The original text of the clause in Georget's will, above quoted from, will be found in *"Rapports et Discussions de l'Academie Royale de Médecine sur le Magnetisme animal,"* by M. P. Foissac, M.D., Paris, 1833, p. 289. The exact words of his avowal are, " À peine avais-je mis au jour la ' Physiologie du Système Nerveux,' que de nouvelles méditations sur un phénomène bien extraordinaire, le somnambulisme, ne me permirent plus de douter de l'existence, en nous et hors de nous, d'un principe intelligent, tout-à-fait différent des existences materielles."

Husson, a member of the Paris Academy of Medicine, in a report to that body made in 1825, speaks of Georget as " notre estimable, laborieux, et modeste collègue."—*Foissac's Rapports et Discussions,* p. 28.

openly professed materialism, he says, "I had scarcely published the 'Physiologie du Système Nerveux,' when additional reflections on a very extraordinary phenomenon, somnambulism, no longer allowed me to doubt of the existence, in us and out of us, of an intelligent principle, differing entirely from any material existence." He adds, "This declaration will see the light when my sincerity can no longer be doubted nor my intentions suspected." And he concludes by an earnest request, addressed to those who may be present at the opening of his will, that they will give to the declaration in question all the publicity possible.

Thus we find an able man, living in a Christian country, where he had access to all the usual evidences of our religion, who remains during the greater part of his life a materialist, and toward its close finds, in a psychological phenomenon, proof sufficient to produce a profound conviction that his life's belief had been an error, and that the soul of man *has* an immortal existence.

The Bible had failed to convince him of his error. But ought not every believer in the soul's immortality to rejoice, that the unbelief which scriptural testimony had proved insufficient to conquer yielded before evidence drawn from examination of one of the many wonders, exhibited by what every one but the atheist declares to be the handiwork of God?

And since that wonder belongs to a class of phenomena the reality of which is denied by many and doubted by more, should not every friend of religion bid God-speed the inquirer who pushes his researches into regions that have produced fruits so valuable as these?

Nor is he a true friend to religion or to his race who does not desire that men should obtain the strongest possible evidence which exists of the soul's immortality, and the reality of a future life. But if there actually be physical evidence, cognizable by the senses, of these great truths, it is, and ever must be, stronger than any which can possibly result from scriptural testimony. Intelligent Christians, even the most orthodox, admit this; Tillotson, for example. It forms, indeed, the staple of his argument against the *real presence*. Says that learned prelate, "Infidelity were hardly possible to men, if all men had the same evidence for the Christian religion which they have against transubstantiation; that is, the clear and irresistible evidence of sense."*

Scripture and common sense alike sustain this doctrine; nay, our every-day language assumes its truth. If a friend, even the most trusted, relate to us some incident which he has witnessed, in what terms do we express our conviction that he has told us the truth? Do we say, "I know his testimony"? There is no such expression in the English language. We say, "I believe his testimony."† It is true that such evidence, subject, however, to cross-examination, decides, in a court of justice, men's lives and fortunes; but only from the necessity of the case; only because the judges and jury could not themselves be eye or ear witnesses of the facts to be proved : and, with every care to scrutinize such testimony, it has ere now brought innocent men to the scaffold. Nor, save in extraordinary or exceptional cases,

---

* *"The Works of the Most Reverend Dr. John Tillotson, late Lord Archbishop of Canterbury,"* 8th ed., London, 1720. Sermon XXVI.

† In the present volume I shall have occasion to testify as to many things which I have heard and seen. Nor do I imagine that men, themselves candid, will suspect in me lack of candor; for when a man of honest motive, seeking only the truth, plainly and impartially narrates his experience, that which he says usually bears with it to the upright mind an internal warrant of sincerity. But yet my testimony is, and ever must be, to the reader, evidence of far lower grade and far less force than that he would have obtained if he had himself personally witnessed what I narrate   The difference is inherent in the nature of things.

is it under our system ever taken in court at second hand.* And when a witness begins to repeat that which others have seen and related, what is the common phrase employed to recall him to his proper sphere of duty? —"Do not tell us what others have said to you: keep to what you can depose of your own *knowledge.*"

So, also, when in Scripture reference is made to persons having faith or lacking it, how are they designated? As *knowers* and *unknowers?* No: but as *believers* and *unbelievers.* "He that believeth"—not he that knoweth —"shall be saved." As to things spiritual the Bible (with rare exceptions) speaks of our belief on this side the grave, our knowledge only on the other. "Then shall we know, even as also we are known."

But to argue at length such a point as this is mere supererogation. There are some truths the evidence for which no argument can strengthen, because they appeal directly to our consciousness and are adopted unchallenged and at once. A pious mother loses her child,—though the very phrase is a falsity: she but parts with him for a season,—but, in the world's language and in her heart's language, she loses her only child by death. If, now, just when her bereavement is felt the most despairingly,—in the bitter moment, perhaps, (the winter's storm raging without,) when the thought flashes across her that the cold sleet is beating on her deserted darling's new-made grave; if in that terrible moment there should reach her suddenly, unexpectedly, a token visible to the senses, an appearance in bodily form, or

---

* I speak of the principles of evidence recognized by the common law; a system under which personal rights and guards to the liberty of the citizen are probably better assured than under any other; though as to some rights of property the civil law system may claim the superiority.

Evidence at second hand is admissible in the case of a dying man, conscious of the near approach of death, or as to what has been said, uncontradicted, in the presence and within the hearing of a prisoner; but these are the exceptions establishing the general rule.

an actual message perhaps, which she *knew* came that instant direct from her child; that appearance or that message testifying that he whom she had just been thinking of as lying, wrested from her loving care, under the storm-beaten turf, was not there, was far happier than even she had ever made him, was far better cared for than even in her arms: in such a moment as that, how poor and worthless are all the arts of logic to prove that the sunshine of such unlooked-for assurance, breaking through the gloomy tempest of the mother's grief, and lighting up her shrouded hopes, has added nothing to the measure of her belief in immortality, has increased not the force of her convictions touching the Great Future, has raised not from faith to knowledge the degree of credence with which she can repeat to her soul the inspiring words, that, though the dust has returned to the earth as it was, the spirit is in the hands of God who gave it!

Then, if it *should* happen that the "unknown Dark" may, in a measure, even here become known; if it *should* be that the Great Dramatist inaptly described the next world, when he called it

> " The undiscovered country, from whose bourn
> No traveler returns;"

if it *should* prove true that occasions sometimes present themselves when we have the direct evidence of our senses to demonstrate the continued existence and affection of those friends who have passed that bourn; if it *should* be the will of God that, at this stage of man's constant progress, more clearly distinguishing phenomena which, in modern times at least, have been usually discredited or denied, he should attain a point at which *Belief*, the highest species of conviction which Scripture or analogy can supply, may rise to the grade of *Knowledge*;—if all this be, in very deed, a *Reality*, is it not a

glorious one, earnestly to be desired, gratefully to be
welcomed?

And should not those who, with a single eye to the
truth, faithfully and patiently question Nature, to discover whether it *is* Reality or Illusion,—should not
such honest and earnest investigators be cheered on
their path, be commended for their exertions? If it be
a sacred and solemn duty to study the Scriptures in
search of religious belief, is it a duty less sacred, less
solemn, to study Nature in search of religious knowledge?

In prosecuting that research, if any fear to sin by
overpassing the limits of permitted inquiry and tres-
passing upon unholy and forbidden ground, let him be
reminded that God, who protects His own mysteries,
has rendered that sin impossible; and let him go, reverently indeed, but freely and undoubtingly, forward.
If God has closed the way, man cannot pass thereon.
But if He has left open the path, who shall forbid its
entrance?

It is good to take with us through life, as companion,
a great and encouraging subject; and of this we feel the
need the more as we advance in years. As to that
which I have selected, eminently true is the happy expression of a modern writer, that "in journeying with
it we go toward the sun, and the shadow of our burden
falls behind us."*

Some one has suggested that, if we would truly determine whether, at any given time, we are occupying
ourselves after a manner worthy of rational and immortal beings, it behooves us to ask our hearts if we are
willing death should surprise us in the occupation.
There is no severer test. And if we apply it to such
researches as these, how clearly stands forth their high

---

* *"Essays written during the Intervals of Business,"* London, 1853, p. 2.

character! If, in prosecuting such, the observer be overtaken by death, the destroyer has no power to arrest his observations. The fatal fiat but extends their field. The torch is not quenched in the grave. It burns far more brightly beyond than ever it did or can in this dim world of ours. Here the inquirer may grope and stumble, seeing but as through a glass darkly. Death, that has delivered so many millions from misery, will dispel his doubts and resolve his difficulties. Death, the unriddler, will draw aside the curtain and let in the explaining light. That which is feebly commenced in this phase of existence will be far better prosecuted in another. Will the inquiry be completed even there? Who can tell?

CHAPTER II.

THE IMPOSSIBLE.

"He who, outside of pure mathematics, pronounces the word *impossible*, lacks prudence."—ARAGO: *Annuaire du Bureau des Longitudes*, 1853.*

THERE was enacted, in April of the year 1493, and in the city of Barcelona, one of those great scenes which occur but a few times in the history of our race.

A Genoese mariner, of humble birth and fortune, an enthusiast, a dreamer, a believer in Marco Polo and Mandeville and in all their gorgeous fables,—the golden shores of Zipango, the spicy paradise of Cathay,—had conceived the magnificent project of seeking out what proved to be an addition to the known world of another hemisphere.

He had gone begging from country to country, from monarch to monarch, for countenance and means. His proposals rejected by his native city, he had carried them to Spain, then governed by two of the ablest sovereigns she ever had. But there the usual fortune of the theorist seemed to pursue him. His best protector the humble guardian of an Andalusian convent, his doctrine rejected by the queen's confessor as savoring of heresy, his lofty pretensions scouted by nobles and archbishops as those of a needy foreign adventurer, his scheme pronounced by the learned magnates of the

---

* The original, with its context, is, "Le *doute* est une preuve de modestie, et il a rarement nui aux progrès des sciences. On n'en pourrait pas dire autant de *l'incrédulité*. Celui qui, en dehors des mathématiques pures, prononce le mot *impossible*, manque de prudence. La réserve est surtout un devoir quand il s'agit de l'organisation animale."—*Annuaire*, p. 445.

Salamanca council (for when was titled Science ever a pioneer?) to be "vain, impracticable, and resting on grounds too weak to merit the support of the government,"—he had scantily found at last, even in the enlightened and enterprising Isabella, tardy faith enough to adventure a sum that any lady of her court might have spent on a diamond bracelet or a necklace of pearl.*

And now, returned as it were from the dead, survivor of a voyage overhung with preternatural horrors, his great problem, as in despite of man and nature, triumphantly resolved, the visionary was welcomed as the conqueror; the needy adventurer was recognized as Admiral of the Western Ocean and Viceroy of a New Continent; was received, in solemn state, by the haughtiest sovereigns in the world, rising at his approach, and invited (Castilian punctilio overcome by intellectual power) to be seated before them.   He told his wondrous story, and exhibited, as vouchers for its truth, the tawny savages and the barbaric gold.   King, queen, and court sunk on their knees; and the Te Deum sounded, as for some glorious victory.

That night, in the silence of his chamber, what thoughts may have thronged on Columbus's mind! What exultant emotions must have swelled his heart! A past world had deemed the Eastern Hemisphere the entire habitable earth.   Age had succeeded to age, century had passed away after century, and still the interdict had been acquiesced in, that westward beyond the mountain pillars† it belonged not to man to explore.

---

* Seventeen thousand florins was the petty amount which the fitting-out of Columbus's first expedition cost the crown of Castile.   How incommensurate, sometimes, are even our successful exertions with the importance of some noble but novel object of research!

† —— quella foce stretta
Ov' Ercole segnò li suoi riguardi,
Acciochè l'uom più oltre non si metta.
                              DANTE, *Inferno*, Canto XVI.

And yet he, the chosen of God to solve the greatest of terrestrial mysteries, affronting what even the hardy mariners of Palos had regarded as certain destruction,—he, the hopeful one where all but himself despaired,—had wrested from the Deep its mighty secret,—had accomplished what the united voice of the Past had declared to be an impossible achievement.

But now, if, in the stillness of that night, to this man, enthusiast, dreamer, believer as he was, there had suddenly appeared some Nostradamus of the fifteenth century, of prophetic mind instinct with the future, and had declared to the ocean-compeller that not four centuries would elapse before that vast intervening gulf of waters—from the farther shore of which, through months of tempest, he had just groped back his weary way—should interpose no obstacle to the free communication of human thought; that a man standing on the western shore of Europe should, within three hundred and seventy years from that day, engage in conversation with his fellow standing on the eastern shore of the new-found world; nay,—marvel of all marvels!—that the same fearful bolt which during his terrible voyage had so often lighted up the waste of waters around him should itself become the agent of communication across that storm-tossed ocean; that mortal creatures, un-aided by angel or demon, without intervention of Heaven or pact with hell, should bring that lightning under domestic subjection, and employ it, as they might some menial or some carrier-dove, to bear their daily messages;—to a prediction so wildly extravagant, so surpassingly absurd, as that, what credence could even Columbus lend? What answer to such a prophetic vision may we imagine that he, with all a life's experience of man's short-sightedness, would have given? Probably some reply like this: that, though in the future many strange things might be, such a tampering with

Nature as *that*—short of a direct miracle from God—was IMPOSSIBLE!

Arago was right. With exact truths we may deal in a positive manner. Of a hexagon inscribed within a circle each side is of the same length as the radius of that circle: it is *impossible* it should be either longer or shorter. The surface contained within the square of the hypothenuse is exactly of the same extent as the squares, taken together, of the two other sides of the same right-angled triangle: it is *impossible* it should be either greater or less. These things we declare to be impossible with the same assurance and the same propriety with which we assert that we exist; and there is no more presumption in declaring the one than in asserting the other. But, outside the domain of pure mathematics, or kindred regions of abstract or intuitive truth, cautious and modest in his pronouncings should be fallible and short-sighted man. By what warrant does he assume to determine what God's laws permit and what they deny? By what authority does he take upon himself to assert that to him *all* these laws are known? The term of his life but a day, the circumference of his ken but a spot, whence derives he his commission, groping about in his little span of the Present, arrogantly to proclaim what is and what is not to be in the illimitable Future? Does not History bear on every page a condemnation of the impiety? Does not Experience daily rise up and testify aloud against such egregious presumption?

Not thus is it that those speak and reason whom deep research has taught how little they know. It occurs to the humble wisdom of such men that laws of nature may exist with which they are wholly unacquainted;*

* I translate from La Place's "*Théorie analytique des Probabilités:*"—"We are so far from knowing all the agents of nature and their various modes of action, that it would not be philosophical to deny any phenomena

nay, some, perhaps, which may never, since man was first here to observe them, have been brought into operation at all.

Sir John Herschel has aptly illustrated this truth. "Among all the possible combinations," says that enlightened philosopher, "of the fifty or sixty elements which chemistry shows to exist on the earth, it is likely, nay, almost certain, that *some* have never been formed; that some elements, in some proportions and under some circumstances, have never yet been placed in relation with one another. Yet no chemist can doubt that it is *already fixed* what they will do when the case does occur. They will obey certain laws, of which we know nothing at present, but which must *be* already fixed, or they would not be laws."*

And what is true as to rules of chemical affinity is equally true of physiological and psychological laws. Indeed, it is more likely to be a frequent truth as to the

---

merely because in the actual state of our knowledge they are inexplicable. This only we ought to do: in proportion to the difficulty there seems to be in admitting them should be the scrupulous attention we bestow on their examination."—*Introd.*, p. 43.

From a widely-accepted authority still better known among us I extract, in the same connection, the following, in the last line of which, however, the word *possibility* might have been more strictly in place than *probability*:—

"An unlimited skepticism is the part of a contracted mind, which reasons upon imperfect data, or makes its own knowledge and extent of observation the standard and test of probability. . . .

"In receiving upon testimony statements which are rejected by the vulgar as totally incredible, a man of cultivated mind is influenced by the recollection that many things at one time appeared to him marvelous which he now knows to be true, and he thence concludes that there may still be in nature many phenomena and many principles with which he is entirely unacquainted. In other words, he has learned from experience not to make his own knowledge his test of probability."—*Abercrombie's Intellectual Powers*, pp. 55 and 60.

* "*Preliminary Discourse on the Study of Natural Philosophy*" by Sir John F. W. Herschel, Bart., K.H., F.R.S. London, 2d ed., 1851, p. 36.

laws of mind than as to those of matter, because there is nothing in the world so constantly progressive as the intelligence of man. His race alone, of all the animated races with which we are acquainted, changes and rises from generation to generation. The elephant and the beaver of to-day are not, that we know, more intelligent or further developed than were the elephant and the beaver of three thousand years ago. Theirs is a stationary destiny, but man's an advancing one,—advancing from savage instincts to civilized sentiments, from unlettered boorishness to arts and sciences and literature, from anarchy to order, from fanaticism to Christianity.

But it is precisely in the case of a being whose progress is constant, and whose destiny is upward as well as onward, that we may the most confidently look, at certain epochs of his development, for the disclosure of new relations and the further unfolding of laws till then but imperfectly known.

There is, it is true, another view to take of this case. To some it will seem an unwarranted stretch of analogical inference that because in the department of chemistry we may anticipate combinations never yet formed, to be governed by laws never yet operating, we should therefore conclude that in the department of mind, also, similar phenomena may be expected. Mind and matter, it may be objected, are separated by so broad a demarkation-line, that what is true of the one may be false of the other.

Are they so widely separated? Distinct they are; nothing is more untenable than the argument of the materialist; but yet how intimately connected! A pressure on the substance of the brain, and thought is suspended; a sponge with a few anesthetic drops applied to the nostrils, and insensibility supervenes; another odor inhaled, and life is extinct.

And if such be the action of matter on mind, no less

striking is the control of mind over matter. The influence of imagination is proverbial; yet it has ever been
underrated. The excited mind can cure the suffering
body. Faith, exalted to ecstasy, has arrested disease.*
The sway of will thoroughly stirred into action often
transcends the curative power of physic or physician.

But it is not in general considerations, such as these,
that the argument rests touching the intimate connection between material influences and mental phenomena.
The modern study of the imponderables, already pro-
ductive of physical results that to our ancestors would
have seemed sheer miracles, has afforded glimpses of
progress in another direction, which may brighten into
discoveries before which the spanning of the Atlantic
by a lightning-wire will pale into insignificance. Galvani's first hasty inferences as to animal electricity were
to a certain extent refuted, it is true, by Volta's stricter
tests. But in Italy, in Prussia, and in England, experiments of a recent date, following up the just though
imperfect idea of the Bolognese professor, have established the fact that the muscular contractions, voluntary
or automatic, which produce action in a living limb,
correspond to currents of electricity existing there in
appreciable quantities.† The discoverer of creosote has

---

* These opinions find ample confirmation—to select one among many
sources—in a branch of study equally interesting to the physician and the
psychologist; the history, namely, of the great mental epidemics of the
world. The reader will find these briefly noticed further on in these pages.

† Galvani's first eventful observation on an electrical agency producing
muscular contractions in animals, made on the 20th of September, 1786,
was, after all, the starting-point of the recent interesting researches by Du
Bois-Reymond, Zantedeschi, Matteucci, and others, on the continent of Europe, and by Rutter and Leger, in England. Du Bois-Reymond himself,
member of the Academy of Sciences of Berlin, very candidly admits this
fact. In a historical introduction to his work on Animal Magnetism
(" *Untersuchungen über thierische Elektricität,*" Berlin, 1848–49) that writer
says, "Galvani really discovered not only the fundamental physiological
experiment of galvanism properly so called, (the contraction of the frog

given to the world the results of a ten years' labor, it may be said, in the same field; distinguishing, however, what he terms the *Odic* from the electric force.* Arago thought the case of Angélique Cottin (well known under the name of the "Electric Girl") worthy of being brought under the notice of the Paris Academy of Sciences;† and, speaking, seven years afterward, of "the actual power which one man may exert over another without the intervention of any known physical agent," he declares that even Bailly's report against Mesmer's crude theory shows "how our faculties ought to be studied

when touched with dissimilar metals,) but also that of the electricity inherent in the nerves and muscles. Both of these discoveries were, however, hidden in such a confusion of circumstances that the result in both cases appeared equally to depend on the limbs or tissues of the animals employed."

The reader, desiring to follow up this subject, may consult a work by H. Bence Jones, M.D., F.R.S., entitled "*On Animal Electricity: being an Abstract of the Discoveries of Emil Du Bois-Reymond,*" London, 1852. Also, "*Traité des Phénomènes électro-physiologiques des Animaux,*" by Carlo Matteucci, Professor in the University of Pisa, 1844. Also, Baron Humboldt's work on Stimulated Nervous and Muscular Fibers, ("*Versuche über die gereizte Muskel- und Nervenfaser, u. s. w.*")

In England experiments in this branch have been pushed further than in any other country; chiefly by Rutter of Brighton, and by Dr. Leger, whose early death was a loss alike to physiological and psychological science. I had an opportunity, through the kindness of Mr. Rutter, of personally witnessing the extraordinary results to which his patient research has led, and which I regret that space does not permit me here to notice at large. I can but refer to his work, "*Human Electricity: the Means of its Development, illustrated by Experiments,*" London, 1854; and to another brief treatise on the same subject, by Dr. T. Leger, entitled "*The Magnetoscope: an Essay on the Magnetoid Characteristics of Elementary Principles, and their Relations to the Organization of Man,*" London, 1852.

The whole subject is singularly interesting, and will richly repay the study that may be bestowed upon it.

* I here refer to Baron Reichenbach's elaborate treatises on what he calls the "Odic Force," without expressing any opinion as to the accuracy of the author's conclusions. Reichenbach discovered creosote in 1833.

† Arago's report on the subject was made on the 16th of February, 1846. It is much to be regretted that an observer so sagacious should have had no opportunity, in this case, to follow up his first hasty experiments.

experimentally, and by what means psychology may one day obtain a place among the exact sciences."* Cuvier, more familiar than Arago with the phenomena of animated nature, speaks more decidedly than he on the same subject. "It scarcely admits of further doubt," says that eminent naturalist, "that the proximity of two living bodies, in certain circumstances and with certain movements, has a real effect, independently of all participation of the imagination of one of the two;" and he further adds that "it appears now clearly enough that the effects are due to some communication established between their nervous systems."† This is conceding the principle lying at the base of Mesmerism,—a concession which is sustained by countless observations, little reliable in some cases, but in others, especially of late, carefully made by upright and capable experimentalists, on the contested ground of artificial somnambulism and kindred phenomena.

Without pausing here to inquire to what extent these various startling novelties need confirmation, or how far the deductions therefrom may be modified or disproved by future observations, enough of indisputable can be found therein, if not to indicate that we may be standing even now on the shores of a Great Ocean, slowly unvailing its wonders, and the exploration of

---

* "*Biographie de Jean-Sylvain Bailly,*" by M. Arago, originally published in the "Annuaire du Bureau des Longitudes" for 1853, pp. 345 to 625.

† "*Leçons d'Anatomie comparée,*" de G. Cuvier, Paris; An. viii. vol. ii. pp. 117, 118. The original text, with its context, is as follows:—

"Les effets obtenus sur des personnes déjà sans connaissance avant que l'opération commençât, ceux qui ont lieu sur les autres personnes après que l'opération leur a fait perdre connaissance, et ceux que présentent les animaux, ne permettent guère de douter que la proximité de deux corps animés, dans certaines positions et avec certains mouvements, n'ait un effet réel, indépendant de toute participation de l'imagination d'une des deux. Il paraît assez clairement, aussi, que les effets sont dus à une communication quelconque qui s'établit entre leurs systèmes nerveux."

which is to bring us richer reward than did that of the
Atlantic to Columbus, at least to convince us that Herschel's philosophical remark may have a wider range
than he intended to give it; that in physiology and in
psychology, as in chemistry, there may be possible combinations that have never yet been formed under our
eyes; new relations, new conditions, yet to exist or
appear; all to be governed, when they do occur, by
laws that have obtained, indeed, from the creation of
the world, but have remained until now, not, indeed,
inoperative, but concealed from general observation.

From *general* observation; for, though unrecognized
by science, they are not therefore to be set down as unknown. It is one of the objects proposed in the pages
which follow, to glean, from the past as well as the
present, scattered intimations of the existence of laws
under which it has been alleged that man may attain,
from sources other than revelation and analogy, some
assurance in regard to the world to come. And since
it is evident that no abstract truth is violated by the
hypothesis of the existence of such laws, may I not
adduce such names as Arago and Herschel to sustain
me in asserting, that they lack prudence who take upon
themselves to pronounce, in advance, that whoever
argues such a theme has engaged in a search after the
impossible?

CHAPTER III.

THE MIRACULOUS.

The universal cause
Acts, not by partial but by general laws.—Pope.

Men are very generally agreed to regard him as
stricken with superstition or blinded by credulity who
believes in any miracle of modern days. And as the
world grows older this disbelief in the supernatural
gradually acquires strength and universality.

The reason seems to be, that the more searchingly
science explores the mechanism of the universe and
unvails the plan of its government, the more evidence
there appears for the poet's opinion that it is by general,
not by partial, laws that the universe is governed.

In such a doctrine the question of God's omnipotence
is not at all involved. It is not whether He *can* make
exceptions to a system of universal law, but whether
He *does*. If we may permit ourselves to speak of God's
choice and intentions, it is not whether, to meet an incidental exigency, He has the power to suspend the
order of those constant sequences which, because of
their constancy, we term laws; but only whether, in
point of fact, He chooses to select that occasional mode
of effecting His objects, or does not rather see fit to
carry them out after a more unvarying plan, by means
less exceptional and arbitrary. It is a question of fact.

But modern Science, in her progress, not only strikes
from what used to be regarded as the list of exceptions
to the general order of nature one item after another:
she exhibits to us, also, more clearly day by day, the

70

simplicity of natural laws, and the principle of unity under which detached branches are connected as parts of one great system

Thus, as applied to what happens in our day, accumulating experience discredits the doctrine of occasional causes and the belief in the miraculous. If a man relate to us, even from his own experience, some incident clearly involving supernatural agency, we listen with a shrug of pity. If we have too good an opinion of the narrator's honesty to suspect that he is playing on our credulity, we conclude unhesitatingly that he is deceived by his own. We do not stop to examine the evidence for a modern miracle: we reject it on general principles.

But, in assenting to such skepticism, we shall do well to consider what a miracle is. Hume, in his well-known chapter on this subject, adduces a useful illustration. The Indian prince, he says, who rejected testimony as to the existence of ice, refused his assent to facts which arose from a state of nature with which he was unacquainted, and which bore so little analogy to those events of which he had had constant and uniform experience. As to these facts, he alleges, "Though they were not contrary to his experience, they were not conformable to it."* And, in explanation of the distinction here made, he adds, in a note, "No Indian, it is evident, could have experience that water did not freeze in cold climates."†

Is the above distinction a substantial one? If so, it leads much further than Hume intended it should.

Not only had the Indian prince never seen water in a solid state; until now, he had never heard of such a thing. Not only was his own unvarying experience

* Hume's "Essays and Treatises on Various Subjects," 2d ed., London, 1784, vol. ii. p. 122.

† Hume's Essays, vol. ii., Note K, p. 479.

opposed to the alleged fact, but the experience of his fathers, the traditions of his country, all declared that water ever had been, as now it was, a fluid. Had he no right to say that solid water was a thing contrary to his experience? Or ought he, with philosophic moderation, to have restricted his declaration to this, that the phenomenon of ice, if such phenomenon had actual existence, "arose from a state of nature with which he was unacquainted."

We, who have so often walked upon solid water, find no difficulty in deciding that this last is what he ought to have said. Let us forgive the ignorant savage his presumptuous denial, as we would ourselves, in similar case, be forgiven!

Let us reflect how much cautious wisdom, that we find not among the best informed and most learned among ourselves, we are expecting from an unlettered barbarian. Let us inquire whether Hume, calm and philosophic as he is, does not himself fail in the very wisdom he exacts. He says, in the same chapter,—

"A miracle is a violation of the laws of Nature; and, as a firm and unalterable experience has established these laws, the proof against a miracle, from the very nature of the fact, is as entire as any argument from experience can possibly be imagined."[*]

Here are two propositions: one, that what a firm and unalterable experience establishes is a law of nature; and the other, that a variation from such a law is a miracle.

But no human experience is *unalterable*. We may say it has hitherto been *unaltered*. And even that it is always hazardous to say.

If any one has a right thus to speak of his experience and that of his fellows, was not the Indian prince justified in considering it to be proved, by unalterable

* Hume's Essays, vol. ii. p. 122.

experience, that a stone placed on the surface of a sheet of water would sink to the bottom? Was he not fully justified, according to Hume's own premises, in setting down the traveler's allegation to the contrary as the assertion of a miracle, and, as such, in rejecting it as impossible?

"No Indian," says Hume, "could have experience that water did not freeze in cold countries." Of course not. That was a fact beyond his experience. Are there no facts beyond ours? Are there no states of nature with which we are unacquainted? Is it the Indian prince alone whose experience is limited and fallible?

When a man speaks of the experience of the past as a regulator of his belief, he means—he *can* mean—only so much of that experience as has come to his knowledge mediately or immediately. In such a case, then, to express himself accurately, he ought not to say, "the experience of the past,"—for that would imply that he knows all that has ever happened,—but only, "my past experience."

Then Hume's assertion, in the paragraph above quoted, is, that *his* past experience, being firm and unalterable,* enables him to determine what are invariable laws of nature, and, consequently, what are miracles.

Nor is this the full extent of the presumption. Elsewhere in this chapter the author says "that a miracle supported by any human testimony is more properly a subject of derision than of argument."†

Taken in connection with the paragraph above cited, what a monstrous doctrine is here set up! Let it be

---

* In another place (p. 119) Hume employs the word *infallible* in a similar connection, thus:—"A wise man proportions his belief to the evidence. In such conclusions as are founded on an infallible experience, he expects the event with the last degree of assurance, and regards his past experience as a full *proof* of the future existence of that event." (The italics are his.)

† Hume's Essays, vol. ii. p. 133.

stated in plain terms. "I regard my past experience as firm and unalterable. If a witness, no matter how credible, testifies to any occurrence which is contrary to that experience, I do not argue with such a man: he is only worthy of derision."

Though, in our day, hundreds who ought to know better act out this very doctrine, I would not be understood as asserting that Hume intended to put it forth. We often fail to perceive the legitimate issue of our own premises.

But let us proceed a step further. Let us inquire under what circumstances we have the right to say, "such or such an occurrence is incredible, for it would be miraculous."

The question brings us back to our first inquiry,—as to what a miracle is. Let us examine Hume's definition :—

"A miracle may be accurately defined, a transgression of a law of nature by a particular volition of the Deity, or by the interposition of some invisible agent."* I remark, in passing, that the expression " by the interposition of some invisible agent" is an inaccuracy. Cold is an invisible agent: it is not even a positive agent at all, being only the withdrawal or diminution of heat. Yet cold suspends what the Indian prince had strong reason for regarding as a law of nature.

But the main proposition remains. "A miracle is a transgression of a law of nature by a particular volition of the Deity."

Here again the language seems unhappily chosen. When we speak of a thing as happening by the will of God, we rationally intend, by the expression, only that it is the act of God; for God's intentions are inscrutable to us, except as they appear in His acts. Can we say

---

* Hume's Essays, vol. ii., Note K, p. 480.

of any thing which occurs at all, that it does not occur by volition of the Deity?

The word "transgression," too, seems not the best that could have been employed.* It must, of course, be taken in its original sense of a going or passing beyond. The author evidently meant a suspension for the time to suit a particular emergency; and that would have been the more appropriate phrase.

Hume's idea, then, would seem to be more fittingly expressed in these terms:—"A miracle is a suspension, in a special emergency and for the time only, of a law of nature, by the direct intervention of the Deity." We might add, to complete the ordinary conception of a miracle, the words, "in attestation of some truth."

And now arises the chief question, already suggested. How are we to know, as to any unusual phenomenon presented to us, that it *is* an effect of the special intervention of God? in other words, whether it is miraculous?

But I will not even ask this question as to ourselves, finite and short-sighted as we are. It shall be far more forcibly put. Let us imagine a sage, favored beyond living mortal, of mind so comprehensive, of information so vast, that the entire experience of the past world, century by century, even from man's creation, lay patent before him. Let us suppose the question addressed to him. And would he,—a being thus preternaturally gifted,—would even he have the right to decide,

---

* It would be hypercriticism to object to this expression in a general way. The best authors have employed it as Hume does, yet rather in poetry than in prose, as Dryden:—

> " Long stood the noble youth, oppressed with awe,
> And stupid at the wondrous things he saw,
> Surpassing common faith, transgressing Nature's law."

But a looseness of expression which may adorn a poetic phrase, or pass unchallenged in a literary theme, should be avoided in a strictly logical argument, and more especially in a definition of terms.

would he have the *means* of deciding, as to any event which may happen to-day, whether it is, or is not, a miracle?

He may know, what we never can, that a uniform experience, continued throughout thousands of years and unbroken yet by a single exception, has established, as far as past experience can establish, the existence of a natural law or constant sequence; and he may observe a variation, the first which ever occurred, to this law. But is it given to him to know whether the Deity, to meet a certain exigency, is suspending His own law, or whether this variation is not an integral portion of the original law itself? in other words, whether the apparent law, as judged by an induction running through thousands of years, is the full expression of that law, or whether the exception now first appearing was not embraced in the primary adjustment of the law itself, when it was first made to act on the great mechanism of the Universe?

Has the Creator of the world no power to establish for its progressive government laws of (what we may call) a change-bearing character? preserving, (that is,) through the lapse of many ages, constancy of sequence, and then, at a certain epoch, by virtue of that character, (impressed upon it by the same original ordination which determined the previous long-enduring constancy,) made to exhibit a variation?

We, his creatures, even with our restricted powers, know how to impress upon human mechanism laws of just such a character. The illustration furnished by Babbage's Calculating Machine, familiar though it may be, so naturally suggests itself in this connection, that I may be pardoned for presenting it here.

Mr. Babbage's engine, intended to calculate and print mathematical and astronomical tables for the British Government, offers interesting incidental results. *Of* these, the following, supplied by the inventor himself, is an example; and one of such a character that no knowledge of the mechanism of the machine, nor acquaintance with mathematical science, is necessary to comprehend it.

He bids us imagine that the machine had been adjusted. It is put in motion by a weight, and the spectator, sitting down before it, observes a wheel which moves through a small angle round its axis, and which presents at short intervals to his eye, successively, a series of numbers engraved on its divided surface. He bids us suppose the figures thus seen to be the series of natural numbers, 1, 2, 3, 4, &c.; each one exceeding its antecedent by unity. Then he proceeds:—

"Now, reader, let me ask how long you will have counted before you are firmly convinced that the engine, supposing its adjustments to remain unaltered, will continue, whilst its motion is maintained, to produce the same series of natural numbers? Some minds, perhaps, are so constituted, that after passing the first hundred terms they will be satisfied that they are acquainted with the law. After seeing five hundred terms few will doubt; and after the fifty thousandth term the propensity to believe that the succeeding term will be fifty thousand and one will be almost irresistible. That term *will* be fifty thousand and one: the same regular succession will continue; the five millionth and the fifty millionth term will still appear in their expected order; and one unbroken chain of natural numbers will pass before your eyes, from *one* up to *one hundred million.*

"True to the vast induction which has thus been made, the next term will be one hundred million and one; but after that the next number presented by the rim of the wheel, instead of being one hundred million and two, is one hundred million *ten thousand* and two. The whole series, from the commencement, being thus:—

1
2
3
4

. . .

. . . .

. . .
99,999,999
100,000,000
regularly as far as 100,000,001
100,010,002   :—the law changes
100,030,003
100,060,004
100,100,005
100,150,006
100,210,007

. . . .

. . . .

"The law which seemed at first to govern this series failed at the hundred million and second term. This term is larger than we expected by 10,000. The next term is larger than was anticipated by 30,000; and the excess of each term above what we had expected is found to be 10,000, 30,000, 60,000, 100,000, 150,000, &c.; being, in fact, what are called the series of *triangular numbers*, each multiplied by 10,000."

Mr. Babbage then goes on to state that this new law, after continuing for 2761 terms, fails at the two thousand seven hundred and sixty-second term, when another law comes into action, to continue for 1430 terms; then to give place to still another, extending over 950 terms; which, like all its predecessors, fails in its turn, and is succeeded by other laws, which appear at different intervals.

Mr. Babbage's remarks on this extraordinary phenomenon are as follows:—

"Now, it must be remarked, that the law *that each number presented by the engine is greater by unity than the preceding number,* which law the observer had deduced from *an induction of a hundred million instances,* was not the true law that regulated its action; and that the occurrence of the number 100,010,002 at the 100,000,002d term was *as necessary a consequence* of the original adjustment, and might have been as fully foreknown at the commencement, as was the regular succession of any one of the intermediate numbers to its immediate antecedent. The same remark applies to the next *apparent* deviation from the new law, which was founded on an induction of 2761 terms, and to all the succeeding laws; with this limitation only,—that, whilst their consecutive introduction at various definite intervals is a necessary consequence of the mechanical structure of the engine, our knowledge of analysis does not yet enable us to predict the periods at which the more distant laws will be introduced."*

This illustration must not be taken as suborned to establish more than it strictly proves. It is, doubtless, not only a wise but a necessary provision in our nature, that the constancy of any sequence in the past should inspire us with faith that it will continue in the future. Without such faith, the common economy of life would stand still. Uncertain whether to-morrow's sun would rise as did the sun of to-day, or whether the seasons would continue their regular alternations, our lives would pass amid scruples and hesitations. All calculation would be baffled; all industry would sink under discouragement.

The chances, so incalculably great, in most cases, as

---

* *"Ninth Bridgewater Treatise,"* by Charles Babbage, 2d ed., London, 1838, pp. 34 to 39. The passage has been already quoted by another, in connection with a physiological question.

for all practical purposes to amount to certainty, are in favor of the constancy of natural sequences. The corresponding expectations, common to man with the lower animals, are instinctive.

All this is not only true, but it is palpable to our every-day consciousness,—a truth whereupon is based the entire superstructure of our daily hopes and actions. The wheel, with its divided surface, ever revolving, *does* present, to human eyes, uniformity of sequence, age after age; and when the unbroken chain has run on from thousands to millions, we *are* justified, amply justified, in expecting that the next term will obey the same law that determined its antecedent. All I have sought to do in this argument is to keep alive in our minds the conviction, that there *may* be a hundred million and second term, at which the vast induction fails; and that, if such does appear, we have no right to conclude that the change, unprecedented as it must seem to us, is not as necessary a consequence of an original adjustment as was the seemingly infinite uniformity that preceded it.

The extreme rarity of what I have called change-bearing laws of nature is to be conceded; but not the improbability of their existence. In a world all over which is stamped the impress of progress, and which, for aught we know, may continue to endure through countless ages, laws of such a character, self-adapted to a changeful state of things, may be regarded as of likely occurrence.*

---

* Modern science is revealing to us glimpses that may brighten into positive proof of this hypothesis. Sir John Herschel, writing to Lyell the geologist, and alluding to what he calls that "mystery of mysteries, the replacement of extinct species by others," says,—

"For my own part, I cannot but think it an inadequate conception of the Creator, to assume it as granted that His combinations are exhausted upon any one of the theaters of their former exercise; though in this, as in all

But it suffices for the present argument to establish the possibility of such laws. If they are possible, then, in regard to any alleged occurrence of modern times, (strange in character, perhaps, but coming to us well attested,) we are barred from asserting that, because contrary to past experience, it would be miraculous, and is consequently impossible. We are as strictly barred from this as are the visitors to Mr. Babbage's engine from pronouncing, when the long uniformity of a past sequence is unexpectedly violated, that the inventor has been dealing in the black art and is trenching on the supernatural.*

His other works, we are led by all analogy to suppose that He operates through a series of intermediate causes, and that, in consequence, the origination of fresh species, could it ever come under our cognizance, would be found to be a natural, in contradistinction to a miraculous, process; although we may perceive no indication of any process, actually in progress, which is likely to issue in such a result."—*Herschel's letter of Feb.* 20, 1836, *published in Appendix to Babbage's work above cited*, p. 226.

* Reading this chapter more than a year after it was written—namely, in March, 1859—to a private circle of friends in London, one of them called my attention, in connection with its argument, to an article then just published in the (London) Athenæum, attributed (correctly, I believe) to Professor De Morgan, of the London University. It proved to be a review of that strange self-commitment of an able man, virtually following Hume's false lead, Faraday's extraordinary lecture on "Mental Training," delivered, before Prince Albert, at the Royal Institution. And it was a satisfaction to me, on referring to the article, to find, from the pen of one of the first mathematicians of Europe, such a paragraph as the following:—

"The natural philosopher, when he imagines a *physical impossibility* which is not an inconceivability, merely states that his phenomenon is against all that has been hitherto known of the course of nature. Before he can compass an impossibility, he has a huge postulate to ask of his reader or hearer, a postulate which nature never taught: it is that the future is always to agree with the past. How do you know that this sequence of phenomena always will be? Answer, Because it must be. But how do you know that it must be? Answer, Because it always has been. But then, even granting that it always has been, how do you know that what always has been always will be? Answer, I feel my mind compelled to that conclusion. And how do you know that the leanings of your mind are always toward truth? Because I am infallible, the answer *ought to*

F

Nay, there are far stronger reasons against such presumption in our case than in that of the supposed spectator before the calculating machine. He *has* observed the entire series, even to the hundred millionth term. How insignificant the fraction that has passed before our eyes! How imperfect our knowledge of that portion which has passed before the eyes of our ancestors! How insufficient, then, are the data for a decision that the past uniformity has been unbroken!

And herein, beyond all question, do we find a source of error infinitely more frequent than is the failure to recognize a change-bearing law. I have set forth the existence of such laws as a possibility beyond human denial; yet only as an argument to meet an extreme case,—a case so exceedingly rare that, notwithstanding its certain possibility, it may never present itself to our observation. So far as the scope of our limited experience extends, the argument, how undeniable soever, may have no practical application. It may never be our fortune to stand before the Great Machine at the moment when the hundred million and second term, unexpectedly presenting itself, indicates a departure from all former precedent.

Among the laws which we see at work, it may chance that we shall never observe one which some ancestor has not seen in operation already. Nay, that chance is a probable one. In other words, if a phenomenon actually present itself which we are tempted to regard as a violation of natural law, it is more likely—ten thousand to one—that a similar phenomenon has already shown itself more or less frequently in the past, than that it presents itself now for the first time in the history of our race.

<hr/>

be: but this answer is never given."—*Athenæum*, No. 1637, of March 12, 1859, p. 350.

The source of our error, then, when we mistake the extraordinary for the miraculous, is far more frequently in our ignorance of what has been than in our false conceptions of what may be.

The error itself, from either source arising, is a grave one, entailing important practical consequences, which have varied in their prevailing character at different periods of the world. In our day the usual result is incredulity, in advance of examination, as to all phenomena that seem, to our limited experience, incapable of rational explanation. One or two centuries ago the same error often assumed a different form. When a phenomenon presented itself to the men of that day, the cause of which they did not comprehend, and which seemed to them, for that reason, out of the course of nature, they were wont to take it for granted that it happened either through the agency of the devil, or else by special interposition of the Deity in attestation of some contested truth. Thus, Racine relates what he calls the miraculous cure of Mademoiselle Perrier, the niece of Pascal, and then an inmate of the celebrated Convent of Port Royal; and Pascal himself seeks to prove that this miracle was necessary to religion, and was performed in justification of the nuns of that convent, ardent Jansenists, and for that reason under the ban of the Jesuits. La Place, treating the whole as imposture, adduces it as a lamentable example—"afflicting to see and painful to read"—of that blind credulity which is sometimes the weakness of great men.*

---

* See Introduction to his "*Théorie analytique des Probabilités*," (7th vol. of his works, Paris, 1847,) p. 95.

For the story itself the reader is referred to Racine's "*Abrégé de l'Histoire de Port Royal*," Paris, 1693. The alleged miracle occurred in 1656. The young girl, Perrier, had been afflicted with a lachrymal fistula. To the diseased eye was applied a relic,—said to be a thorn from the crown which the Jewish soldiers in mockery placed on the head of Christ. The

The truth in this case, as in many others, may rationally be sought between these extremes of opinion. We cannot, at this distance of time, assume to decide what the precise facts were; but, without impeaching the good faith of a crowd of respectable witnesses, we may deem it probable that the cure really was an extraordinary one, due, it may be, to the influence of the excited mind over the body, or to some magnetic or other occult agency hitherto unrecognized by science; at all events, to some natural, though hidden, cause. Pascal and La Place are doubtless equally in error; the latter in denying that a wonderful cure was effected, the former in seeking its cause in the special intervention of a supernatural power; in imagining that God had

---

girl declared that the touch had cured her. Some days afterward she was examined by several physicians and surgeons, who substantiated the fact of her cure, and expressed *the opinion* that it had not been brought about by medical treatment, or by any natural cause. Besides this, the cure was attested not only by all the nuns of the convent,—celebrated over Europe for their austerity,—but it is further fortified by all the proof which a multitude of witnesses of undoubted character—men of the world as well as physicians—could bestow upon it. The Queen Regent of France, very much prejudiced against Port Royal as a nest of Jansenists, sent her own surgeon, M. Felix, to examine into the miracle; and he returned an absolute convert. So incontestable was it regarded, even by the enemies of the nuns, that it actually saved their establishment for a time from the ruin with which it was threatened by the Jesuits,—who ultimately succeeded, however, some fifty-three years later, in suppressing the convent; it being closed in October, 1709, and razed to the ground the year after.

To Racine—writing in 1673, and therefore unacquainted with these facts—the argument could not occur, that God does not suffer Himself to be baffled by man, and that it is difficult to imagine Him interfering one day in support of a cause which, the next, He suffers to go down before the efforts of its enemies.

But here we approach a subject vailed from finite gaze, the intentions of the Infinite. We are as little justified in asserting that God had no special purpose in permitting an extraordinary phenomenon, which to the ignorance of that day seemed a miracle, as in assuming to decide what that purpose may have been.

suspended for the occasion a great law of nature, for the purpose of indorsing the five propositions of Jansenius, of reprehending a certain religious order, and of affording a momentary triumph to a few persecuted nuns

Similar errors have been of frequent occurrence. Perhaps the most striking example on record is contained in that extraordinary episode in the instructive history of the mental epidemics of Europe, the story of what have been called the *Convulsionists* of St. Médard. It is to this that Hume alludes, in a paragraph of the chapter from which I have already quoted, when he says,—

"There surely never was a greater number of miracles ascribed to one person than those which were lately said to have been wrought in France upon the tomb of the Abbé Pâris, the famous Jansenist, with whose sanctity the people were so long deluded. The curing of the sick, giving hearing to the deaf and sight to the blind, were everywhere talked of as the usual effects of that holy sepulcher. But, what is more extraordinary, many of the miracles were immediately proved upon the spot, before judges of unquestioned integrity, attested by witnesses of credit and distinction, in a learned age, and on the most eminent theater that is now in the world. Nor is this all: a relation of them was published and dispersed everywhere; nor were the Jesuits, though a learned body, supported by the civil magistrates, and determined enemies to those opinions in whose favor the miracles were said to have been wrought, ever able distinctly to refute or detect them. Where shall we find such a number of circumstances agreeing to the corroboration of one fact? And what have we to oppose to such a cloud of witnesses but the absolute impossibility or miraculous nature of the events which they relate? And this, surely, in the eyes of all reasonable people, will alone be regarded as a sufficient refutation."*

Hume here places himself in the category of those whom Arago considers deficient in prudence. He pronounces certain events to be impossible, because they are contrary to his experience. He is misled by the pretensions of those who relate them. The eminent magistrate to whose elaborate work we are indebted for a narrative of the events in question (Carré de Montgéron) assumes that they were brought about by the special intervention of God, exerted, at the intercession of the deceased Abbé, to sustain the cause of the Jansenist Appellants and condemn the doctrines of the Bull Unigenitus.† Hume cannot admit the reason or justice of such pretensions. Nor can we. But here we must distinguish. It is one thing to refuse credit to the reality of the phenomena, and quite another to demur to the interpretation put upon them. We may admit the existence of comets, yet deny that they portend the

---

* *Hume's Essays*, vol. ii. p. 133.

† *"La Vérité des Miracles opérés par l'intercession de M. de Pâris et autres Appellans,"* par M. Carré de Montgéron, Conseiller au Parlement de Paris. 3 vols. 4to, 2d ed., Cologne, 1745.

I copy from the advertisement, p. 5 :—"Il s'agit de miracles qui prouvent evidemment l'existence de Dieu et sa providence, la vérité du Christianisme, la sainteté de l'église Catholique, et la justice de la cause des Appellans de la bulle UNIGENITUS."

The weight of evidence brought to bear, in this extraordinary work, in proof of each one of the chief miracles there sought to be established, would be sufficient, in a court of justice, to convict twenty men. I doubt whether such an overwhelming mass of human testimony was ever before thrown together to sustain any class of contested facts.

I had prepared, and had intended to give in the present volume, a chapter containing a condensed narrative of this marvelous epidemic, and the phenomena it brought to light; also to devote several other chapters to the details of other historical episodes somewhat similar in character. But the subject grew under my hands to such dimensions that I was compelled to exclude it.

birth or death of heroes. The first is a question of fact, the second only of inference or imagination.

This view of the case does not appear to have suggested itself at the time either to friend or foe. The Jesuit inquisitors, unable to contest the facts, found nothing for it but to ascribe them to witchcraft and the devil. Nor did any better mode occur to them of refuting Montgéron's work than to have it burned by the hands of the common hangman, on the 18th of February, 1739.

Modern science is more discriminating. The best medical writers on insanity and kindred subjects, after making due allowance for the exaggerations incident to the heat of controversialism, and for the inaccuracies into which an ignorance of physiology was sure to betray inexperienced observers, still find sufficient evidence remaining to prove, beyond cavil, the reality of certain cures, and other wonderful phenomena exhibited; but they seek the explanation of these in natural causes.* They do not imagine that the Deity suspended the laws of nature in order to disprove a papal bull; but neither do they declare, with Hume, the impossibility of the facts claimed to be miraculous.

---

* Consult, for example, Dr. Calmeil's excellent work, "*De la Folie, considérée sous le point de vue pathologique, philosophique, historique, et judiciaire,*" 2 vols., Paris, 1845. It will be found vol. ii. pp. 313 to 400, in the chapter entitled "*Théomanie Extato-Convulsive parmi les Jansénistes,*" in which the subject is examined in detail, from a medical point of view, and natural explanations offered of the phenomena in question, many of which phenomena are of so astounding a character that Hume, ignorant as he was of the effects produced in somnambulism, during catalepsy, and in other abnormal states of the human system, may well be pardoned for his incredulity.

Calmeil believes—and it seems probable enough—that these convulsions constituted a nervous malady of an aggravated character, probably hysteria complicated with ecstatic and cataleptic symptoms. He says, "Dès 1732, l'hystérie se compliqua de phénomènes extatiques, de phénomènes cataleptiformes."—Vol. ii. p. 395.

A judgment similar to that which the Scottish historian, more than a century ago, passed on the miracles of St. Médard, is passed in our day, by a large majority of the world, on all alleged appearances or agencies of an ultramundane character. The common opinion is, that such things cannot happen except miraculously; that is, by special intervention of the Deity, and a temporary suspension by Him, in favor of certain persons, of one or more of the laws which govern the universe. And, as they cannot believe in miracles, they reject, unexamined, all evidence tending to establish the reality of such phenomena.

I am not here asserting that such phenomena do occur. I am but adducing evidence for the opinion that, if they do, they are as much the result of natural law as is a rainbow or a thunder-clap. I am seeking to show cause to the believers in their existence why they should cease to attach to them any inkling of the supernatural.

Numerous examples of these alleged phenomena will be found in succeeding chapters. Meanwhile, assuming for a moment the affirmative on this point, I might found, on mere general principles, an argument in connection with it. To a question naturally suggesting itself, namely, to what end God permits (if He does permit) ultramundane intercourse, I might reply, that it is doubtless for a purpose as comprehensive as benevolent; that we may reasonably imagine Him to be opening up to our race a medium of more certain knowledge of another world, in order to give fresh impulse to our onward progress toward wisdom and goodness in this, and more especially to correct that absorbing worldliness, the besetting sin of the present age, creeping over its civilization and abasing its noblest aspirings. And, if these be admitted as rational surmises, I might go on to ask how we may suppose that God would be likely to carry out such an intent;—whether, after a partial and exceptional fashion, by an obtrusive suspension of His own laws for the benefit of a few favored children of preference, or, under the operation of the universal order of Nature, to the common advantage of all His creatures, in silent impartiality and harmony, as He causes the morning sun to rise and the evening dews to fall.

I might proceed a step further, and inquire whether, if such an extension of our earthly horizon enter into God's design, it can rationally be imagined that the Great Framer should find His purpose thwarted by the laws Himself had framed; or whether it does not far better comport with just ideas of God's omnipotence and ·omniprescience to conclude that, in the original adjustment of the world's economy, such a contingency was foreseen and provided for, as surely as every other human need has been.

Such arguments might not unfairly be made. Yet all *a priori* reasoning touching God's intentions, and the means we imagine He may select to effect these, seem to me hazarded and inconclusive. I think we do better to take note of God's doings than to set about conjecturing His thoughts, which, we are told, are not as ours. It is safer to reason from our experience of His works than from our conceptions of His attributes; for these are wrapped in mystery, while those are spread open before us.

I rest the case, therefore, not on the vagueness of general induction, but on the direct evidence of phenomena observed. That evidence will be adduced in its proper place. Suffice it for the present to express my conviction, based on experimental proof, that, *if* the Deity is now permitting communication between mortal creatures in this stage of existence and disembodied spirits in another, He is employing natural causes and general laws to effect His object; not resorting for that purpose to the occasional and the miraculous.

NOTE.

It will be evident, to the reflecting reader, that the argument running through the preceding chapter applies only in so far as we may accept the popular definition of a miracle; the same adopted by Hume. Some able theologians have assumed a very different one; Butler, for example, in his well-known "Analogy of Religion," in which he favors a view of the subject not very dissimilar to that taken by myself. "There is a real credibility," says he, "in the supposition that it might be part of the original plan of things that there should be miraculous interpositions." And he leaves it in doubt whether we ought "to call every thing in the dispensations of Providence not discoverable without Revelation, nor like the known course of things, miraculous."*

Another distinguished prelate speaks more plainly still. In one of his sermons Archbishop Tillotson says, "It is not the essence of a miracle (as many have thought) that it be an immediate effect of the Divine Power. It is sufficient that it exceed any natural power that we know of to produce it."†

This is totally changing the commonly-received definition. If we are not to regard it as "the essence of a miracle that it be an immediate effect of the Divine Power,"—if we may properly call any occurrence miraculous which is not "like the known course of things,"—if we may declare each and every phenomenon a miracle which "exceeds any natural power that we know of to produce it,"—then it is evident that the miracle of one age may be the natural event of the succeeding. In this sense we are living, even now, among miracles.

Nor, if in this we follow Butler and Tillotson, are we

* "Analogy of Religion to the Constitution and Course of Nature," Part II., chap. 2.   † Sermon CLXXXII.

at all invalidating the efficacy of the early Christian miracles. Their influence on the minds of men was the same whether they were the result of partial or of general laws. In point of fact, they *did* attract attention and add force to the teachings of a system, the innate beauty and moral grandeur of which was insufficient to recommend it to the semi-barbarism of the day. Whatever their character, they did their work. And the mistake as to that character, if mistake it is to be termed, may have been the very means ordained by Providence to cherish and advance, in its infancy, a religion of peace and good will springing up in an age of war and discord. Nor, in one sense, was the error, if as such we are to regard it, one of essence, but rather of manner. The signs and wonders which broke in upon the indifference and awoke the belief of Jew and Gentile, whether they were produced by momentary suspension of law or by its preordained operation, were equally His work from whom all law proceeds. And shall we appreciate God's handiwork the less because, in the progress of His teachings, He gradually unfolds to us the mode in which He moves to perform it? Then in heaven we should less venerate Him than upon earth.

Is it an unreasonable surmise that it may be God's purpose to raise the vail of eighteen hundred years, in proportion as our eyes can bear the light; in proportion as our minds can take in the many things which Christ taught not, in His day, to those who could not bear them; in proportion as we are prepared to receive Christianity, for its intrinsic excellence and on its internal evidence, without the aid of extraneous warrant?

But I put forth these suggestions, touching, as they do, on matters beyond our ken, incidentally and hypothetically only. They are not essential to my argument, nor strictly included in its purpose; that being to treat of modern, not of ancient, miracles.

CHAPTER IV.

THE IMPROBABLE.

"It may be said, speaking in strictness, that almost all our knowledge consists of possibilities only."—LA PLACE: *Théorie des Probabilités*, Introd. p. 1.

IN quest of truth there are two modes of proceeding: the one, to sit down, draw upon one's stock of preconceptions; settle, before we enter upon an inquiry, what may be, or ought to be, or must be; make to ourselves, in advance, what we call clear ideas of the naturally possible and impossible; then sally forth, armed against all non-conforming novelties, and with a fixed purpose to waste no time in their examination. The other plan, more modest and Baconian, is to step out into the world, eyes and ears open, an unpledged spectator, our fagot of opinions still unbound and incomplete; no such screen as a *must be* set up to prevent our seeing and hearing whatever presents itself; no ready-made impossibility prepared to rule out reliable testimony; no prejudgment barring the way against evidence for improbabilities.

Few persons realize how arbitrary and unreliable may be the notions they keep on hand of the improbable. We laugh at Jack's mother, who, when her sailor son sought to persuade her there were flying-fish, resented the attempt as an insult to her understanding, but accepted, unquestioned, the young rogue's story about one of Pharaoh's chariot-wheels brought up on the anchor-fluke from the bottom of the Red Sea. Yet the old lady is one of a large class, numbering learned and

92

lettered celebrities among its members, who have their flying-fish, insulting to the understanding, as well as she. These are a frequent phenomenon within the precincts of scientific academies and royal institutions.

We forget, after a time, what have been the flying-fish of the past. It needs official reference to convince us now that for nearly half a century after Harvey's brilliant discovery the Paris Academy of Medicine listened to those who classed it among the impossibilities.* We have almost forgotten that, until the commencement of the present century, the old ladies of the scientific world rejected, as resentfully as their prototype of the story, all allegations going to prove the reality of aerolites.†

Meteoric stones and the circulation of the blood have now lost their piscatory character, are struck off the

---

* In the records of the Paris Royal Society of Medicine we read that, as late as the year 1672, a candidate for membership, François Bazin, sought to conciliate the favor of that learned body by selecting as his theme the *impossibility* of the circulation of the blood; (*" ergo sanguinis motus circularis impossibilis."*) Harvey had given to the world his great discovery in the year 1628; but forty-four years sufficed not to procure for it the sanction of official medical authority in the French capital.

† The fall of larger or smaller mineral masses, usually called meteoric stones, was long set down by the scientific world as among popular fables, notwithstanding the testimony of all antiquity in its favor. Stones alleged to have dropped from heaven were preserved in various ancient temples, as at Cybele. Plutarch, in his life of Lysander, describes a celebrated aerolite which fell in Thrace, near the mouth of the Ægos Potamos. But these and a hundred other analogous cases, recorded throughout the past, failed to dispel scientific incredulity, until Chladni, a naturalist of Wurtemberg, verified the fall of a meteorite at Sienna, in Tuscany, on the 16th of June, 1794. His report of the marvel staggered the skepticism of many. Yet it was not till nine years afterward—when, to wit, on the 26th of April, 1803, an aerolite fell in broad daylight at L'Aigle, in Normandy—that all doubt was removed. The Paris Academy of Sciences appointed a commission to institute inquiries into this case; and their report settled the question. Howard, an English naturalist, afterward prepared a list of all the aerolites known to have fallen on our earth up to the year 1818; and Chladni continued the list to the year 1824.

list of impossibilities, and inserted in the accredited catalogue of scientific truths. It used to be vulgar and ridiculous to admit them; now the vulgarity and absurdity consist in denying their existence.

Mesmeric phenomena, on the other hand, are an example of improbabilities that have not yet passed muster.

"When I was in Paris," says Rogers, (the poet,) in his "Table-Talk," "I went to Alexis, and desired him to describe my house in St. James Place. On my word, he astonished me! He described most exactly the peculiarities of the staircase; said that not far from the window in the drawing-room there was a picture of a man in armor, (the painting by Giorgone,) and so on. Colonel Gurwood, shortly before his death, assured me that he was reminded by Alexis of some circumstances that had happened to him in Spain, and which he could not conceive how any human being except himself should know. Still, I cannot believe in clairvoyance,—*because the thing is impossible.*"*

Not because the opportunities for observation were too few, and the experiments needed repetition: that would have been a valid objection. Not because the evidence was imperfect and lacked confirmation: Rogers's difficulty was a more radical one. *No* evidence would suffice. Fish cannot have wings: the thing is impossible.†

---

* Let us deal fairly by Science, and give her the credit of this quotation. I found it in the (London) Medical Times and Gazette, No. 444, new series; and the italics are not mine, but those of the medical editor.

† Rogers evidently had never read La Place's celebrated work on Probabilities, or else he did not agree with its doctrine. Witness this passage:— "It is exceedingly unphilosophical to deny magnetic phenomena merely because they are inexplicable in the present state of our knowledge."— *Calcul des Probabilités,* p. 348.

It is remarkable enough that in a matter like this, usually deemed to savor of imagination, the mathematician should reprove the incredulity of the poet.

An example of graver character and more influential effect is to be found in a lecture, delivered in 1854, at the Royal Institution, before Prince Albert and a select audience, by England's first electrician. Rogers's flying-fish was clairvoyance; Faraday's is table-moving.

But if great men fall into one extreme, let us not, for that reason, be betrayed into another. Let us bear in mind that, antecedent to sufficient proof adduced to establish them, the circulation of the blood, the fall of meteorites, the phenomena of clairvoyance, the reality of table-moving,—all are, or were, improbabilities.

But there are few propositions to which the common sense of mankind, indorsing the most accredited scientific authority,* assents more readily, or with greater justice, than this: that in proportion as an event or phenomenon is in its nature improbable is greater weight of evidence required to produce a rational belief in its reality.

The converse of this proposition, it is true, has been plausibly argued, sometimes where one would least expect to find an apology for credulity;† but men have been so frequently deceivers, and so much more frequently themselves deceived, that, when their testimony is adduced to prove something of a marvelous and unexampled nature, every dictate of experience warns us against its reception, except after severest scrutiny, or the concurrence, when that can be had, of many disinterested witnesses, testifying independently of each other.

The argument, however, in regard to the weight of evidence which may be procured through such concurrence of testimony to one and the same fact, has, in my

---

* "Plus un fait est extraordinaire, plus il a besoin d'être appuyé de fortes preuves. Car ceux qui l'attestent pouvant ou tromper, ou avoir été trompés, ces deux causes sont d'autant plus probables que la réalité du fait l'est moins en elle-même."—LA PLACE: *Théorie analytique des Probabilités*, Introd. p. 12.

† As in the French Encyclopedia, article "*Certitude.*"

judgment, sometimes been pushed beyond what it will bear. Where human testimony enters as an element into the calculation, its disturbing agency may be such as to weaken, almost to the point of overthrowing, the force of all strictly mathematical demonstration.

Thus, in substance, has the argument been put.* Let us suppose two persons, A. and B., of such a character for veracity and clear-sightedness that the chances are that they will speak the truth, and will avoid being deceived, in nine cases out of ten. And let us suppose that these two persons, absolutely unknown to and unconnected with each other, are about to testify in regard to any fact. What are the chances that, if their testimony shall agree, the fact has happened?

Evidently, a hundred to one. For if their testimony agree and the fact has not happened, there must be a concurrent lie or self-deception. But, as, in the first place, the chances are ten to one against A. lying or being deceived, and then, in the contingency that he should be, the chances are again ten to one against B. failing to relate the truth, it is evident that the chances against the double event are ten times ten (or one hundred) to one.

Pursuing the same calculation, we find that, in the event of three such witnesses concurring, the chances are a thousand to one against the falsehood of their testimony; if four such concur, ten thousand to one; and so on. So that it requires but a small number of such witnesses to establish a degree of probability which, in practice, is scarcely short of certainty itself.

---

* The reader may consult La Place's "*Théorie analytique des Probabilités*," where all the calculations connected with this argument are given in detail; or, if unprepared for the difficulties of Calculus, he will find the matter set out in more condensed and popular form, by Babbage, in his "*Ninth Bridgewater Treatise*," 2d ed., pp. 124 to 131; and in *Note E of Appendix* to the same work.

And, following out this principle, it will be found that, if we can but procure witnesses of such a character that it is more probable that their testimony is true than that it is false, we can always assign a sufficient number of such to establish the occurrence of any event or the reality of any phenomenon, no matter how improbable or marvelous such event or phenomenon, in itself considered, may be.

If the postulates be granted, these conclusions clearly follow; and they have been employed by Dr. Chalmers* and others, in treating of miracles, to illustrate the great accumulation of probability which arises from the concurrence of independent witnesses.

The difficulty lies in the postulates. It seems, at first, a very easy matter to find witnesses of such moderate veracity and intelligence that we are justified in declaring it to be more probable that their testimony shall be true than that it shall be false.

As to willful falsehood, the matter is beyond doubt. Let cynicism portray the world as it will, there is far more of truth than of falsehood in it. But as to freedom from self-deception, that is a condition much more difficult to obtain. It depends to a great extent upon the nature of the event witnessed or the phenomenon observed.

An extreme case may assure us of this. If two independent witnesses of good character depose to having seen a market-woman count out six dozen eggs from a basket which was evidently of capacity sufficient to contain them, we deem the fact sufficiently proved. But if two thousand witnesses of equally good character testify that they saw Signor Blitz or Robert-Houdin take that number of eggs out of an ordinary-sized hat, they fail to convince us that the hat really contained

---

* *"Evidences of Christian Revelation,"* vol. i. p. 129.

them. We conclude that they were deceived by sleight of hand.

Here, therefore, the postulates must be rejected. And, without speaking of mathematical impossibilities, in regard to which, of course, no imaginable number of concurrent witnesses avail in proof, the character of the event or phenomenon testified to must ever count for much; and, whatever theorists may say, it will always greatly influence our opinion, not perhaps of the honesty, but of the freedom from delusion, of the testifiers. So that, in a case where proof of some marvel is in question, the assumed condition, namely, that we shall find witnesses whom we believe more likely to speak the truth than to lie or be deceived, may not be capable of fulfillment.

And the difficulty of procuring such may, under certain circumstances, greatly increase. There are mental as well as physical epidemics, and during their prevalence men's minds may be so morbidly excited, and their imaginations so exalted, that entire masses may become incapacitated to serve as dispassionate witnesses.

There is another consideration, noticed by Hume in his chapter on Miracles, which should not be overlooked. "Though we readily reject," says he, "any fact which is unusual and incredible in an ordinary degree, yet, in advancing further, the mind observes not always the same rule." We sometimes accept, he thinks, a statement made to us, for the very reason which should cause us to reject it; on account of its ultra-marvelous character. The reason is shrewdly assigned:—"The passion of surprise and wonder arising from miracles, being an agreeable emotion, gives a sensible tendency toward the belief of those events from which it is derived."* In a word, we should be on

---

* *Hume's Essays*, vol. ii. p. 125.

our guard against that love of the marvelous which we find inherent in our nature.

These and similar considerations will ever weigh with the prudent and reflecting observer. Yet it is to be conceded, that the principle above referred to, of the vast accumulation of evidence from the concurrence of reliable witnesses, is not only just, mathematically considered, but, in a variety of cases, strictly applies in practice.

If we find, for instance, at different periods of the world and in various nations, examples constantly recurring of men testifying to certain phenomena of the same or a similar character, then, though these alleged phenomena may seem to us highly improbable, we are not justified in ascribing the concurrence of such testimony to chance. We are not justified in setting down the whole as idle superstition; though in these modern days it is very much the fashion of the world, proud of having outgrown its nursery-tales, so to do. Disgusted by detecting a certain admixture of error and folly, we often cast aside an entire class of narrations as wholly baseless and absurd; forgetting that when, at remote periods, at distant points, without possibility of collusion, there spring up, again and again, the same or similar appearances, such coincidence ought to suggest to us the probability that something more enduring than delusion may be mixed in to make up the producing cause.*

---

* "Take any one of what are called popular errors or popular superstitions, and on looking at it thoroughly we shall be sure to discover in it a firm, underlying stratum of truth. There may be more than we suspected of folly and of fancy; but when these are stripped off there remains quite enough of that stiff, unyielding material which belongs not to persons or periods, but is common to all ages, to puzzle the learned and silence the scoffer."—RUTTER: *Human Electricity*, Appendix, p. vii.

To the same effect is the expression of a celebrated French philosopher:—

"In every error there is a kernel of truth: let us seek to detach that kernel from the envelop that hides it from our eyes."—BAILLY.

It is truth only that is tenacious of life, and that rises, with recurring effort, throughout the lapse of ages, elastic under repression and contempt.

Let us take, as an example, that description of popular stories which relate to haunted houses, the universal prevalence of which is admitted by those who the most ridicule the idea that they prove any thing save the folly and credulity of mankind.*   Is it the part of Philosophy contemptuously to ignore all evidence that may present itself in favor of the reality of such alleged disturbances?

It may be freely conceded, that for many of the stories in question no better foundation can be found than those panic terrors which are wont to beset the ignorant mind; that others, doubtless, are due to a mere spirit of mischief seeking to draw amusement

---

* "Who has not either seen or heard of some house, shut up and uninhabitable, fallen into decay and looking dusty and dreary, from which at midnight strange sounds have been heard to issue,—aerial knockings, the rattling of chains and the groaning of perturbed spirits?—a house that people have thought it unsafe to pass after dark, that has remained for years without a tenant, and which no tenant would occupy, even were he paid to do so?   There are hundreds of such houses in England at the present day, hundreds in France, Germany, and almost every country of Europe; which are marked with the mark of fear,—places for the pious to bless themselves at, and ask protection from, as they pass,—the abodes of ghosts and evil spirits.   There are many such houses in London; and if any vain boaster of the march of intellect would but take the trouble to find them out and count them, he would be convinced that intellect must yet make some enormous strides before such old superstitions can be eradicated."—*Mackay's Popular Delusions*, vol. ii. p. 113.   The author does not deem the hypothesis that there is any thing real in such phenomena worth adverting to, even as among possible things.

Nor was the idea of haunted houses less commonly received in ancient times than among us.   Plautus has a comedy entitled *Mostellaria*, from a specter said to have shown itself in a certain house, which on that account was deserted.   The particular story may have been invented by the dramatist; but it suffices to indicate the antiquity of the idea.—·*Plaut. Mostell.*, Act ii. v. 67.

from these very terrors; and, finally, that there are instances where the mystification may have covered graver designs.* But because there are counterfeits, is there therefore no true coin? May there not be originals to these spurious copies?

In another part of this work I shall bring up the evi-

---

* One such is related by Garinet, in his *"Histoire de la Magie en France,"* (p. 75;) a clever trick played off by certain monks on that king whose piety has procured for him the title of *" The Saint."*

Having heard his confessor speak in high terms of the goodness and learning of the monks of St. Bruno, the king expressed a desire to found a community of them near Paris. Bernard de la Tour, the superior, sent six of the brethren; and Louis assigned to them, as residence, a handsome dwelling in the village of Chantilly. It so happened that from their windows they had a fine view of the old palace of Vauvert, originally erected for a royal residence by King Robert, but which had been deserted for years. The worthy monks, oblivious of the tenth commandment, may have thought the place would suit them; but ashamed, probably, to make a formal demand of it from the king, they seem to have set their wits to work to procure it by stratagem. At all events, the palace of Vauvert, which had never labored under any imputation against its character till they became its neighbors, began, almost immediately afterward, to acquire a bad name. Frightful shrieks were heard to proceed thence at night; blue, red, and green lights were seen to glimmer from its casements and then suddenly disappear. The clanking of chains succeeded, together with the howlings of persons as in great pain. Then a ghastly specter, in pea-green, with long, white beard and serpent's tail, appeared at the principal windows, shaking his fists at the passers-by. This went on for months. The king, to whom of course all these wonders were duly reported, deplored the scandal, and sent commissioners to look into the affair. To these the six monks of Chantilly, indignant that the devil should play such pranks before their very faces, suggested that if they could but have the palace as a residence they would undertake speedily to clear it of all ghostly intruders. A deed, with the royal sign-manual, conveyed Vauvert to the monks of St. Bruno. It bears the date of 1259. From that time all disturbances ceased; the green ghost, according to the creed of the pious, being laid to rest forever under the waters of the Red Sea.

Another instance, occurring in the Chateau d'Arsillier, in Picardy, will be found in the *"Causes Célèbres,"* vol. xi. p. 374; the bailiff having dressed himself up as a black phantom, with horns and tail, and guaranteed himself against the chance of a pistol-shot by a buffalo's hide fitted tightly to his body. He was finally detected, and the cheat exposed.

dences which present themselves to one who seriously seeks an answer to the above queries.* Let those who may decide, in advance, that the answer is not worth seeking, be reminded that there are twenty allegations which are worthy to be examined, for every one that may be unhesitatingly received.

Again, there is a class of phenomena, as widely spread as the disturbances above alluded to,—probably somewhat allied to them, but more important than they,—to which the same principle in regard to the concurrence of testimony in various ages and countries eminently applies; those strange appearances, namely, which, for lack of a more definite term, may be grouped together as *mesmeric.*

Without seeking, amid the obscurity of remote antiquity, a clew to all that we read of the so-called Occult Arts,—as among the magicians of Egypt, the soothsayers and diviners of Judea, the sibyls and oracles of Greece and Rome,†—we shall find, in later times, but commencing long before the appearance of Mesmer, a succession of phenomena, with resemblance sufficient to substantiate their common origin, and evidently referable to the same unexplained and hidden causes, operating during an abnormal state of the human system, whence spring the various phases of somnambulism and other analogous manifestations, physical and mental, observed by animal magnetizers.

Time after time throughout the psycho-medical his-

---

* See further on, under title "*Disturbances popularly termed Hauntings.*"

† The curious in such matters may consult the "*Geschichte der Magie,*" by Dr. Joseph Ennemoser, Leipzig, 1844,—of which, if he be not familiar with German, he will find an English translation, by William Howitt, "*History of Magic,*" London, 1854.

Also, the "*Cradle of the Twin Giants, Science and History,*" by the Rev. Henry Christmas, M.A., F.R.S., F.S.A., London, 1849.

Both are works of great research.

tory of the Middle Ages and of modern Europe—sometimes among Catholics, sometimes among Protestants
—recur these singular episodes in the history of the
human mind, usually epidemical in their character
while they last, each episode, however, independent of
the others and separated from them widely by time
and place; all narrated by writers who take the most
opposite views of their nature and causes, yet all, no
matter by whom narrated, bearing a family likeness,
which appears the more striking the more closely they
are studied.

Examples are numerous: as the alleged obsession
(1632 to 1639) of the Ursuline Nuns of Loudun, with
its sequel, in 1642, among the Sisters of St. Elizabeth
at Louviers; the mental aberrations of the Prophets or
Shakers (Trembleurs) of the Cevennes, (1686 to 1707,)
caused by the persecutions which followed the revoca-
tion of the Edict of Nantes; and the pseudo-miracles
of the Convulsionists of St. Médard (1731 to 1741) at
the tomb of the Abbé Pâris.*

All this occurred, it will be observed, before the very
name of Animal Magnetism was known, or any natural
explanation of these strange manifestations was suspected; at a time when their investigation was considered the province of the ecclesiastical tribunals, not

* For details touching the disturbances at Loudun, consult *"La Démonomanie de Loudun,"* by La Flèche, 1634; *"Cruels Effets de la Vengeance du Cardinal de Richelieu; ou, Histoire des Diables de Loudun,"* Amsterdam, 1693; *"Examen et Discussions Critiques de l'Histoire des Diables
de Loudun,"* by M. de la Ménardaye, Paris, 1747; *"Histoire Abrégée de la
Possession des Ursulines de Loudun,"* by the Père Tissot, Paris, 1828. For
those of Louviers, see *"Réponse à l'Examen de la Possession des Religieuses
de Louviers,"* Rouen, 1643. As to the Prophets of the Cevennes, see
"Théatre Sacré des Cevennes," by M. Misson, London, 1707; *"An Account
of the French Prophets and their Pretended Inspirations,"* London, 1708;
"Histoire des Troubles des Cevennes," by M. Court, Alais, 1819. The works
on the St. Médard disturbances are elsewhere noticed.

of the medical profession or of the psychological inquirer.

And for that very reason, inasmuch as many of the phenomena in question, and running through almost all the above examples, resemble, more or less closely, others alleged to have been observed by modern magnetizers, the remarkable concurrence of testimony among the narrators in regard to these becomes the more convincing of the reality, in some shape or other, of the facts narrated.

For, as soon as we find, in a succession of examples, a *class* of phenomena, no matter how extraordinary or inexplicable they may seem, the chance of their being genuine is very greatly increased. A phenomenon may be deemed improbable so long as it appears to be the only one of its class. But so soon as we have grouped around it others similar in nature, we have brought to bear one of the strongest arguments to sustain the probability of its existence.

But, besides the inherent probability or improbability of any alleged phenomenon, and besides the general considerations, universally admitted, touching the number and concurrence of witnesses, their usual character for veracity, their freedom from interest in what they affirm,—besides all this, the manner of each individual deposition or narration has, very properly, much to do with the confidence we repose in the narrator. There is, if the testimony be oral, a look and an accent of truth, which inspires instinctive confidence. And though in a written statement simulation is easier, yet even in that case an air of candor, or a sense of the lack of it, commonly attaches so strongly to an author's writing, that we are enabled, if we have some experience of the world, to form a shrewd judgment in regard to his honesty of purpose.

Modesty and moderation in narrative justly enlist our credence. We incline to believe most that which is least arrogantly asserted. Earnestness of conviction in the testifier is, indeed, necessary to produce a corresponding confidence in his audience; but no two things are more distinct than earnestness and dogmatism. We lose trust in a man who, if you will but take his own word for it, is always in the right,—who makes no calculation that is not verified, attempts no experiment that does not succeed. A partial failure often inspires us with more confidence than a complete success.

Nor does it materially weaken the probability of an observation in itself reliable, that some other experimentalists in search of similar results have not yet obtained them. One successful experiment, sufficiently attested, is not to be rebutted by twenty unsuccessful ones. It cannot disprove what I have seen that others have not seen it. The conditions of success may be difficult and precarious, especially where living beings are the subjects of experiment. And even as to inanimate substances, there is not a naturalist who has reached at last some important discovery who may not have failed a hundred times on the road to it. If even numerous intelligent observers report unobtained results, their negative testimony, unless it approach universality, can amount to no more than an adverse presumption, and may only prove the rarity of the quested phenomenon.*

---

* In a subsequent portion of this work (on *"Disturbances popularly termed Hauntings"*) will be found a notice of Glanvil's celebrated story usually entitled "The Drummer of Tedworth." It attracted so much attention at the time that the king sent some gentlemen of his court to examine into the matter, who spent a night in the house reputed to be haunted, but heard nothing; and this has been adduced as a complete refutation of the narrative. Glanvil (in the third edition of his *" Sadducismus Triumphatus,"* p. 337) justly remarks thereon,—

"'Tis true, that when the gentlemen the king sent were there the house

If to some it seem that this remark is so evident as scarcely to be needed, eminent examples can be adduced to show that it touches upon an error to which men are sufficiently prone.

On the 28th of February, 1826, a commission was appointed from among its members by the Royal Academy of Medicine, of Paris, to examine the subject of Animal Magnetism. After an investigation running through more than five years, to wit, on the 21st of June, 1831, this commission reported, through their president, Dr. Husson, at great length, in favor of the reality of certain somnambulic phenomena; among them, insensibility, vision with the eyes closed, prescience during sickness, and, in one case, perception of the diseases of others: the report being signed unanimously. Some years later, namely, on the 14th of February, 1837, the same Academy appointed a second commission for the same purpose; and they, after nearly six months, (on the 7th of August, 1837,) reported, also unanimously, through their chairman, Dr. Dubois, expressing their conviction that not one of these phenomena had any foundation except in the imagination of the observers. They reached this conclusion by examining two somnambules only.

..was quiet, and nothing seen or heard that night, which was confidently and with triumph urged by many as a confutation of the story. But 'twas bad logic to conclude in matters of fact from a single negative, and such a one against numerous affirmatives, and so affirm that a thing was never done because not at such a particular time, and that nobody ever saw what this man or that did not. By the same way of reasoning, I may infer that there were never any robberies done on Salisbury Plain, Hounslow Heath, or the other noted places, because I have often traveled all those ways, and yet was never robbed; and the Spaniard inferred well that said, 'There was no sun in England, because he had been six weeks there and never saw it.'"

Glanvil properly reminds us that "the disturbance was not constant, but intermitted sometimes several days, sometimes weeks." Under these circumstances, it is quite evident that its non-appearance during a single night proves nothing.

Dr. Husson, commenting before the Academy* on the conclusions of this last report, truly observes that "the negative experiences thus obtained can never destroy the positive facts observed by the previous commission; since, though diametrically opposed to each other, both may be equally true."†

It is a fact curious, and worth noticing in this connection, that the same dogmatic skepticism which often acts as a clog to advancement in knowledge may be betrayed, in certain contingencies, into an error the very opposite.

For there are some men who run from the excess of unbelief to the extreme of credulity. Once convinced of their error in obstinately denying one startling fact, they incontinently admit, not that only, but twenty other allegations, unchallenged, in its company. They defend to the last extremity the outer line of fortification; but, that once forced, they surrender, without further effort, the entire citadel. "Such," says Buffon, "is the common tendency of the human mind, that when it has once been impressed by a marvelous object it takes pleasure in ascribing to it properties that are chimerical, and often absurd." Against this temptation we should be constantly on our guard.

There remains to be touched upon, in connection with the observation of phenomena in themselves improbable, a consideration of some importance. To what extent, and under what circumstances, is it reasonable to distrust the evidence of our senses?

There are a hundred examples of the manner in which

* During their session of August 22, 1837. M. Husson's discourse is reported verbatim in Ricard's *"Traité du Magnetisme animal,"* précis historique, pp. 144 to 164.

† I forget who relates the anecdote of a clown who proposed to rebut the testimony of a trustworthy gentleman, who had sworn to the use of certain language, by producing ten men to swear that they had not heard it.

one or other of our senses may, for the time, testify only to deceive us.* The most familiar, perhaps, are what are usually termed conjuring tricks. Those who, like myself, have sat through an evening with Robert-Houdin, preserve, probably, a vivid recollection how that wonderful artist enacted what seemed sheer impossibilities, before the very eyes of his mystified audience. But this was on his own theater, with months or years to prepare its hidden machinery and manufacture its magical apparatus; with the practice of a lifetime, too, to perfect his sleight of hand. There is little analogy between such professional performances and phenomena presenting themselves spontaneously, or at least without calculated preparation, in the privacy of a dwelling-house, or in the open air, often to persons who neither expect nor desire them.

But there suggests itself, further, the contingency of hallucination. This subject will be treated of in a subsequent chapter.† Suffice it here to say that, according to the doctrine contained in the most accredited works on the subject, if two or more persons, using their senses independently, perceive, at the same time and place, the same appearance, it is not hallucination; that is to say, there is *some* actual foundation for it. Both may, indeed,

---

* Each sense may, in turn, mislead us. We are constantly impressed with the conviction that the moon just after it rises appears of a greater magnitude than when seen on the meridian. Yet if, by means of a frame with two threads of fine silk properly adjusted, we measure the moon's apparent magnitude on the horizon and again on the meridian, we shall find them the same. So of the sense of touch. If, while the eyes are closed, two fingers of the same hand, being crossed, be placed on a table, and a single marble, or pea, be rolled between them, the impression will be that two marbles, or two peas, are touched.

A popular review of the fallacies of the senses will be found in Lardner's "*Museum of Science and Art*," vol. i. pp. 81 to 96.

† See Chapter 1 of Book IV., on "*Appearances commonly called Apparitions.*"

mistake one thing for another; but there *is* something to mistake.

On the other hand, if but one person perceive some prodigy, it may be a pure hallucination only, especially if the person be under the influence of great agitation or of a nervous system unduly excited. If such a person perceive what others around him do not, it may be taken as *prima facie* evidence that he is the subject of hallucination. Yet we can imagine circumstances that would rebut such a presumption. If, for example, it should be satisfactorily proved, in any given case, that a certain appearance, perceived by one witness only out of many present, conveyed to that witness, with unmistakable accuracy, correct information touching the distant or the future, which it was impossible by ordinary means to acquire, we should needs conclude that there was something other than hallucination in the case. The alleged second-sight in Scotland, and especially in the island of Skye,* if perfectly authenticated in any one

---

* The curious will find many details of the pretensions touching the Scottish second-sight, and particularly in the Hebrides, recorded in *"Description of the Western Islands of Scotland,"* by M. Martin, London, 1706. The author regards this phenomenon as sufficiently proved, especially among the inhabitants of the island of Skye. He alleges that the gift of second-sight is usually hereditary; that animals are wont to distinguish, at the same time as the seer, the apparition which he alone of all the human beings present perceives, and to be violently affected by it. He adds that the gift seems endemical, since natives of Skye noted as seers, if they pass into a distant country, lose the power, but recover it as soon as they return to their native land.

The subject is mentioned, also, in Dr. Johnson's *"Journey to the Western Islands of Scotland,"* p. 247, and in Boswell's *"Journal of a Tour to the Hebrides with Samuel Johnson,"* 1785, p. 490.

Scheffer, too, in his History of Lapland, adduces various examples which he considers as indicating the existence of second-sight among the people of that country. But it appears to differ in its form from the second-sight of Scotland, and more nearly to approach somnambulism; for the seer is, according to Scheffer, plunged into a deep sleep, or lethargy, during which his prophecies are uttered. See his work translated from the original Latin

example where chance prediction or conjecture could not be imagined, would be a case in point. Beyond all question, however, such cases ought to be scrupulously scanned. That one unlikely prediction, for instance, should be fulfilled, while a hundred fail, may be a rare coincidence, only, fairly to be ascribed to what we call chance. Cicero relates that Diagoras, when at Samothrace, being shown in a temple, as evidence of the power of the god there adored, the numerous votive offerings of those who, having invoked his aid, were saved from shipwreck, asked how many persons, notwithstanding such invocation, had perished.* Predictions, however, may be of such a nature, and so circumstantial in their details, that the probabilities against their accidental fulfillment suffice to preclude altogether that supposition.

In a general way, it may be said that where a phenomenon observed by several persons, however extraordinary and unexampled it may be, is of a plain and evident character, palpable to the senses, especially to the sight, we are not justified in distrusting the evidence of sense in regard to it.†

Suppose, for example,‡ that, sitting in one's own well-lighted apartment, where no concealed machinery or other trickery is possible, in company with three or four

---

into French by the Geographer of the King, and entitled "*Histoire de Laponie*," Paris, 1778, vol. iv. p. 107 *et seq.*

* Cicero "De naturâ deorum," lib. iii.

† It is the remark of a distinguished theologian, "In some circumstances our senses may deceive us; but no faculty deceives us so little or so seldom; and when our senses do deceive us, even that error is not to be corrected without the help of our senses."—*Tillotson's Works*, Sermon XXVI.

‡ The case supposed is not an imaginary one. It occurred in my apartments at Naples, on the 11th of March, 1856, and, with slight variations, on two subsequent occasions. I had the table and the lamp which were used on these occasions weighed. The weight of the former was seventy-six pounds and of the latter fourteen,—together, ninety pounds.

friends, all curious observers like oneself, around a large center-table, weighing eighty or a hundred pounds, the hands of all present resting upon it, one should see and feel this table, the top maintaining its horizontal, rise suddenly and unexpectedly to the height of eight or ten inches from the floor, remain suspended in the air while one might count six or seven, then gently settle down again; and suppose that all the spectators concurred in their testimony as to this occurrence, with only slight variations of opinion as to the exact number of inches to which the table rose and the precise number of seconds during which it remained suspended: ought the witnesses of such a seeming temporary suspension of the law of gravitation to believe that their senses are playing them false?

Mr. Faraday says that, unless they do, they are not only " ignorant as respects education of the judgment," but are also " ignorant of their ignorance."* An educated judgment, he alleges, knows that " it is impossible to create force." But " if we could, by the fingers, draw a heavy piece of wood upward without effort, and then, letting it sink, could produce, by its gravity, an effort equal to its weight, that would be a creation of power,

---

* The assertion occurs in Mr. Faraday's lecture at the Royal Institution, already referred to, delivered on the 6th of May, 1854. It may be supposed to embody the author's deliberate opinion, since, after five years, it is republished by him in his " *Experimental Researches in Chemistry and Physics*," London, 1859. The passage quoted, with its essential context, is as follows:—

"You hear, at the present day, that some persons can place their fingers on a table, and then, elevating their hands, the table will rise and follow them; that the piece of furniture, though heavy, will ascend, and that their hands bear no weight, or are not drawn down to the wood." . . . "The assertion finds acceptance in every rank of society, and among classes that are esteemed to be educated. Now, what can this imply but that society, generally speaking, is not only ignorant as respects the education of the judgment, but is also ignorant of its ignorance?"—p. 470.

and *cannot be.*"* His conclusion is, that tables never rise. The thing is impossible.

That is a very convenient short-cut out of a difficulty. The small objection is, that the facts are opposed to it. It is all very well for Mr. Faraday to bid the witnesses carry with them an educated judgment. The recommendation does not reach the case. Unless this educated judgment could persuade them that they did not see what they actually saw and did not feel what they actually felt, it would certainly never convince them, as Mr. Faraday proposes it should, that what happened before their eyes *cannot be.*

They might very properly doubt whether what they saw and felt *was* a suspension of a law universal as that of gravitation. They would do quite wrong in asserting, as Mr. Faraday takes it for granted they must, that " by the fingers they draw a heavy piece of wood upward without effort :"† that might be mistaking the *post*

---

* *Work cited,* p. 479. The italics are Faraday's.

That gentleman is among the number of those who believe that "before we proceed to consider any question involving physical principles, we should set out with clear ideas of the naturally possible and impossible."—p. 478. But it avails nothing to set out with what we cherish as clear ideas, if on the way we encounter phenomena which disprove them. Mr. Faraday is one of those imprudent persons spoken of by Arago. (See motto to chap. ii. Book I.)

† The imposition of hands is not a necessary condition. In the dining-room of a French nobleman, the Count d'Ourches, residing near Paris, I saw, on the 1st day of October, 1858, in broad daylight, at the close of a *déjeuner à la fourchette,* a dinner-table seating seven persons, with fruit and wine on it, rise and settle down, as already described, while all the guests were standing around it, *and not one of them touching it at all.* All present saw the same thing. Mr. Kyd, son of the late General Kyd, of the British army, and his lady, told me (in Paris, in April, 1859) that, in December of the year 1857, during an evening visit to a friend, who resided at No. 28 Rue de la Ferme des Mathurins, at Paris, Mrs. Kyd, seated in an arm-chair, suddenly felt it move, as if some one had laid hold of it from beneath. Then slowly and gradually it rose into the air, and remained there suspended for the space of about thirty seconds, the lady's feet being four or

hoc for the *propter hoc.* All they would be justified in saying is, that they placed their hands on the table, *and the table rose.*

If still Mr. Faraday should reply that it did *not* rise, because it could not, he would afford an eminent example of a truth as old as the days of Job, that "great men are not always wise." That which *does* happen *can* happen; and the endeavor by argument to persuade men to the contrary is labor lost.

I make no assertion that tables are raised by spiritual agency. But suppose Mr. Faraday, by disproving every other hypothesis, should drive one to this:* it would be

---

five feet from the ground; then it settled down gently and gradually, so that there was no shock when it reached the carpet. No one was touching the chair when it rose, nor did any one approach it while in the air, except Mr. Kyd, who, fearing an accident, advanced and touched Mrs. Kyd. The room was at the time brightly lighted, as a French *salon* usually is; and of the eight or nine persons present all saw the same thing, in the same way. I took notes of the above, as Mr. and Mrs. Kyd narrated to me the occurrence; and they kindly permitted, as a voucher for its truth, the use of their names.

Here is no drawing up of a heavy object, without effort, with the fingers, the concomitant which Mr. Faraday speaks of as indispensable. And the phenomenon occurred in a private drawing-room, among persons of high social position, educated and intelligent. Thousands, in the most enlightened countries of the world, can testify to the like. Are they all to be spoken of as "ignorant of their ignorance"?

* He scorns the idea. In his letter on Table-Turning, published in the London "Times" of June 30, 1853, he says, "The effect produced by table-turners has been referred to electricity, to magnetism, to attraction, to some unknown or hitherto unrecognized physical power able to affect inanimate bodies, to the revolution of the earth, and even to diabolical or supernatural agency. The natural philosopher can investigate all these supposed causes out the last: that must, to him, be too much connected with credulity or superstition to require any attention on his part."— *Work cited,* p. 382.

This is a summary and convenient disclaimer,—more convenient than satisfactory. Mr. Faraday thinks of ultramundane agency as Hume did of miracles, that "supported by human testimony it is more properly a subject of derision than of argument." The time is coming when, in this world or another, he may discover his mistake.

H　　　　10*

much more philosophical to adopt it than to reject the clear and palpable evidence of sense.

For, if we assume any other principle, all received rules of evidence must be set at naught;* nay, our very lives would be made up of uncertainty and conjecture. We might begin to doubt the most common events of daily occurrence,† and perhaps, at last, to dream, with Berkeley, that the external world exists only in our sensations. Indeed, if the senses of an entire community of men were to concur in imposing on them unreal sights and sounds, appearing to all the same, who would there be to declare it a delusion, and what means would remain to prove it such?

Nor is it irrational to trust the evidence of our senses in cases so marvelous that we may reject hearsay testimony of an ordinary character when brought to prove

---

* The reader will find in Reid's excellent work on the Mind (*Essay 2, "Perception"*) some remarks much in point. He says, "No judge will ever suppose that witnesses may be imposed upon by trusting to their eyes and ears; and if skeptical counsel should plead against the testimony of witnesses that they had no other evidence for what they declared but the testimony of their eyes and ears, and that we ought not to put so much faith in our senses as to deprive men of life and fortune upon their testimony, surely no upright judge would admit a plea of this kind. I believe no counsel, however skeptical, ever dared to offer such an argument; and if it were offered it would be rejected with disdain."

† The legal records of the Middle Ages furnish examples, scarcely credible, of such skepticism. During the thousand trials for witchcraft which occurred in France throughout the sixteenth century, the women suspected were usually accused of having joined the witches' dance at midnight under a blasted oak. "The husbands of several of these women (two of them were young and beautiful) swore positively that, at the time stated, their wives were comfortably asleep in their arms; but it was all in vain. Their word was taken; but the archbishop told them they were deceived by the devil and their own senses. It is true they might have had the semblance of their wives in their beds, but the originals were far away at the devil's dance under the oak."—*Mackay's Popular Delusions; chapter on the Witch-Mania.*

them. "I must see that to believe it," is often the expression of no unreasonable scruple.*

La Place puts the case, that we should not trust the testimony of a person who would allege that, having thrown a hundred dice into the air, they all fell with the same side up; while if we saw the thing happen, and carefully inspected the dice, one after the other, we should cease to doubt the fact. He says, "After such an examination we should no longer hesitate to admit it, notwithstanding its extreme improbability; and no one would be tempted, by way of explaining it, to resort to the hypothesis of an illusion caused by an infraction of the laws of vision. Hence we may conclude that the probability of the constancy of natural laws is, for us, greater than the probability that the event referred to should not occur."

So it may be, fairly enough, as to the phenomena witnessed by myself and others, to which allusion has just been made; the moving, namely, without apparent physical agency, of tables and other material substances. These are of a character so extraordinary, that the evidence of testimony, credible though it be regarded, may bring home to the reader no conviction of their reality. If that should be so, he will but find himself in the same position in which I myself was before I witnessed them. Like him whom La Place supposes to be listening to the story of the hundred dice, I doubted hearsay evidence, even from persons whose testimony in any ordinary case I should have taken without hesitation. But I doubted only: I did not deny. I resolved, on the first opportunity, to examine for myself; and the

---

* "I have finally settled down to the opinion that, as to phenomena of so extraordinary a character, one may, by dint of discussion, reach the conviction that there are sufficient reasons for believing them, but that one really *does* believe them only after having seen them."—BERTRAND: "*Traité du Somnambulisme*," p. 165.

evidence of my senses wrought a conviction which testimony had failed to produce. If the reader, doubting like me, but seek the same mode of resolving his doubts, I may have rendered him a service. Let him demand, like Thomas, to see and to feel; let him inspect the dice one after the other; let him avoid, as in the preceding pages I have sought to induce him, the extremes of credulity and unbelief; but let him not imagine that the senses his Creator has given him are lying witnesses, merely because they testify against his preconceptions.

And thus, it may be, shall he learn a wholesome lesson; a lesson of warning against that wisdom in his own conceit which, we are told, is more hopeless than folly itself.

Thus, too, perhaps he may be induced, as I was, patiently to listen to the testimony of others, as contained in many of the following pages, touching what I once considered, and what he may still consider, mere fanciful superstitions. And thus he may be led, as I have been, as to these strange phenomena, carefully to weigh the contending probabilities. I assume not to have reached absolute certainty. How seldom, in any inquiry, is it attained! Where the nature of the case admits but more or less probable deductions, it suffices to show a fair balance of evidence in favor of the conclusions we infer. Nor is it unreasonable to act on such an inference though it fall short of infallible proof. Of all the varied knowledge which regulates our daily actions, how overwhelming a portion, as La Place reminds us, appertains, strictly speaking, to the various shades of the possible only!

And of that knowledge how much has been gradually drawn forth from the obscurity where for ages it lay, vailed by the mists of incredulity, under the ban of the Improbable!

BOOK II.

TOUCHING CERTAIN PHASES OF SLEEP.

CHAPTER 1.

SLEEP IN GENERAL.

"Half our days we pass in the shadow of the earth, and the brother of death exacteth a third part of our lives."—Sir Thomas Browne.

If we sit down to make clear to ourselves what is, and what is not, marvelous,—to define, with precision, the *wonderful,*—we may find the task much more difficult than we apprehend. The extraordinary usually surprises us the most; the ordinary may be not only far more worthy of our attention, but far more inexplicable also.

We are accustomed to call things *natural* if they come constantly under our observation, and to imagine that that single word embodies a sufficient explanation of them. Yet there are daily wonders, familiar household marvels, which, if they were *not* familiar, if they were *not* of daily recurrence, would not only excite our utmost astonishment, but would also, beyond question, provoke our incredulity.

Every night, unless disease or strong excitement interpose, we become ourselves the subjects of a phenomenon which, if it occurred but once in a century, we should regard—if we believed it at all—as the mystery of mysteries. Every night, if blessed with health and tranquillity, we pass, in an unconscious moment, the threshold of material existence; entering another world,

117

where we see, but not with our eyes; where we hear, when our ears convey no perception; in which we speak, in which we are spoken to, though no sound pass our lips or reach our organs of hearing.

In that world we are excited to joy, to grief; we are moved to pity, we are stirred to anger; yet these emotions are aroused by no objective realities. There our judgment is usually obscured, and our reasoning faculties are commonly at fault; yet the soul, as if in anticipation of the powers which the last sleep may confer upon it, seems emancipated from earthly trammels. Time has lost its landmarks. Oceans interpose no barrier. The Past gives back its buried phantoms. The grave restores its dead.

We have glimpses into that world. A portion of it is revealed to us dimly in the recollections of some sleeping thoughts. But a portion is inscrutable,—almost as inscrutable as that other world beyond the tomb.

What means have we of knowing that which passes through our minds in sleep? Except through our memory, (unless, indeed, we are sleep-talkers, and our sleep-talking is overheard,) none whatever. Sleeping thoughts not remembered are, for us in our waking state, as if they had never existed. But it is certain that many such thoughts are wholly forgotten before we awake. Of this we have positive proof in the case of persons talking in sleep, and thus indicating the subject of their dreams. It constantly happens that such persons, interrogated as to their dreams the next morning, deny having had any; and even if the subject of their sleep-talking be suggested to them, it awakens no train of memory.*

---

* Abercrombie's "*Intellectual Powers*," 15th ed., p. 112.

But all physiologists are agreed as to this phenomenon. In some cases, however, two mental states seem to be indicated; the memory of the dream being not so wholly lost that it cannot be revived, at a future time, in sleep.

The question whether we ever sleep without dreaming—as old as the days of Aristotle—is equally curious and difficult of solution. In support of the theory that no moment of sleep is void of dreaming thoughts or sensations, we have such names as Hippocrates, Leibnitz, Descartes, Cabanis. The most formidable authority on the opposite side is Locke. But that eminent man evidently had not before him all the phenomena necessary to afford a proper understanding of this subject. His definition of dreaming is faulty,[*] and the argument with which he supports his views, namely, that "man cannot think at any time, waking or sleeping, without being sensible of it,"[†] evidently does not reach the case.

Of more modern writers, Macnish and Carpenter conclude that perfectly sound sleep is dreamless; while Holland, Macario, and (as far as they express themselves) Abercrombie and Brodie, assume the opposite ground. Plausible reasons may be adduced for either opinion.

Whatever be the conditions of that mysterious mechanism which connects the immaterial principle in man with the brain, this we know: that throughout waking life cerebral action of some kind is the necessary antecedent, or concomitant, of thought. This action, in some modified form, appears to continue at least during those periods of sleep when there occur dreams of such a character that they are remembered, or that their presence is testified by outward signs of emotion in the sleeper.

Dr. Perquin, a French physician, has reported the

---

[*] His definition is, " Dreaming is the having of ideas, whilst the outward senses are stopped, not suggested by any external object or known occasion, nor under the rule and conduct of the understanding."

But, while dreaming, the outward senses are, in general, only partially stopped; ideas are often suggested by external objects and by physical sensations; and sometimes the understanding, instead of being dethroned, acquires a power and vivacity beyond what it possesses in the waking state.

[†] *"An Essay concerning Human Understanding,"* Book II. chap. i. p. 10.

case of a female, twenty-six years of age, who had lost by disease a large portion of her skull-bone and dura mater, so that a corresponding portion of the brain was bare and open to inspection. He says, "When she was in a dreamless sleep her brain was motionless, and lay within the cranium. When her sleep was imperfect, and she was agitated by dreams, her brain moved, and protruded without the cranium, forming cerebral hernia. In vivid dreams, reported as such by herself, the protrusion was considerable; and when she was perfectly awake—especially if engaged in lively conversation—it was still greater. Nor did the protrusion occur in jerks alternating with recessions, as if caused by the impulse of the arterial blood. It remained steady while conversation lasted."*

Here we have three separate mental states, with the corresponding cerebral action intimated, so far as external indications are a clew to it: the waking state, in which the brain gives sign of full activity; a state known to be dreaming, during which there is still cerebral action, but in a diminished degree; and a third state, exhibiting no outward proof of dreaming, nor leaving behind any remembrance of dreams, and during which cerebral action is no longer perceptible to the spectator.

But we stretch inference too far if we assert, as some physiologists do,† that in this third state there *is* no cerebral action and there *are* no dreams.

All that we are justified in concluding is, that, during this period of apparent repose, cerebral action, if such

---

* This case was observed in one of the hospitals of Montpellier, in the year 1821. It is by no means an isolated one. Macnish quotes it in his "*Philosophy of Sleep.*"

† Carpenter ("*Principles of Human Physiology,*" p. 634) is of opinion that during profound sleep the cerebrum and sensory ganglia are "in a state of complete functional inactivity."

continue, is much diminished,* and dreams, if dreams there be, are disconnected, by memory or otherwise, from our waking life.

If we push our researches further, and inquire what is the state of the soul, and what the conditions of its connection with the cerebrum, during the quiescent state, we are entering a field where we shall meet a thousand speculations, and perhaps not one reliable truth beyond the simple fact that, while life lasts, *some* connection between mind and matter must be maintained. We may imagine that connection to be intermediate only,—kept up, it may be, directly with what Bichât calls the system of organic life,† and only through the medium of that system, by anastomosis, or otherwise, with the system of animal life and its center, the cerebral lobes; or we may suppose the connection still to continue direct with the brain. All we know is that, at any moment, in healthy sleep, a sound more or less loud, a touch more or less rude, suffices to restore the brain to complete activity, and to re-establish, if it ever was interrupted, its direct communication with the mind.

The Cartesian doctrine that the soul never sleeps is incapable alike of refutation and of practical applica-

---

* Cases of catalepsy, or trance, in which for days no action of the heart or lungs is cognizable by the senses of the most experienced physician, so that actual death has been supposed, are of common occurrence; yet no one concludes that, however deep the trance, the heart *has* ceased to beat, or the lungs to play. Their action is so much enfeebled as to have become imperceptible: that is all.

† See "*Récherches physiologiques sur la Vie et la Mort*," par X. Bichât, 3d ed., Paris, 1805, p. 3.

His division of the animal functions is into two classes: those of organic life and those of animal life; the first including the functions of respiration, circulation, nutrition, secretion, absorption, the instinctive or automatic functions common to animal and vegetable life; the second restricted to animal life alone, and including the functions which connect man and animals with the external world,—as of sensation, volition, vocal expression, and locomotion.

11

tion. If we imagine that the soul has need of rest, we must admit, as a corollary, that sleep is a phenomenon that will be met with in the next world as it is in this. If, on the other hand, we assert that there can be no moment in which an immortal spirit has not thoughts and sensations, it may be replied that the words *thought* and *sensation*, when used by human beings in regard to their present phase of life, properly apply only to mental conditions which presuppose the action of the human brain; and that, as to the action of the soul without the action of the brain, if such a state can be while the soul is connected with the body, it evinces lack of wisdom to occupy ourselves about it. We can predicate nothing in regard to it; not having in our human vocabulary even the words necessary to embody any conceptions of its phenomena.

Thus, even when we admit that it is the bodily organs only, not the spiritual principle, that experience a sense of fatigue and the necessity for intermittence of action, we do not concede, by the admission, that dreams, in the proper acceptation of the term, pervade all sleep.

We approach a solution more closely when we inquire whether, as a general rule, persons who are suddenly awakened from a profound sleep are, at the moment of awaking, conscious of having dreamed. But here physiologists are not agreed as to the facts. Locke appears to have assumed the negative. Macnish declares, as the result of certain experiments made on purpose, that in the majority of cases the sleeper retained at the moment of waking no such consciousness.* This I much doubt. It is certain that, unless such experiments are conducted with scrupulous care, the true results may readily escape us. If, two years ago, I had myself been

---

* Hazlitt, in his *"Round Table,"* alleges the contrary.

asked whether I was in the habit of dreaming, I should have replied that I very rarely dreamed at all; the fact being then, as it still is, that I scarcely ever have a dream which I remember, or could repeat, even at breakfast the next morning. But my attention having been recently attracted to the subject, so that I acquired the habit of taking special note of my sensations at the moment of awaking, I became aware, after repeated observations, that in every instance I was conscious of having dreamed. Yet, with very few exceptions, the memory of my sleeping thought was so vague and fugitive, that even after ten, or perhaps five, seconds, it had faded away, and that so completely that I found it quite impossible to recall or repeat my dream. After that period I remembered nothing, except that I *had* been conscious of having dreamed; and, to obtain in every case the certainty even of this, I had to awake with the *intention* of making the observation. So exceedingly brief and shadowy and fleeting were these perceptions, that in the great majority of cases no effort I could make sufficed to arrest them. They escaped even at the moment I was endeavoring to stamp them on my memory.

It is true that these observations were usually made at the moment of awaking, naturally, from a night's sleep, and that the strongest advocates of the theory of dreamless sleep (as Lord Brougham, in his *"Discourse on Natural Theology"*) admit that the imperfect sleep bordering on the waking state is full of dreams. But yet the reality in connection with sleeping thoughts of a memory so feeble and evanescent that it requires an intentional effort to detect its existence, should induce us to receive with many scruples the assertions of those who declare that they have no dreams.*

---

* As of a young man, mentioned by Locke, (Essay on *"Human Understanding,"* Book II. chap 1. § 14,) a scholar with no bad memory, who de-

Another argument in this connection is the fact, of which almost every one, probably, has taken frequent note, that we seldom awake from brief sleep, no matter how sound and tranquil it may have been, without a consciousness of time elapsed since we fell asleep. But time, or rather human perception of it, can exist only in connection with a series of thoughts or sensations. Hence the probability that such, even during that deep and motionless slumber, affected the mind.

Upon the whole, though we cannot disprove the theory put forth by Locke and other maintainers of dreamless sleep, the probabilities seem to me against it. Since numerous indications assure us that in a thousand cases in which sleep *seems* dreamless, and even insensibility complete, there exists a constant succession of thoughts and sensations, I think there is sufficient reason to agree, with Brodie, that "not to dream seems to be not the rule, but the exception to the rule;"* and, if it be, how many of the phenomena of sleep may have hitherto escaped our observation! How many more may be covered by a vail that will forever remain impenetrable to mortal eyes!

That large class of phenomena occurring during sleep, of which we retain no recollection after sleep, and which are thus disconnected from waking consciousness, have attracted, as they eminently deserve, much more attention in modern times, particularly during the last seventy years, than at any former period. Seventy-five years ago somnambulism (artificially induced) was unknown. But coma, somnambulism, trance, ecstasy, may be properly regarded as but phases of sleep; abnormal, indeed, and therefore varying widely in some respects from natural sleep, yet all strictly hypnotic states;

---

clared that till he had a fever, in his twenty-sixth year, he had never dreamed in his life.

* *"Psychological Inquiries,"* by Sir B. Brodie, 3d ed., p. 149.

which we do well to study in their connection with each other.

We shall find that they have much in common. The same insensibility which often supervenes during somnambulism and during coma presents itself in a degree during ordinary sleep. Children, especially, are often roused from sleep with difficulty; and sound sleepers of adult age frequently remain unconscious of loud noises or other serious disturbances. It has not unfrequently occurred to myself to hear nothing, or at least to retain no recollection of having heard any thing, of a long-continued and violent thunder-storm, that disturbed and alarmed my neighbors; and in the year 1856, being then in Naples, I slept quietly through an earthquake, the shock of which filled the streets with terrified thousands, imploring the compassion of the Madonna.

Some even of the most remarkable phenomena of somnambulism and ecstasy appear in modified form during natural sleep. That exaltation of the mental powers which forms one of the chief features of the above-named states is to be met with, in numerous examples, during simple dreaming. We read that Cabanis, in dreams, often saw clearly the bearings of political events which had baffled him when awake; and that Condorcet, when engaged in some deep and complicated calculations, was frequently obliged to leave them in an unfinished state and retire to rest, when the results to which they led were unfolded to him in dreams.* Brodie mentions the case of a friend of his, a distinguished chemist and natural philosopher, who assured him that he had more than once contrived in a dream an apparatus for an experiment he proposed to make; and that of another friend, a mathematician and a man of extensive general information, who has solved

---

* Macnish's *"Philosophy of Sleep,"* p. 79.

11*

problems when asleep which baffled him in his waking state. The same author mentions the case of an acquaintance of his, a solicitor, who, being perplexed as to the legal management of a case, imagined, in a dream, a mode of proceeding which had not occurred to him when awake, and which he adopted with success.

Carpenter admits that "the reasoning processes may be carried on during sleep with unusual vigor and success," and cites, as an example, the case of Condillac, who tells us that, when engaged in his "Cours d'Étude," he frequently developed a subject in his dreams which he had broken off before retiring to rest. Carpenter supposes this to occur "in consequence of the freedom from distraction resulting from the suspension of external influences."*

Abercrombie, in this connection, adduces the case of Dr. Gregory, who had thoughts occurring to him in dreams, and even the very expressions in which they were conveyed, which appeared to him afterward, when awake, so just in point of reasoning and illustration, and so happily worded, that he used them in his lectures and in his lucubrations. Even our own practical and unimaginative Franklin appears to have furnished an example of this exaltation of the intellect during sleep. "Dr. Franklin informed Cabanis," says Abercrombie, "that the bearings and issue of political events which had puzzled him when awake were not unfrequently unfolded to him in his dreams."†

A still nearer approach to some of the phenomena of artificial somnambulism and ecstasy, and to the involuntary writing of modern mediums, is made when the sleeping man produces an actual record of his dreaming thoughts. Of this a remarkable example is adduced by

---

* "*Principles of Human Physiology*," p. 643.
† Abercrombie's "*Intellectual Powers*," 15th ed., p. 221.

Abercrombie, in the case of a distinguished lawyer of the last century, in whose family records all the particulars are preserved. They are as follows :—

· " This eminent person had been consulted respecting a case of great importance and much difficulty, and he had been studying it with intense anxiety and attention. After several days had been occupied in this manner, he was observed by his wife to rise from his bed in the night and go to a writing-desk which stood in the bedroom. He then sat down and wrote a long paper, which he carefully put by in the desk, and returned to bed. The following morning he told his wife he had had a most interesting dream; that he had dreamed of delivering a clear and luminous opinion respecting a case which had exceedingly perplexed him, and he would give any thing to recover the train of thought which had passed before him in his sleep. She then directed him to the writing-desk, where he found the opinion clearly and fully written out. It was afterward found to be perfectly correct."*

Carpenter admits, during certain phases of sleep, the exaltation not only of the mental powers, but of the senses. Speaking of what Mr. Braid calls *hypnotism*,†—

---

* Abercrombie, Work cited, p. 222.

It is scarcely necessary to remind the reader that the cases above adduced, though numerous, are exceptional. As a general rule, the reasoning powers are enfeebled during sleep. "Sometimes," says Müller, (*Physiology*, Baly's translation, p. 1417,) "we reason more or less accurately in our dreams. We reflect on problems, and rejoice in their solution. But on awaking from such dreams the seeming reasoning is found to be no reasoning at all, and the solution over which we had rejoiced to be mere nonsense."

This, also, is not without its analogy in somnambulism and ecstasy. The opinions expressed and the statements made during these states are often altogether untrustworthy.

† "*Neurypnology ; or, The Rationale of Sleep*," by James Braid, M.R.C.S.E., London, 1843.

which is, in fact, only sleep artificially induced by gazing fixedly on any near object,—he mentions some cases that have come under his observation, thus :—

"The author has witnessed a case in which such an exaltation of the sense of smell was manifested, that the subject of it discovered, without difficulty, the owner of a glove placed in his hands in an assemblage of fifty or sixty persons; and in the same case, as in many others, there was a similar exaltation of the sense of temperature. The exaltation of the muscular sense, by which various actions that ordinarily require the guidance of vision are directed independently of it, is a phenomenon common to the mesmeric, with various other forms of artificial as well as natural somnambulism.

"The author has repeatedly seen Mr. Braid's hypnotized subjects write with the most perfect regularity, when an opaque screen was interposed between their eyes and the paper, the lines being equidistant and parallel; and it is not uncommon for the writer to carry back his pencil or pen to dot an *i*, or cross a *t*, or make some other correction in a letter or word. Mr. B. had one patient who would thus go back and correct with accuracy the writing on a whole sheet of note-paper; but, if the paper was moved from the position it had previously occupied on the table, all the corrections were on the *wrong* points of the paper as regarded the *actual* place of the writing, though on the *right* points as regarded its previous place. Sometimes, however, he would take a fresh departure, by feeling for the upper left-hand corner of the paper; and all his corrections were then made in their right positions, notwithstanding the displacement of the paper."*

Again, Dr. Carpenter informs us that when the atten-

---

* *"Principles of Human Physiology,"* p. 646.

tion of the patient was fixed on a certain train of thought, whatever happened to be spoken in harmony with this was heard and appreciated; but what had no relation to it, or was in discordance with it, was entirely disregarded.

What can be more completely in accordance with certain somnambulic phenomena, of which the existence has been stoutly denied, than all this?

But a little careful search in this field may disclose to us points of resemblance more numerous still. It belongs more properly to the next chapter, on Dreaming, than to this, to inquire whether, in exceptional cases, during natural sleep, there do not present themselves some of the most extraordinary powers or attributes, the alleged and seldom-credited phenomena of somnambulism,—such as clear-sight, (clairvoyance,) far-sight, (*vue à distance,*) and even that most strongly contested of all, the faculty of presentiment, the prophetic instinct.

But there is another point of analogy, connected with the renovating influence of sleep and the causes which render necessary to man such an intermittent action, to which it may be useful here to allude.

It would be very incorrect to say that the continued exercise of any function induces fatigue, and consequently necessitates sleep. It is well known that this is true of some functions only. It is not true of the functions of organic life, the automatic or involuntary functions. We tire of walking, we tire of thinking, we tire of seeing or hearing, or of directing the attention in any way to external objects; but we never tire of breathing, though breathing is a more continued action than any of these.

This obvious fact suggested to physiologists, before Darwin's time, the opinion which was first prominently brought forward by that naturalist, that *the essential*

I

part of sleep is the suspension of volition. And some have gone so far as to assert that the only source of fatigue, and therefore the sole necessitating cause of sleep, is the exercise of volition; adducing in support of this theory the observation, that when the muscles of an arm or a leg are contracted under the influence of the will, fatigue follows in a few minutes; while the same contraction taking place involuntarily (as in catalepsy, whether naturally or mesmerically induced) may continue for a long time without any fatigue whatever.

But we cannot adopt unconditionally such an opinion without assuming that there is no waking state in which the volition is suspended or inactive. For we know of no waking state, no matter how listless and purposeless, the continuance of which obviates the necessity, after a comparatively brief interval, for sleep. Nor is it true that men of strong will and constant activity always require more sleep than the indolent and infirm of purpose. Three or four hours out of the twenty-four are said to have sufficed, for months at a time, to Napoleon, the very embodiment of energetic purpose and unceasing activity of volition.

Not the less, however, must we admit the truth and importance of Darwin's remark, that the essential condition of sleep is the suspension of volition. And in this respect the resemblance is striking between sleep and the various states of the human system during which mesmeric and what have been called spiritual phenomena present themselves. The somnambule, the "medium," are told that the first condition of success in the production of the phenomena sought is, that the subject should remain absolutely passive; that he should implicitly surrender to the action of external influences his will. Indeed, the somnambule is put to sleep, if artificially, not the less absolutely, by the magnetizer. And when a medium joins a circle around the table, or engages in automatic writing, drowsiness, after a brief period, is usually induced.

Upon the whole, the facts seem to justify the assertion that all mesmeric and so-called spiritual phenomena, so far as they depend on a peculiar condition of the human system, are more or less hypnotic in their character. To obtain a proper understanding of their true nature, and a discriminating appreciation of the results obtained, this should constantly be borne in mind.

For the rest, it may be doubted whether the popular opinion that it is only during sleep that there is accumulation in the cerebral lobes of the nervous fluid be a correct one, and whether we ought to consider the expenditure of that fluid as restricted to the waking state.

The better opinion appears to be, that, as a general rule, there are, at all times, both a generation and a consumption; that, whether during the sleeping or waking state, that mysterious process which supplies renovating force to the human system is constantly going on,—the supply falling short of the demand upon it, and therefore gradually diminishing, during our waking hours, but exceeding it, and therefore gradually accumulating, during sleep. In other words, we may suppose the supply regular and constant, both by day and night, as in the case of that other automatic process, as little understood, of assimilation; and the demand never wholly ceasing, nor ever, perhaps, perfectly regular in its requisitions, but intermittent as to quantity, usually every twenty-four hours,—making, so long as the will is in action and the senses are awake, its calls at such a rate as must, after a time, exhaust the supply; and then again, during the comparative inaction of sleep, restricting these calls, so that the nervous fluid can increase in quantity and a surplus accumulate before morning.

That, in all cases, a certain reserve fund remains is evident from the fact that, under circumstances of urgency, we can postpone sleep even for several nights. But this encroachment is usually attended with injurious results. Nor does it appear that the brain can be overloaded with nervous fluid, any more than it can be unduly deprived of it, without injury; for there are diseases induced by excessive sleep.

It would seem, also, that the brain can only deal out its supply of nervous force at a certain rate.

For an exercise of *violent* volition is commonly succeeded, after a brief period, by exhaustion; and rest (which is a very different thing from sleep, being only a cessation from active exertion) becomes necessary before a second such call on the nervous reservoir can be made.

How that reservoir is supplied,—by what precise process there is generated in the cerebrum that store of fluid or force, the most wonderful of all the imponderables, without which, in the human system, there would be neither exercise of volition nor any outward sign of intelligence; whether this mysterious agent is, after all, but a modification of that proteus-showing fluid, the electrical, or, if not electrical, whether it may not be of electroid character:—these various questions how shall we determine?—we who, after the lapse of twenty-five centuries since Thales's first observation on a bit of amber, can scarcely tell, when we speak of positive and negative electricity, which hypothesis is the more correct,—that of a single agent, now in excess, now in deficiency, or that of two electricities, the vitreous and the resinous; we who, indeed, have but learned enough to become conscious that this very agency itself, called by us electrical, must yet be spoken of as unknown,—

unknown in its essence, albeit observed, by thousands of naturalists, in some of its effects.*

Intelligent physiologists and psychologists, it is true, have speculated on this subject; Sir Benjamin Brodie, for example. Speaking of the changes which the nervous system may be supposed to undergo in connection with mental processes, and in reply to the questions, "Are these simply mechanical? or do they resemble the chemical changes in inorganic matter? or do they not rather belong to that class of phenomena which we refer to imponderable agents, such as electricity and magnetism?" he says, "The transmission of impressions from one part of the nervous system to another, or from the nervous system to the muscular and glandular structures, has a nearer resemblance to the effects produced by the imponderable agents alluded to than to any thing else. It seems very probable, indeed, that the nervous force is some modification of that force which produces the phenomena of electricity and magnetism; and I have already ventured to compare the generation of it by the action of the oxygenized blood

---

* A few years since, at the meeting of the British Association for the Advancement of Science held at Swansea, a discussion having arisen as to the essence or nature of electricity, and an appeal having been made to Faraday for his opinion on the subject, what did he, the first electrician perhaps of the age, reply? "There was a time when I thought I knew something about the matter; but the longer I live and the more carefully I study the subject, the more convinced I am of my total ignorance of the nature of electricity."—*Quoted by Bakewell, in his "Electric Science,"* p. 99.

"Some of the conditions which we call the *laws* of electricity and of magnetism are known. These may not improperly be viewed as their habits or modes of action,—the ways in which they manifest themselves to some of our senses. But of what they consist, whether they possess properties peculiar to themselves and independent of the ponderable substances with which we have always found them associated, or in what respects they differ from light and heat and from each other, is beyond the range of our experience and, probably, of our comprehension."—*Rutter's Human Electricity,* pp. 47, 48.

12

on the gray substance of the brain and spinal cord, to the production of the electric force by the action of the acid solution on the metallic plates in the cells of a voltaic battery."[*]

Such a view may assist our insufficient conceptions; yet, in all reasonable probability, when we liken the nervous force or fluid to electricity, and the action of the cerebrum to that of an electric or galvanic apparatus, the comparison should be understood as illustrative and approximating,—as embodying only an adumbration of the truth,—not as indicating a close resemblance, still less a strict and positive identity of action.

That, in some way or other, the blood is an agent in the generation of the nervous force can scarcely be doubted. Sir Henry Holland, speaking of the intimate relations between the nervous and vascular systems, and the obvious structural connection of the nerves and blood-vessels, adds, "We cannot designate a single part in the whole economy of animal life in which we do not find these two great powers conjointly concerned,—their co-operation so essential that no single function can be perfectly performed without it. The blood and the nervous force, so far as we know, are the only agents which actually pervade the body throughout; the connection of the machinery by which they are conveyed becoming closer in proportion as we get nearer to the ultimate limits of observation. Besides those results of their co-operation which have regard to the numerous other objects and phenomena of life, we cannot doubt the existence of a reciprocal action upon each other, necessary to the maintenance and completeness of their respective powers." . . . . "We cannot, indeed, follow, with any clear understanding, the notion

---

[*] *"Psychological Inquiries,"* by Sir Benjamin Brodie, London, 1856, vol. iii. pp. 158, 159.

of the nervous element as evolved by the action of the blood, or as actually *derived* from the blood, and depending for its maintenance and energy on the conditions of this fluid. Yet we can hardly doubt that mutual actions and relations of some such nature really exist. Evidence to this effect is furnished, directly or indirectly, by all the natural phenomena of health, and even more remarkably by the results of disorder and disease. The whole inquiry is of singular importance to the physiology of animal life."*

Taking into view the above remarks, and assuming Brodie's suggestion as to the electroid character of the nervous element,—bearing in mind, too, that hœmatin, one of the constituents of the blood, has seven or eight per cent. of iron, while other portions contain, in smaller quantities, other metals, and that, in consequence, we have *an electroid force or agent* brought into intimate relation with *a metal-bearing fluid*, a condition that may be supposed favorable to something resembling electro-chemical action,—have we not a hint as to the manner in which (to borrow analogous terms in default of accurate ones) the cerebral battery may possibly be charged?

How closely, when we touch on such topics, are we approaching the confines of human knowledge! A step or two further in this direction we may, indeed, some day advance; but what then? "The chain of our knowledge," says Berzelius, "ends ever at last in a link unknown." If even we could discover how this battery is charged, a deeper mystery remains still vailed; the manner, namely, in which the spiritual principle within us avails itself of this wonderful mechanism to produce motion and direct thought.

And another inquiry, more immediately connecting

* *"Chapters on Mental Physiology,"* by Sir Henry Holland, M.D., London, 1852.

the foregoing digression with the subject of this chapter, may be mooted here,—an inquiry which some will dismiss as unworthy even to be entertained, but which, nevertheless, is justified, in my eyes, by its connection with certain psychological phenomena to be presented in subsequent portions of this volume; the inquiry, namely, whether, in certain exceptional conditions of the human system, as occasionally during dreams, or under other circumstances when the will is surrendered, some immaterial principle or occult intelligence other than our own may not, for a time and to a certain extent, possess itself of the power to employ the cerebral mechanism so as to suggest or inspire thoughts and feelings which, though in one sense our own, yet come to us from a foreign source.

Such a hypothesis, though adopted at the present day by not a few sensible men, may, I well know, startle as incredible the majority of my readers. I remind them that the first question is, not whether it be true, but whether it be worth examining. "In the infancy of a science," says Brewster, "there is no speculation so worthless as not to merit examination. The most remote and fanciful explanations of facts have often been found the true ones; and opinions which have in one century been objects of ridicule have in the next been admitted among the elements of our knowledge."*

If still there be among my readers those who are disposed to reject at the threshold the inquiry in question, as savoring of superstition, I pray them to postpone decision in regard to it until they shall have read the chapters which follow, especially the next, treating a subject which it is difficult to disconnect from that of sleep in the abstract; the subject, namely, of dreams.

---

* "*The Martyrs of Science,*" by Sir David Brewster, 3d ed., London, 1856, p. 219.

CHAPTER II.

DREAMS.

"In a dream, in a vision of the night, when deep sleep falleth upon men in slumberings upon the bed; then God openeth the ears of men, and sealeth their instruction."—JOB xxxiii. 14.

MODERN writers on the phenomena of sleep usually concur in the assertion that man's sleeping thoughts are meaningless and inconsequent, and that dreams are, therefore, untrustworthy.

Such was not the opinion of our ancestors, especially in remote times. They attached great importance to dreams and their interpretation. They had resort to them for guidance in cases of difficulty or of great calamity. Thus, when pestilence spread among the Grecian host before Troy, Homer represents Achilles as proposing that method of ascertaining the cause of what was regarded as an evidence of the anger of the gods; and his reason for the proposal is,—

"for dreams descend from Jove."*

Aristotle, Plato, Zeno, Pythagoras, Socrates, Xenophon, Sophocles, have all expressed, more or less distinctly, their belief in the divine or prophetic character of dreams. And even some of the ancient philosophers who denied all other kinds of divination, as some distinguished Peripatetics, admitted those which proceeded from frenzy and from dreams.†

---

* Homer's Iliad, Book I. line 85 of Pope's translation.
† Cicero "De Divinatione," lib. i. ? 3. See also ? 25 et seq.
The analogy between dreams and insanity has been often noticed. Aris-

It does not appear, however, that any of these philosophers went so far as to claim for *all* dreams a divine or reliable character. Many proceeded from the ivory gate. It was usually the vision of some seer, or augur, or priestess, occurring within sacred or consecrated ground, to the warnings of which implicit faith was attached. Plato, however, seems to intimate that all dreams might be trusted if men would only bring their bodies into such a state, before going to sleep, as to leave nothing that might occasion error or perturbation in their dreams.*

Aristotle—whose works, like Bacon's, may be said to have marked out the limits of the knowledge of his day—restricts to certain favored individuals this faculty of prescience. His expression, literally translated, is, "And that, as to some persons, prophecy occurs in dreams, is not to be disbelieved."†

That the modern opinion as to the fantastic and imaginative character of dreams is, in the main, correct; that, when the senses are overcome by slumber, the judgment also, as a general rule, is either entirely in abeyance, or only partially and very obscurely active; these are facts so readily ascertained, usually by a little accurate observation of our own nightly sensations, as to be

---

totle had already surmised that the same cause which, in certain diseases, produces deception of the waking senses, is the origin of dreams in sleep. Brierre de Boismont remarks that waking hallucinations differ chiefly from dreams in their greater vivacity. Macario considers what he calls sensorial dreams as almost identical with hallucination. Holland says that the relations and resemblances of dreaming and insanity are well deserving of notice, and adds, "A dream put into action might become madness, in one or other of its frequent forms; and, conversely, insanity may often be called a waking and active dream."—"*Chapters on Mental Physiology,*" p. 110. Abercrombie declares that "there is a remarkable analogy between the mental phenomena in insanity and in dreaming."—"*Intellectual Powers,*" p. 240.

* Quoted by Cicero, "*De Divinatione,*" lib. i. §§ 29, 30.

† "*De Divinatione et Somniis,*" cap. i.

beyond reasonable doubt.* Whether for the notions of the ancients touching the higher character of some dreams there be not, in exceptional cases, sufficient warrant, is a much more difficult question.†

Certain it is that the framework of many dreams is made up of suggestions derived from waking ideas or desires that have preceded them, or from occurrences that happen during their continuance and are partially perceived by the sleep-bound senses.

The ruling passion of a man's life is not unlikely to shape itself into dreams. The constant thought of the day may encroach on the quiet of the night. Thus, Columbus dreamed that a voice said to him, "God will give thee the keys of the gates of the ocean."‡ And thus any earnest longing, experienced when we compose ourselves to sleep, may pass over into our sleeping consciousness, and be reproduced, perhaps, in some happy

---

* A disregard of these truths has led to fatal results. Aubrey, who will not be suspected of trusting too little to dreams, personally vouches, as will be observed, for the following :—

"Mrs. Cl——, of S——, in the county of S——, had a beloved daughter, who had been a long time ill and received no benefit from her physicians. She dreamed that a friend of hers, deceased, told her that if she gave her daughter a drench of yew pounded she would recover. She gave her the drench, and it killed her. Whereupon she grew almost distracted : her chambermaid, to compliment her and mitigate her grief, said, surely that could not kill her: she would adventure to take the same herself. She did so, and died also. This was about the year 1670 or 1671. I knew the family."—"*Aubrey's Miscellanies,*" *Chapter on Dreams,* p. 64 of Russell Smith's reprint.

† Such ideas are by no means confined to the ancients, but are to be found scattered through writings of repute in all ages. Here is an example :—

" That there are demoniacal dreams we have little reason to doubt. Why may there not be angelical ? If there be guardian spirits, they may not be inactively about us in sleep, but may sometimes order our dreams ; and many strange hints, instigations, and discourses, which are so amazing unto us, may arise from such foundations."—SIR THOMAS BROWNE : *Chapter on Sleep.*

‡ Humboldt's " *Cosmos,*" vol. i. p. 316.

delusion. As true to nature as graceful in art is that beautiful vision of home and its joys, described by the poet as occurring, after the battle, to the war-worn soldier,—

"When sentinel stars set their watch in the sky,
When thousands had sunk on the ground overpowered,
The weary to sleep, and the wounded to die."

But it is worthy of remark that it is not alone dominant emotions, not mental impressions of a vivid character only, that become suggestive of dreams. Trifling occurrences, that have passed from our recollection before composing ourselves to rest, are sometimes incorporated into the visions of the night that succeeds. I find an example in my journal, under date Naples, May 12, 1857 :—

"Last evening my servant informed me that a house, the second from that which I inhabit, and just across a garden on which the windows of my apartments open, was on fire, and that the furniture of several rooms was burning. As, however, the fire did not reach the outside walls, and as, during my four years' residence in Naples, where all buildings are fireproof, I had never heard of such a thing as a house burning down, I gave myself little uneasiness about it. Later I learned that the fire had been subdued; and before I went to sleep the circumstance had ceased to occupy my mind.

"Nevertheless, I had the following dream. I thought I was traversing a small town, in which a house was on fire. Thence I passed out into the open country, and arrived at a point where I had a view over a valley through which a river ran; and on the banks of that river were several large buildings. Of these I observed that two, at some distance from each other, were in flames. The sight instantly suggested to me the idea that the fires must be the work of incendiaries;

since (it was thus I argued in my sleep) it was not likely that three buildings, quite disconnected, yet within a short distance of each other, should be on fire by mere accident at the same time. 'Is it some riot or revolution that is commencing?' was my next thought. And, in my dream, I heard several shots, as from different parts of the country, confirming (possibly creating) my idea of a popular disturbance. At this point I awoke, and, after listening a few moments, became aware that some persons were letting off fire-crackers in the street, —a common Neapolitan amusement."

The causes predisposing to such a dream are evident. I had heard, a short time before going to rest, of a house on fire; and the idea, in a modified form, was continued in my sleep. I was in a country where one lives amid daily rumors of a revolutionary outbreak: hence, probably, the suggestion as to the cause of the fires. This received confirmation from the actual detonation of the fire-crackers, which my dreaming fancy construed into a succession of musket-shots.

It is to be remarked, however, that these suggestive circumstances were by no means of a character to make much impression on my waking thoughts. I was not under the slightest apprehension about the fire; and I had lived so long amid daily reports of an impending revolution that I had ceased to ascribe to them any credit or probability. The inference seems to be, that even feeble waking impressions may become incentives to dreams.

Occasionally it has been found that dreams may be actually framed by the suggestions of those who surround the bed of the sleeping man. A remarkable example in the case of a British officer is given by Dr. Abercrombie, in which "they could produce in him any kind of dream by whispering in his ear, especially if this was done by a friend with whose voice he was familiar."* In this way they conducted him through the whole course of a quarrel, which ended in a duel; and finally, a pistol being placed in his hand, he discharged it, and was awakened by the report. Similar examples have been elsewhere noticed, as one of a medical student, given by Smellie, in his "Natural History;" and another, mentioned by Dr. Beattie, of a man in whose case any kind of dream could be induced by his friends gently speaking in his presence on the particular subject they wished him to dream about.

The same power seems, at times, to be exercised by a magnetizer over one whom he has been in the habit of magnetizing. Foissac relates of his somnambule, Mademoiselle Cœline, that, *in her natural sleep*, he could not only lead her on to dream whatever he pleased, but also cause her to remember the dream when she awoke from it.† In the case mentioned by Abercrombie, the subject preserved no distinct recollection of what he had dreamed.

There is another remarkable phenomenon connected with the suggestion of dreams, which is well worth

---

* *"Intellectual Powers,"* pp. 202, 203.

† *"Rapports et Discussions,"* Paris, 1833, p. 438. In actual somnambulism artificially induced, this power of suggestion is more frequent and more marked. Dr. Macario, in his work on Sleep, relates a striking example, as having occurred in his presence. It was in the case of a certain patient of a friend of his, Dr. Gromier,—a married lady, subject to hysterical affections. Finding her one day a prey to settled melancholy, he imagined the following plan to dissipate it. Having cast her into a magnetic sleep, he said to her, *mentally*, "Why do you lose hope? You are pious: the Holy Virgin will come to your assistance: be sure of it." Then he called up in his mind a vision, in which he pictured the ceiling of the chamber removed, groups of cherubim at the corners, and the Virgin, in a blaze of glory, descending in the midst. Suddenly the somnambule was affected with ecstasy, sunk on her knees, and exclaimed, in a transport of joy, "Ah, my God! So long—so very long—I have prayed to the Holy Virgin; and now, for the first time, she comes to my aid!"

I adduce this example in evidence how closely the phenomena of natural sleep and artificial somnambulism sometimes approach each other. It may afford a clew, also, to the true origin of many ecstatic visions.

noticing. It would seem that as, in what Braid calls the hypnotic condition, there is sometimes an exaltation of the intellect and of the senses, so in dreams there is occasionally a sort of refreshening and brightening of the memory. Brodie gives an example from his own experience. He says, "On one occasion I imagined I was a boy again, and that I was repeating to another boy a tale with which I had been familiar at that period of my life, though I had never read it nor thought of it since. I awoke, and repeated it to myself at the time, as I believe, accurately enough; but on the following day I had forgotten it again." When, therefore, in sleep something is recalled to us which in our waking state we had forgotten, we ought not, on that account, to conclude that there is any thing more mysterious about it than there is in many other familiar, if unexplained, operations of the mind.

We should be on our guard, also, against another class of dreams, sometimes spiritually interpreted, which lie open to the hypothesis that they may have been the result of earnest longing and expectation in the dreamer. Such a one is given in the biography of William Smellie, author of the "Philosophy of Natural History." Intimately acquainted with the Rev. William Greenlaw, they had entered into a solemn compact, in writing, signed with their blood, that whoever died first should return, if possible, and testify to the survivor regarding the world of spirits; but if the deceased did not appear within a year after the day of his death, it was to be concluded that he could not return. Greenlaw died on the 26th of June, 1774. As the first anniversary of his death approached and he had made no sign, Smellie became extremely anxious, and even lost rest during several successive nights, in expectation of the reappearance of his friend. At last, fatigued with watching, and having fallen asleep in his armchair, Greenlaw appeared to him, stating that he was now in another and a better world, from which he had found great difficulty in communicating with the friend he had left behind, and adding, as to that world, that "the hopes and wishes of its inhabitants were by no means satisfied, for, like those of the lower world, they still looked forward in the hope of eventually reaching a still happier state of existence."*

Those who believe that they have sufficient evidence, in other examples, of the reality of such revisitings, will probably conclude, as the biographer states Smellie himself to have believed even to the day of his death, that his friend Greenlaw had actually appeared to him; but it is evident that a different interpretation may be put on the incident; for it is clearly supposable, in this case, as in that of the war-worn soldier in Campbell's ballad, that the longing of the day may have engendered the vision of the night.

But while we admit, what the facts abundantly prove, that, in a great majority of instances, dreams are, or may be, either the breaking forth in sleep of a strong desire, or the offspring of fancy running riot beyond the control of the judgment, or else the result of suggestion, sometimes direct and intentional, more frequently proceeding, apparently by accident, from antecedent thoughts or emotions, there remain to be dealt with certain exceptional cases, which do not seem to be properly included in any of the above categories. To judge understandingly of these, it behooves us to examine them somewhat in detail.

We may dispose, preliminarily, of one class, as evidently susceptible of simple and natural explanation; those, namely, which, more or less distinctly, bring about their own fulfillment.

---

* *"Memoirs of the Life, Writings, and Correspondence of William Smellie, F.R.S. and F.A.S.,"* by Robert Kerr, F.R.S., Edinburgh, 1811, p. 187.

Such, for example, is an old story, mentioned by several Italian authors, of a merchant, traveling between Rome and Sienna, who dreamed that he was murdered on the road. His host, to whom he told his dream, advised him to pray and confess. He did so, and was afterward assassinated on the way by the very priest to whom, in confession, he had communicated the knowledge of his wealth and his apprehensions.

A case of similar character, occurring a few years since near Hamburg, was given at the time in the newspapers of the day. The apprentice of a certain locksmith of that city, named Claude Soller, one day informed his master that the night before he had dreamed that he had been murdered on the road between Hamburg and Bergsdorff. His master laughingly told him he had just then a hundred and forty rix-dollars to send to his brother-in-law in Bergsdorff; and, to prove to him how ridiculous it was to believe in such omens, he (the apprentice) should be the bearer of it. The young man, after vainly remonstrating, was compelled to set out, which he did, about eleven o'clock in the day. Arrived half-way, at the village of Billwaerder, and recollecting, with terror, the particulars of his dream, he called upon the baillie of the village, found him engaged with some workmen, related to him, in their presence, his dream, mentioned the sum of money he had with him, and begged that some one might be allowed to accompany him through a small wood that lay in his way. The baillie, smiling at his fears, bade one of the workmen go with him as he desired. The next day the body of the apprentice was found, his throat cut, and a bloody reaping-hook near the body. It was afterward proved that the man who accompanied him had used that very reaping-hook some time before, to cut willows. He was apprehended, confessed his crime, and declared that it

K   13

was the recital of the dream which had prompted him to its commission.

In some cases the connection between the influence of the dream and its fulfillment, though we may admit its possibility, is not so clearly made out. A romantic example—perfectly authenticated, however—I here translate from Macario's work on Sleep.

HOW A PARIS EDITOR OBTAINED A WIFE.

In a small town of Central France, Charité-sur-Loire, in the Department of Nièvre, there lived a young girl, of humble rank, being the daughter of a baker, but remarkable for her grace and beauty. There were several aspirants for her hand, of whom one, on account of his fortune, was favored by her parents. The girl, however, not liking him, rejected his proposals of marriage. The parents insisted; and finally the daughter, pressed by their importunities, repaired to the church, prostrated herself before the image of the Virgin, and earnestly prayed for counsel and guidance in the choice of a husband.

The following night she dreamed that there passed before her a young man, in a traveler's dress, with spectacles, and wearing a large straw hat; and a voice from within seemed to tell her that he was to be her husband. As soon as she awoke, she sought her parents, told them, respectfully, but firmly, that she had positively decided not to accept the man of their choice; and from thenceforward they no longer pressed the matter.

Some time afterward, at a village ball, she recognized the young traveler, just as he had appeared in her dream. She blushed. He was attracted by her appearance, fell in love, as the phrase is, at first sight, and after a brief interval they were married. Her husband is M. Émile de la Bédollière, one of the editors of the Paris journal the "Siècle;" and, in a letter to Dr.

Macario, dated Paris, 13th December, 1854, he certifies to the accuracy, in every particular, of the above relation, adding other details. He states that it was at a subscription ball, held in August, 1833, at the house of a man named Jacquemart, which he visited in company with his friend, Eugène Lafaure, that he first saw his future wife, Angèle Bobin; that her emotion on seeing him was apparent, and that he ascertained from the lady at whose pension the young girl then was, Mademoiselle Porcerat by name, that she who afterward became Madame de la Bédollière had given to her teacher, long before his own accidental appearance for the first time at La Charité, an accurate description of his person and dress.*

In this case, though the coincidence seems remarkable, we may, as to the matter of personal resemblance, allow something to chance and something to latitude of imagination in an enthusiastic young girl. For the rest, the conscious blush of a village beauty was sufficient to attract the attention and interest the heart of a young traveler, perhaps of ardent and impressible temperament. It would be presumptuous positively to assert that these considerations furnish the true explanation. But the possibility is to be conceded that they may do so.

So in another case, the dream or vision of Sir Charles Lee's daughter, in which, however, it was death, not marriage, that was foreshadowed. Though it occurred nearly two hundred years ago, it is very well authenticated, having been related by Sir Charles Lee himself to the Bishop of Gloucester, and by the Bishop of Gloucester to Beaumont, who published it, soon after he

---

* "*Du Sommeil, des Rêves, et du Somnambulisme,*" by Dr. Macario, Ex-Deputy of the Sardinian Parliament, Lyons, 1857, pp. 80, 81.

heard it, in a postscript to his well-known "Treatise of Spirits." Thence I transcribe it.

THE BISHOP OF GLOUCESTER'S STORY.

"Having lately had the honor to hear a relation of an apparition from the Lord Bishop of Gloucester, and it being too late for me to insert it in its proper place in this book, I give it you here by way of postscript, as follows:—

"Sir Charles Lee, by his first lady, had only one daughter, of which she died in childbirth; and, when she was dead, her sister, the Lady Everard, desir'd to have the education of the child; and she was by her very well educated till she was marriageable; and a match was concluded for her with Sir William Perkins, but was then prevented in an extraordinary manner. Upon a Thursday night, she, thinking she saw a light in her chamber after she was in bed, knock'd for her maid, who presently came to her; and she asked why she left a candle burning in her chamber. The maid said she left none, and there was none but what she brought with her at that time. Then she said it was the fire; but that, her maid told her, was quite out, and said she believed it was only a dream; whereupon she said it might be so, and compos'd herself again to sleep. But about two of the clock she was awaken'd again, and saw the apparition of a little woman between her curtain and her pillow, who told her she was her mother, that she was happy, and that by twelve o'clock that day she should be with her. Whereupon she knock'd again for her maid, called for her clothes, and, when she was dress'd, went into her closet, and came not out again till nine, and then brought out with her a letter sealed to her father, brought it to her aunt, the Lady Everard, told her what had happen'd, and desir'd that, as soon as she was dead, it might be sent to him. But the lady thought she was suddenly fall'n mad, and thereupon sent presently away to Chelmsford for a physician and surgeon, who both came immediately; but the physician could discern no indication of what the lady imagin'd, or of any indisposition of her body. Notwithstanding, the lady would needs have her let blood, which was done accordingly. And when the young woman had patiently let them do what they would with her, she desir'd that the chaplain might be called to read prayers; and when the prayers were ended she took her gittar and psalm-book, and sate down upon a chair without arms, and play'd and sung so melodiously and admirably that her musick-master, who was then there, admired at it. And near the stroke of twelve she rose, and sate herself down in a great chair with arms, and presently, fetching a strong breathing or two, immediately expired; and was so suddenly cold as was much wondered at by the physician and surgeon. She dyed at Waltham, in Essex, three miles from Chelmsford; and the letter was sent to Sir Charles, at his house in Warwickshire; but he was so afflicted with the death of his daughter, that he came not till she was buried; but, when he came, caus'd her to be taken up and to be buried by her mother at Edminton, as she desir'd in her letter. This was about the year 1662 or 1663. And that relation the Lord Bishop of Gloucester had from Sir Charles Lee himself."*

In the case here narrated, though it be doubtless an extraordinary and unusual thing for any one, not reduced by sickness to an extreme state of nervous weakness, to be so overcome by imagination that a confident

---

* *"An Historical, Physiological, and Theological Treatise of Spirits,"* by John Beaumont, Gent., London, 1705, pp. 398 to 400.

expectation of death at a particular hour should cause it, even within a few minutes after the patient was, to all appearance, in good health, yet, as such things may possibly be, we cannot in this case, any more than in the preceding example, absolutely deny that the dream itself may have been instrumental in working out its fulfillment.

There are many other dreams, however, as to the fulfillment of which no such explanation can be given. One of the best known and most celebrated is that of Calphurnia, on the night before the Ides of March. We read that she almost succeeded in imparting to her husband the alarm which this warning of his death created in herself, and that Cæsar was finally confirmed in his original intention to proceed to the Senate-chamber by the ridicule of one of the conspirators, who made light of the matron's fears.*

Those fears, natural in one whose husband, through a thousand perils, had reached so dangerous a height, might, indeed, have suggested the dream; and its exact time may possibly have been determined by the prediction of that augur, Spurina, who had bidden the dictator beware of the Ides of March. So that here again, though the dream had no effect in working out its fulfillment, apparent causes may be imagined to account for it.

A dream of somewhat similar character, occurring in modern times, is cited in several medical works, and

* Plutarch tells us that the arguments which Calphurnia used, and the urgent manner in which she expressed herself, moved and alarmed her husband, especially when he called to mind that he had never before known in her any thing of the weakness or superstition of her sex; whereas now she was affected in an extraordinary manner, conjuring him not to go to the Senate that day. And, he adds, had it not been for the suggestions of Decius Brutus Albinus, one of the conspirators, but a man in whom Cæsar placed much confidence, these arguments would have prevailed.

vouched for, as "entirely authentic," by Abercrombie.*
It is as follows:—

THE FISHING-PARTY.

Major and Mrs. Griffith, of Edinburgh, then residing in
the Castle, had received into their house their nephew,
Mr. Joseph D'Acre, of Kirklinton, in the county of Cum-
berland,—a young gentleman who had come to the
Scottish capital for the purpose of attending college,
and had been specially recommended to his relatives'
care. One afternoon Mr. D'Acre communicated to
them his intention of joining some of his young com-
panions on the morrow in a fishing-party to Inch-Keith;
and to this no objection was made. During the ensuing
night, however, Mrs. Griffith started from a troubled
dream, exclaiming, in accents of terror, "The boat is
sinking! Oh, save them!" Her husband ascribed it to
apprehension on her part; but she declared that she had
no uneasiness whatever about the fishing-party, and
indeed had not thought about it. So she again composed herself to sleep. When, however, a similar dream
was thrice repeated in the course of the night, (the last
time presenting the image of the boat lost and the
whole party drowned,) becoming at last seriously alarmed,
she threw on her wrapping-gown and, without waiting
for morning, proceeded to her nephew's room. With
some difficulty she persuaded him to relinquish his
design, and to send his servant to Leith with an excuse.
The morning was fine, and the party embarked; but
about three o'clock a storm suddenly arose, the boat
foundered, and all on board were lost.†

* *"Intellectual Powers,"* 15th ed., p. 215. Abercrombie condenses the story
and omits the names.

† Independently of Abercrombie's voucher, this narrative is perfectly

Here it may be alleged, that, as the aunt, in her waking state, experienced no apprehension for her nephew's safety, it is not at all likely that alarm on her part should have suggested the dream. I have shown, however, from my own experience, that dreams may be suggested by incidents that have made but trifling impression, and that had ceased to occupy the mind at the time of going to sleep. And, inasmuch as the risk attending sailing-parties on the Firth of Forth to young people, careless, probably, and thoughtless of danger, is considerable, the chances against a fatal result, in any particular case, cannot be regarded as so overwhelmingly great that we are precluded from adopting the hypothesis of an accidental coincidence. Cicero says, truly enough, "What person who aims at a mark all day will not sometimes hit it? We sleep every night, and there are few on which we do not dream: can we wonder, then, that what we dream sometimes comes to pass?"*

Yet, if such examples should be found greatly multiplied, and particularly if details, as well as the general result, correspond accurately with the warning, the probabilities against a chance coincidence increase.

But it is very certain that such instances are much

---

well authenticated. The late Mary Lady Clerk, of Pennicuik, well known in Edinburgh during a protracted widowhood, was a daughter of Mr. D'Acre; and she herself communicated the story to Blackwood's Magazine, (vol. xix. p. 73,) in a letter dated "Princes Street, May 1, 1826," and commencing thus:—"Being in company the other day when the conversation turned upon dreams, I related one, of which, as it happened to my own father, I can answer for the perfect truth." She concludes thus:—"I often heard the story from my father, who always added, 'It has not made me superstitious; but with awful gratitude I never can forget that my life, under Providence, was saved by a dream.'—M. C."

In the Magazine (of which I have followed, but somewhat abridged, the version) the names are initialized only. Through the kindness of an Edinburgh friend, I am enabled to fill them up from a copy of the anecdote in which they were given in full by Lady Clerk in her own handwriting.

* "De Divinatione," lib. ii. § 59.

more numerous throughout society than those who have given slight attention to the subject imagine. Men usually relate with reluctance that which exposes them to the imputation of credulity. It is to an intimate friend only, or to one known to be seriously examining the question, that such confidences are commonly made. In the three or four years last past, during which I have taken an interest in this and kindred subjects, there have been communicated to me so many examples of dreams containing true warnings, or otherwise strangely fulfilled, that I have become convinced there is a very considerable proportion of all the persons we meet in our intercourse with the world, who could relate to us, if they would, one or more such, as having occurred either in their own families or to some of their acquaintances. I feel assured that among those who may read this book there will be few who could not supply evidence in support of the opinion here expressed.

I proceed to furnish, from among the narratives of this character which have thus recently come to my knowledge, a few specimens, for the authenticity of which I can vouch.

In the year 1818, Signor Alessandro Romano, the head of an old and highly-respected Neapolitan family, was at Patu, in the province of Terra d'Otranto, in the kingdom of Naples. He dreamed one night that the wife of the Cavaliere Libetta, Counselor of the Supreme Court, and his friend and legal adviser, who was then in the city of Naples, was dead. Although Signor Romano had not heard of the Signora Libetta being ill, or even indisposed, yet the extreme vividness of the dream produced a great impression on his mind and spirits; and the next morning he repeated it to his family, adding that it had disturbed him greatly, not only on account of his friendship for the family, but also because the Cavaliere had then in charge for him a lawsuit of importance, which he feared this domestic affliction might cause him to neglect.

Patu is two hundred and eighty miles from Naples; and it was several days before any confirmation or refutation of Signor Romano's fears could be obtained. At last he received a letter from the Cavaliere Libetta, informing him that he had lost his wife by death; and, on comparing dates, it was found that she died on the very night of Signor Romano's dream.

This fact was communicated to me by my friend Don Giuseppe Romano,* son of the gentleman above referred to, who was living in his father's house when the incident took place, and heard him relate his dream the morning after it occurred.

Here is another, which was narrated to me, I remember, while walking, one beautiful day in June, in the Villa Reale, (the fashionable park of Naples, having a magnificent view over the bay,) by a member of the A—— legation, one of the most intelligent and agreeable acquaintances I made in that city.

On the 16th of October, 1850, being then in the city of Naples, this gentleman dreamed that he was by the bedside of his father, who appeared to be in the agonies of death, and that after a time he saw him expire. He awoke in a state of great excitement, bathed in cold perspiration; and the impression on his mind was so strong that he immediately rose, though it was still night, dressed himself, and wrote to his father, inquiring after his health. His father was then at Trieste, distant from Naples, by the nearest route, five days' journey; and the son had no cause whatever, except the above dream, to be uneasy about him, seeing that

---

* On the 25th of April, 1858, at his villa, near Naples. I took notes of the occurrence at the time, which were then and there examined and corrected by the narrator.

his age did not exceed fifty, and that no intelligence of his illness, or even indisposition, had been received. He waited for a reply with some anxiety for three weeks, at the end of which time came an official communication to the *chef* of the mission, requesting him to inform the son that it behooved him to take some legal measures in regard to the property of his father, who had died at Trieste, after a brief illness, *on the sixteenth of October.*

It will be observed that in this instance the agitation of mind in the dreamer was much greater than commonly occurs in the case of an ordinary dream. The gentleman rose, dressed himself in the middle of the night, and immediately wrote to his father, so great was his anxiety in regard to that parent's fate. The same may usually be noticed in the record of cases in which the dream is fulfilled, even if the person to whom it occurs is a skeptic in all such presentiments.

Such a skeptic is Macnish, author of the "Philosophy of Sleep;"* yet he admits the effect which such a dream, occurring to himself in the month of August, 1821, produced upon his spirits. I quote the narrative in his own words:—

"I was then in Caithness, when I dreamed that a near relation of my own, residing three hundred miles off, had suddenly died; and immediately thereafter awoke in a state of inconceivable terror, similar to that produced by a paroxysm of nightmare. The same day, happening to be writing home, I mentioned the circumstance in a half-jesting, half-earnest way. To tell the truth, I was afraid to be serious, lest I should be laughed

---

* Speaking of the hypothesis that dreams may at times give us an insight into futurity, Macnish says, "This opinion is so singularly unphilosophical that I would not have noticed it, were it not advocated by persons of good sense and education."—*Philosophy of Sleep*, p. 129.

But, after all, it avails nothing to allege that an opinion is unphilosophical if it should happen that facts attest its truth.

at for putting any faith in dreams. However, in the interval between writing and receiving an answer I remained in a state of most unpleasant suspense. I felt a presentiment that something dreadful had happened or would happen; and, though I could not help blaming myself for a childish weakness in so feeling, I was unable to get rid of the painful idea which had taken such rooted possession of my mind. Three days after sending away the letter, what was my astonishment when I received one written the day subsequent to mine, and stating that the relative of whom I had dreamed had been struck with a fatal shock of palsy the day before,— that is, the very day on the morning of which I had beheld the appearance in my dream! I may state that my relative was in perfect health before the fatal event took place. It came upon him like a thunderbolt, at a period when no one could have the slightest anticipation of danger."*

Here is a witness disinterested beyond all possible doubt; for he is supplying evidence against his own opinions. But are the effects he narrates such as are usually produced by a mere dream on the mind of a person not infected with superstition? Inconceivable terror, though there was no nightmare; a presentiment lasting for days, taking rooted possession of the feelings, and which he strove in vain to shake off, that something dreadful had happened or would happen! Yet, with all this alarm, unnatural under ordinary circumstances, how does the narrator regard the case? He sets down his terrors as a childish weakness, and declares, as to the coincidence which so excited his astonishment, that there is nothing in it to justify us in referring it to any other origin than chance. Taking the case as an isolated one, it would be illogical positively to deny this;

* *"Philosophy of Sleep,"* 6th ed., pp. 134–136.

yet may we not fairly include Dr. Macnish in the category of those to whom Dr. Johnson alludes when, speaking of the reality of ultramundane agency, he says that "some who deny it with their tongues confess it with their fears"?

The next example I shall cite came, in part, within my own personal knowledge. A colleague of the diplomatic corps, and intimate friend of mine, M. de S——, had engaged for himself and his lady passage for South America in a steamer, to sail on the 9th of May, 1856. A few days after their passage was taken, a friend of theirs and mine had a dream which caused her serious uneasiness. She saw, in her sleep, a ship in a violent storm founder at sea; and an internal intimation made her aware that it was the same on board which the S——s proposed to embark. So lively was the impression that, on awaking, she could scarcely persuade herself the vision was not reality. Dropping again to sleep, the same dream recurred a second time. This increased her anxiety; and the next day she asked my advice as to whether she ought not to state the circumstances to her friends. Having, at that time, no faith whatever in such intimations, I recommended her not to do so, since it would not probably cause them to change their plans, yet might make them uncomfortable to no purpose. So she suffered them to depart unadvised of the fact. It so happened, however, as I learned a few weeks later, that fortuitous circumstances induced my friends to alter their first intention, and, having given up their places, to take passage in another vessel.

These particulars had nearly passed from my memory, when, long afterward, being at the Russian Minister's, his lady said to me, "How fortunate that our friends the S——s did not go in the vessel they had first selected!" "Why so?" I asked. "Have you not heard," she replied, "that that vessel is lost? It must have perished at sea; for, though more than six months have elapsed since it left port, it has never been heard of."

In this case, it will be remarked, the dream was communicated to myself some weeks or months before its warning was fulfilled. It is to be conceded, however, that the chances against its fulfillment were not so great as in some of the preceding examples. The chances against a vessel about to cross the Atlantic being lost on that particular voyage, are much less than are the chances against a man, say of middle age and in good health, dying on any one particular day.

In the next example we shall find a new element introduced. Mrs. S—— related to me, that, residing in Rome in June, 1856, she dreamed, on the 30th of that month, that her mother, who had been several years dead, appeared to her, gave her a lock of hair, and said, " Be especially careful of this lock of hair, my child, for it is your father's; and the angels will call him away from you to-morrow." The effect of this dream on Mrs. S——'s spirits was such that, when she awoke, she experienced the greatest alarm, and caused a telegraphic notice to be instantly dispatched to England, where her father was, to inquire after his health. No immediate reply was received; but, when it did come, it was to the effect that her father had died that morning at nine o'clock. She afterward learned that, two days before his death, he had caused to be cut off a lock of his hair, and handed it to one of his daughters, who was attending on him, telling her it was for her sister in Rome. He had been ill of a chronic disease; but the last accounts she received of his health had been favorable, and had given reason to hope that he might yet survive for some years.*

---

* Read over to Mrs. S—— on the 25th of April, 1858, and its accuracy assented to by her.

The peculiarity in this example is, that there is a double coincidence: first, as to the exact day of death; and, secondly, as to the lock of hair. The chances against that double event are very much greater than against a single occurrence only.

Abercrombie relates and vouches for the following, in which, in a similar manner, a double event was truly foreshadowed.

A clergyman, who had come to Edinburgh from a short distance, being asleep at an inn, dreamed of seeing a fire, and one of his children in the midst of it. He awoke with the impression, and instantly started out on his journey home. Arrived within sight of his house, he found it in flames, and reached it just in time to rescue one of his children, who in the confusion had been left in a situation of great danger.*

On this Abercrombie remarks, that, "without calling in question the possibility of supernatural communication in such cases," he thinks the incident may be explained on natural principles; as originating, namely, in paternal anxiety, coupled, perhaps, with experience of carelessness in the servants left in charge. We may admit this; but it is evident that the fortuitous fulfillment of the two incidents witnessed in the dream (the fire itself, and the special danger therefrom to one of his children) is a contingency much more unlikely than would have been a single coincidence.

There may, on the other hand, be peculiar circumstances which increase, in particular instances, the chances in favor of fortuitous fulfillment. One such is given by Macnish, which, he says, may be confidently relied upon. It is the case of a young lady, a native of Ross-shire in Scotland, who was devotedly attached to an officer, then with Sir John Moore in the

---

* "Intellectual Powers," p. 213.

Spanish war. The constant danger to which he was exposed preyed on her spirits. She pined, and fell into ill health. Finally, one night, in a dream, she saw her lover, pale, bloody, and wounded in the breast, enter her apartment. He drew aside the curtains of the bed, and, with a mild look, told her he had been slain in battle, bidding her, at the same time, to be comforted, and not take his death to heart. The consequences of this dream were fatal to the poor girl, who died a few days afterward, desiring her parents to note down the date of her dream, which she was confident would be confirmed. It was so. The news shortly after reached England that the officer had fallen at the battle of Corunna, on the very day on the night of which his mistress had beheld the vision.*

Dr. Macnish considers this "one of the most striking examples of identity between the dream and the real circumstances with which he is acquainted." Such an opinion is a proof how little exact men sometimes are in testing the character of phenomena like this. In itself, and without reference to numerous other analogous cases in which the dead are said to have appeared to some dear friend soon after the moment of decease, this incident is far less striking than Dr. Macnish's own dream, given in a previous part of this chapter. Let us compare the cases. In the one, the young lady's constant thought was of her lover placed in continual daily peril. What so natural as that she should dream of him? The wonder would have been, if she had not. That he should appear to her pale and wounded, was but a reflection of the picture which in her sad daily reveries had doubtless a hundred times suggested itself. The coincidence as to the day remains. But it is to be remembered that the incident occurred during one of the most disastrous episodes of the

---

* "*Philosophy of Sleep*," pp. 132 to 134.

Peninsular War, when each hour was expected to bring news of a bloody battle. It was at a time when every officer and soldier under the gallant and unfortunate Moore's command might be said to go forth each morning with his life in his hand. The chances of death to any one of these officers on any one particular day were perhaps twenty, thirty, fifty fold greater than to an individual engaged in the ordinary pursuits of peaceful life. The chances against the fortuitous coincidence as to the day were diminished in a corresponding ratio.

How different the circumstances in Dr. Macnish's own case! His relative, as he informs us, was in perfect health and at three hundred miles' distance. There does not appear to have been any thing to direct the doctor's thoughts specially to him,—certainly nothing to make him anxious as to his fate; nothing, therefore, to induce a dream about him, still less to suggest a vision of his death. Yet, under all these improbabilities, Macnish dreams that his relative is dead. Nor is this all. Without apparent cause except what he regards as a feeling of childish superstition, there clings to him a panic terror, a presentiment of evil so deep-rooted that for days his reason is powerless to eradicate it. Then follows the coincidence of the day, also under circumstances in which, according to every human calculation, the improbability of the event was extreme; seeing that there were no grounds for the slightest anticipation of danger.

Yet, such is the power of romantic incident on the imagination, our author passes lightly over his own most remarkable case, and declares, as to that of the young lovers, that it is one of the most striking on record. The managers of any insurance-company would be found more clear-sighted. Suppose they had been asked to insure, for a month or two, the two lives; that of the officer daily exposed to shot or shell, and that of the country gentleman in a quiet home. The

vastly-increased premium which they would be certain
to demand in the former case as compared to the latter
would sufficiently mark their estimate of the comparative chances of death.

Such considerations should be borne in mind in judging
all cases of dreams fulfilled, when the fulfillment happens
to depend upon an event which, though usually unlikely, may, from peculiar circumstances of danger or
otherwise, have been brought within the range of probability. An instance is supplied by a curious custom
still prevalent at Newark-upon-Trent, in England, on
the 11th of March of every year. On that day penny
loaves are given away to any poor persons who apply
for them at the Town Hall. The origin of the custom
is this. During the bombardment of Newark by Oliver
Cromwell's forces, a certain Alderman Clay dreamed,
three nights successively, that his house had taken fire;
and so much was he impressed thereby that he removed
his family to another residence. A few days afterward,
on the 11th of March, his house was burned down by
the besiegers. In gratitude for what he regarded as a
miraculous deliverance, he left by his will, dated 11th December, 1694, to the Mayor and Aldermen, two hundred
pounds; the interest of half that sum to be paid to the
vicar annually, on condition of his preaching an appropriate sermon, and with the interest of the other half
bread to be yearly purchased for distribution to the
poor.

Here the coincidence was remarkable, but certainly
less so than if the alderman's house, through the casual-
ties incident to a siege, had not been placed under circumstances of extra risk.

Let us pass on to another class of dreams, usually regarded as depending on the revival of old associations
One of the most remarkable examples is given by Aber

crombie, who states that it occurred to a particular friend of his, and that it "may be relied upon in its most minute particulars." It is in these words:—

"The gentleman was at the time connected with one of the principal banks in Glasgow, and was at his place at the teller's table where money is paid, when a person entered, demanding payment of a sum of six pounds.

"There were several persons waiting, who were in turn entitled to be served before him; but he was extremely impatient and rather noisy, and, being besides a remarkable stammerer, he became so annoying that another gentleman requested my friend to pay him his money and get rid of him. He did so, accordingly, but with an expression of impatience at being obliged to attend to him before his turn; and he thought no more of the transaction. At the end of the year, which was eight or nine months after, the books of the bank could not be made to balance, the deficiency being exactly six pounds. Several days and nights had been spent in endeavoring to discover the error, but without success; when, at last, my friend returned home much fatigued, and went to bed. He dreamed of being at his place in the bank, and the whole transaction with the stammerer, as now detailed, passed before him, in all its particulars. He awoke under a full impression that the dream was to lead him to the discovery of what he was so anxiously in search of; and, on investigation, he soon discovered that the sum paid to this person, in the manner now mentioned, had been neglected to be inserted in the book of interests, and that it exactly accounted for the error in the balance."*

Commenting on this case, Abercrombie says, "The fact upon which the importance of the case rested was not his having paid the money, but having neglected to insert

* "Intellectual Powers," p. 205.

the payment. Now, of this there was no impression made upon his mind at the time, and we can scarcely conceive upon what principle it could be recalled. The deficiency being six pounds, we may indeed suppose the gentleman endeavoring to recollect whether there could have been a payment of this sum made in any irregular manner, that might have led to an omission or an error; but in the transactions of an extensive bank, in a great commercial city, a payment of six pounds, at a distance of eight or nine months, could have made but a very faint impression. And, upon the whole, the case presents, perhaps, one of the most remarkable mental phenomena connected with this curious subject."

The difficulty in the above case is, not that something was recalled which, in the waking state, had passed from the memory; for this, as in the example already cited from Brodie, is a phenomenon known to show itself, occasionally, in dreams': the true difficulty is that the fact of which the teller was in search, namely, the omission to enter a sum of six pounds, was *not* recalled by the dream at all. The dream, indeed, *did* recall and present again to his memory, in all its details, a certain forgotten circumstance, namely, that he had made a payment eight or nine months before, in a somewhat irregular manner, to a certain troublesome stammerer; and the impression was produced on his mind "that the dream was *to lead him to the discovery* of what he was so anxiously in search of;" nothing more. It was only a hint given; a mere suggestion, as if some one had said, "See if that affair of the stammerer be not in some way connected with the error that has so long escaped you." And we are expressly told that it was only *on investigation* the teller discovered that the payment to the annoying customer was the one actually omitted. If this be not an example of a suggestion made from some foreign source, instead of being a mere instance of old associations revived, it has, at least, very much the appearance of it.

Other examples, apparently more extraordinary and more closely trenching on what is usually deemed the supernatural, are more susceptible of natural explanation. For instance, a story related by Sir Walter Scott,* as follows:—

THE ARREARS OF TEIND.

"Mr. Rutherford of Bowland,† a gentleman of landed property in the Vale of Gala, was prosecuted for a very considerable sum, the accumulated arrears of teind, (or tithe,) for which he was said to be indebted to a noble family, the titulars (lay impropriators of the tithes). Mr. Rutherford was strongly impressed with the belief that his father had, by a form of process peculiar to the law of Scotland, purchased these teinds from the titular, and, therefore, that the present prosecution was groundless. But, after an industrious search among his father's papers, an investigation among the public records, and a careful inquiry among all persons who had transacted law business for his father, no evidence could be recovered to support his defense. The period was now near at hand when he conceived the loss of his lawsuit to be inevitable; and he had formed the determination to ride to Edinburgh next day and make the best bargain he could in the way of compromise. He went to bed with this resolution, and, with all the circumstances of the case floating upon his mind, had a dream to the following purpose. His father, who had been many years dead, appeared to him, he thought, and asked him

---

* In that edition of the Waverley Novels to which Sir Walter himself supplied notes. It is given in a note to the "Antiquary," in Volume V.

† Sir Walter gives the initial and final letters only of the name, (Mr. R——d.) I am indebted for the filling up, and for many other obligations, to an Edinburgh friend, whom I wish that I might here thank by name.

why he was disturbed in his mind. In dreams men are not surprised at such apparitions. Mr. Rutherford thought that he informed his father of the cause of his distress, adding that the payment of a considerable sum of money was the more unpleasant to him because he had a strong consciousness that it was not due, though he was unable to recover any evidence in support of his belief. 'You are right, my son,' replied the paternal shade: 'I did acquire right to these teinds, for payment of which you are now prosecuted. The papers relating to the transaction are in the hands of Mr. ——, a writer, (or attorney,) who is now retired from professional business and resides at Inveresk, near Edinburgh. He was a person whom I employed on that occasion for a particular reason, but who never, on any other occasion, transacted business on my account. It is very possible,' pursued the vision, 'that Mr. —— may have forgotten a matter which is now of a very old date; but you may call it to his recollection by this token, that, when I came to pay his account, there was difficulty in getting change for a Portugal piece of gold, and we were forced to drink out the balance at a tavern.'

"Mr. Rutherford awoke, in the morning, with all the words of the vision imprinted on his mind, and thought it worth while to walk across the country to Inveresk, instead of going straight to Edinburgh. When he came there, he waited on the gentleman mentioned in the dream,—a very old man. Without saying any thing of the vision, he inquired whether he ever remembered having conducted such a matter for his deceased father. The old gentleman could not, at first, bring the circumstance to his recollection; but, on mention of the Portugal piece of gold, the whole returned upon his memory. He made an immediate search for the papers, and recovered them; so that Mr. Rutherford carried to Edinburgh the documents necessary to gain the cause which he was on the verge of losing."

Sir Walter adds, as to the authenticity of the above narration, "The author has often heard this story told by persons who had the best access to know the facts, who were not likely themselves to be deceived, and who were certainly incapable of deception. He cannot, therefore, refuse to give it credit, however extraordinary the circumstances may appear."

The hypothetical explanation which Scott offers is, "that the dream was only the recapitulation of information which Mr. Rutherford had really received from his father while in life, but which, at first, he merely recalled as a general impression that the claim was settled."

The possibility that this may be the true theory cannot be denied; and it is easier to imagine it in this case than in that of the bank-teller. Yet serious difficulties present themselves in opposition. We cannot assign to these their exact weight, because, as unfortunately too often happens in such narrations, some of the essential particulars are omitted. We do not know how old Mr. Rutherford was at the time of the purchase of the teinds. We merely learn that it was a transaction "of a very old date." The chances are that he was a child. If so, it is very unlikely that his father would have related to him all the minute details connected with such a transaction, as the difficulty about getting change for a Portuguese coin, and the adjournment to a tavern. If, on the other hand, he was already of adult age, it is not probable that a matter of so much importance should have so completely faded from his memory that it could not be (as to the recollection of the aged attorney it was) consciously recalled. And it is evident that it was not so recalled. The son firmly believed that it was no revival of recollection, but that he had actually conversed with his parent's spirit; for, Scott tells us, "This remarkable circumstance was attended with bad consequences to Mr. Rutherford, whose health and spirits were afterward impaired by the attention which he thought himself obliged to pay to the visions of the night."

There is yet another difficulty; the coincidences, namely, between the suggestions of the (alleged) spirit and what actually happened during the visit to the attorney at Inveresk. He *had* forgotten the transaction. Was that circumstance anticipated by chance? His memory *was* refreshed by allusion to the incident of the Portugal piece of gold. Was that a purely fortuitous selection?

Unless we assume it as a point settled that there *is* no such thing as ultramundane communication, the simple and natural conclusion in such a case surely is, that the father really appeared, in dream, to the son. And an argument against this which Scott adduces in his comments on the story has little weight. He says, "Few will suppose that the laws of nature were suspended, and a special communication from the dead to the living permitted, for the purpose of saving Mr. Rutherford a certain number of hundred pounds." It is quite true that these would be unreasonable suppositions. Little as we can safely predicate in regard to the ways of God, we may still give weight to the ancient maxim, "Nec Deus intersit, nisi dignus vindice nodus." But, assuming for a moment that it was the paternal spirit who conveyed intelligence to the son, it does not by any means follow that there was a suspension of the laws of nature, or any special permission required, in the case. I have already* given my reasons for believing that if there be occasional communication between the dead and the living, it occurs under certain fixed conditions, perhaps

* Book I. chapter iii., on "The Miraculous."

physical, at all events governed by laws as constant and unchangeable as are those which hold the planets to their appointed course. And if, as Scripture intimates* and poets have sung,† the spirits of the departed still take an interest in the well-being of those friends they have left behind upon earth, and if they may sometimes, by virtue of these laws, evince that interest, why may we not imagine a father availing himself of such opportunity to avert an injustice about to overtake his son? And why should we admit and adopt extreme improbabilities in order, at all hazards, to escape from such a conclusion?

Mr. Rutherford seems to have fallen into the same error as Sir Walter; though in the case of the latter it resulted in skepticism, and of the former, in superstition. A more enlightened view of the case might have benefited both. It might have induced the author of Waverley to doubt the propriety of denying (if indeed he did in his heart deny) the occasional reality of ultra-mundane agency; and it might have spared Mr. Ruther-

---

* Luke xvi. 27.

"They that tell us that such as Dives retain no love to their brethren on earth, speak more than they can prove, and are not so credible as Christ, that seemeth to say the contrary."—BAXTER: *World of Spirits*, p. 222.

† "And is there care in Heaven? And is there love
    In heavenly spirits to these creatures base,
    That may compassion of their evils move?
    There is!"—SPENSER.

When a beloved child is taken from us, there is, perhaps, no idea to which the bereaved heart turns more eagerly and naturally than to this. In the Protestant cemetery at Naples lie the remains of a young girl, the beautiful and gifted daughter of an American clergyman; and upon her tombstone I had inscribed, by the father's instructions, the well-known stanza,—who has not admired it?—

"Fold her, O Father, in thine arms,
    And let her henceforth be
A messenger of love between
    Our human hearts and thee."

15

ford the delusion of imagining, as he seems to have done, that he was the favored subject of a special and miraculous intervention from God.

Let us proceed a step further. Supposing that we are willing to regard the two last-mentioned cases, beset with difficulties though they be, as mere examples of old associations recalled, let us inquire whether no cases are to be found in which there is presented to the mind of the sleeper a reality which could not have been drawn from the forgotten depths of the memory, because it never existed there. What shall we do, for example, with such a case as this, occurring to William Howitt, and recorded by that author himself? It occurred during his voyage to Australia, in 1852.

"Some weeks ago, while yet at sea, I had a dream of being at my brother's at Melbourne, and found his house on a hill at the farther end of the town, next to the open forest. His garden sloped a little way down the hill to some brick buildings below; and there were green-houses on the right hand by the wall, as you looked down the hill from the house. As I looked out from the windows in my dream, I saw a wood of dusky-foliaged trees, having a somewhat segregated appearance in their heads; that is, their heads did not make that dense mass like our woods. 'There,' I said, addressing some one in my dream, 'I see your native forest of Encalyptus!' This dream I told to my sons, and to two of my fellow-passengers, at the time; and, on landing, as we walked over the meadows, long before we reached the town, I saw this very wood. 'There,' I said, 'is the very wood of my dream. We shall see my brother's house there!' And so we did. It stands exactly as I saw it, only looking newer; but there, over the wall of the garden, is the wood, precisely as I saw it, and now see it as I sit at the dining-room window writing. When I look on this scene, I seem to look into my dream."*

Unless we imagine that Mr. Howitt is confounding ideas originally obtained from a minute description of the scene from his brother's windows with impressions here represented as first received by him in dream, (a supposition which in the case of so intelligent a writer is inadmissible,) how can we explain this dream by the theory of past memories revived? And here the hypothesis of mere accidental coincidence is clearly out of place. Indeed, the case is difficult of explanation according to any theory heretofore commonly received.

Equally so is the following, a personal experience, given by Mrs. Howitt in the Appendix to her husband's translation of Ennemoser just cited. "On the night of the 12th of March, 1853," she says, "I dreamed that I received a letter from my eldest son. In my dream I eagerly broke open the seal, and saw a closely-written sheet of paper; but my eye caught only these words, in the middle of the first page, written larger than the rest, and underdrawn:—*My father is very ill.* The utmost distress seized me, and I suddenly woke to find it only a dream; yet the painful impression of reality was so vivid that it was long before I could compose myself. The first thing I did, the next morning, was to commence a letter to my husband, relating this distressing dream. Six days afterward, on the 18th, an Australian mail came in and brought me a letter,—the only letter I received by that mail, and not from any of my family, but from a gentleman in Australia with whom we were acquainted. This letter was addressed on the outside *Immediate;* and, with a trembling hand,

---

* Given in Appendix to "*History of Magic*," by Ennemoser, translated by William Howitt, London, 1854, vol. ii. p. 416.

I opened it; and, true enough, the first words I saw and those written larger than the rest, in the middle of the paper, and underdrawn, were, '*Mr. Howitt is very ill.*' The context of these terrible words was, however, 'If you hear that *Mr. Howitt is very ill,* let this assure you that he is better;' but the only emphatic words were those which I saw in my dream, and these, nevertheless, slightly varying, as, from some cause or other, all such mental impressions, spirit-revelations, or occult dark sayings, generally do, from the truth or type which they seem to reflect."

What are we to make of such a case as this, directly testified to by a lady of the highest character and intelligence, and resting upon her own personal experience? In dream, opening a letter from her son, then in Australia, she sees, *written in the middle of the first page, in characters larger than the rest, and underlined,* the words, "My father is very ill." Six days afterward she actually receives a letter from Australia, not indeed from her son, but from a friend, and therein, *in the middle of the page, and in characters larger than the rest, and underlined,* the first words that meet her eye on opening it are, "Mr. Howitt is very ill." Is this chance? What! all of it? First, the words, almost literally corresponding, and in sense exactly so; next, the position in the center of the paper; then, the larger size of the characters; and, finally, the underlining? The mind instinctively, and most justly, rejects such a conclusion. Whatever else it is, it is *not* chance. Mesmerists would call it a case of clear-sight (clairvoyance) or far-sight (*vue à distance*) characterized by somewhat imperfect lucidity.

Lest the reader should imagine that in accounting on ordinary principles for the preceding examples he has reached the limit of the difficulties attending the present subject, I shall here cite, from a multitude of similar examples of what might not inaptly be termed natural clairvoyance, one or two additional cases, with which the reader may find it still more embarrassing to deal on the theory of fortuitous coincidence.

The truth of the first is vouched for by Dr. Carlyon, author of a work from which I extract it, who had it from the main witness, and who adduces, in attestation, every particular of name, place, and date.

THE MURDER NEAR WADEBRIDGE.

"On the evening of the 8th of February, 1840, Mr. Nevell Norway, a Cornish gentleman, was cruelly murdered by two brothers of the name of Lightfoot, on his way from Bodmin to Wadebridge, the place of his residence.

"At that time his brother, Mr. Edmund Norway, was in the command of a merchant-vessel, the 'Orient,' on her voyage from Manilla to Cadiz; and the following is his own account of a dream which he had on the night when his brother was murdered:—

"Ship 'Orient,' from Manilla to Cadiz,
"February 8, 1840.

"About 7.30 P.M. the island of St. Helena N.N.W., distant about seven miles; shortened sail and rounded to with the ship's head to the eastward; at eight, set the watch and went below; wrote a letter to my brother, Nevell Norway. About twenty minutes or a quarter before ten o'clock, went to bed; fell asleep, and dreamt I saw two men attack my brother and murder him. One caught the horse by the bridle, and snapped a pistol twice, but I heard no report; he then struck him a blow, and he fell off the horse. They struck him several blows, and dragged him by the shoulders across the road and left him. In my dream, there was a house on the left-hand side of the road. At four o'clock I was called, and went on deck to take charge of the ship. I
15*

told the second officer, Mr. Henry Wren, that I had had
a dreadful dream,—namely, that my brother Nevell
was murdered by two men on the road from St. Columb
to Wadebridge, but that I felt sure it could not be there,
as the house there would have been on the right-hand
side of the road; so that it must have been somewhere
else. He replied, 'Don't think any thing about it; you
west-country people are so superstitious! You will make
yourself miserable the remainder of the voyage.' He
then left the general orders and went below. It was
one continued dream from the time I fell asleep until I
was called, at four o'clock in the morning.

" EDMUND NORWAY,

"*Chief Officer Ship ' Orient.'*

"So much for the dream. Now for the confession of
William Lightfoot, one of the assassins, who was executed, together with his brother, at Bodmin, on Monday, April 13, 1840.

"'I went to Bodmin last Saturday week, the 8th inst.,
(February 8, 1840,) and in returning I met my brother
James at the head of Dummeer Hill. It was dim like.
We came on the turnpike-road all the way till we came
to the house near the spot where the murder was committed. We did not go into the house, but hid ourselves in a field. My brother knocked Mr. Norway
down; he snapped a pistol at him twice, and it did not
go off. He then knocked him down with the pistol. I
was there along with him. Mr. Norway was struck
while on horseback. It was on the turnpike-road, between Pencarrow Mill and the directing-post toward
Wadebridge. I cannot say at what time of the night it
was. We left the body in the water, on the left side of
the road coming to Wadebridge. We took some money
in a purse, but I did not know how much. My brother
drew the body across the road to the watering.'

"At the trial, Mr. Abraham Hambly deposed that he left Bodmin ten minutes before ten, and was overtaken by Mr. Norway about a quarter of a mile out of Bodmin. They rode together for about two miles from Bodmin, where their roads separated.

"Mr. John Hick, a farmer of St. Minver, left Bodmin at a quarter-past ten, on the Wadebridge road. When he got to within a mile of Wadebridge, he saw Mr. Norway's horse galloping on before him, without a rider. The clock struck eleven just before he entered Wadebridge.

"Thomas Gregory, Mr. Norway's wagoner, was called by Mr. Hick about eleven o'clock, and, going to the stable, found his master's horse standing at the gate. Two spots of fresh blood were on the saddle. He took the pony and rode out on the road. Edward Cavell went with him. They came to a place called North Hill. There is a lone cottage there, by the right-hand side of the road going to Bodmin, which is unoccupied. On the Wadebridge side of the cottage there is a small orchard belonging to it, and near the orchard a little stream of water coming down into the road. They found the body of Mr. Norway in the water.

"The evidence of the surgeon, Mr. Tickell, showed that the head was dreadfully beaten and fractured.

"It will be seen that Mr. Edmund Norway, in relating his dream the following morning to his shipmate, observed that the murder could not have been committed on the St. Columb road, because the house, in going from thence to Wadebridge, is on the right hand, whereas the house was in his dream (and in reality is) on the left. Now, this circumstance, however apparently trivial, tends somewhat to enhance the interest of the dream, without in the least impugning its fidelity; for such fissures are characteristic of these sensorial impressions, which are altogether involuntary, and bear a

much nearer relation to the productions of the daguer-
reotype than to those of the portrait-painter, whose
lines are at his command.

"I asked Mr. Edmund Norway whether, supposing
that he had not written a letter to his brother, Mr. N.
Norway, on the evening of the 8th February, and had
nevertheless dreamt the dream in question, the impression made by it would have been such as to have prevented his writing to him subsequently. To which he
replied, that it might not have had that effect; but he
could not say with any precision whether it would or
not.

"At all events, the dream must be considered remarkable, from its unquestionable authenticity, and its perfect
coincidence in time and circumstances with a most horrible murder."*

So far the statement of Dr. Carlyon. Let us briefly
review the case it presents.

The coincidence as to time is exact, the murder occurring on the same night as the dream. The incident is
not an ordinary accident, but a crime of rare occurrence.
The precise correspondence between the dream and the
actual occurrences is not left to be proved by recollections
called up weeks or months after the dream; for the evidence is an extract taken *verbatim* from the ship's log,
—the record of the moment, when every thing was fresh
on the memory.

It is very true that Mr. Norway had been writing
to his brother just before he retired to rest; and the
chances are that he fell asleep thinking of him. It is
possible that, but for this direction of his thoughts, he
might not have had the dream at all; for who shall de-

---

* "*Early Years and Late Reflections,*" by Clement Carlyon, M.D., Fel
low of Pembroke College, in 2 vols., vol. i, p. 219.

termine the power of sympathy, or assign to that power its limit?

It was natural, then, that he should dream of his brother. But was it (in the usual acceptation of the term) natural, also, that every minute particular of that night's misdeeds, perpetrated in England, should be seen at the time, in a vision of the night, by a seaman in a vessel off the island of St. Helena?

The minuteness of the correspondence can best be judged by placing the various incidents seen in the dream in juxtaposition with those which were proved, on the trial, to have happened.

Mr. Edmund Norway dreamed that his brother Nevell was attacked by two men, and murdered.	Mr. Nevell Norway *was* attacked, the same night, by William Lightfoot and his brother James, and was murdered by them.
Mr. Edmund Norway dreamed that "it was on the road from St. Columb to Wadebridge."	"It was on the turnpike-road between Pencarrow Mill and the directing-post toward Wadebridge."
Mr. Edmund Norway dreamed that "one of the men caught the horse by the bridle, and snapped a pistol twice, but he heard no report; he then struck him a blow, and he fell off his horse."	James Lightfoot "snapped a pistol at Mr. Norway twice, and it did not go off; he then knocked him down with the pistol." . . . "Mr. Norway was struck while on horseback."
Mr. Edmund Norway dreamed that the murderers "struck his brother several blows, and dragged him by the shoulders across the road, and left him."	James Lightfoot "drew the body across the road to the watering.". . . The murderers "left the body in the water, on the left side of the road coming to Wadebridge."

A more complete series of correspondences between dream and reality can hardly be imagined. The incident of the pistol twice missing fire is in itself conclusive. The various coincidences, taken together, as proof that chance is not the true explanation, have all the force of a demonstration in Euclid.

M

There *was* an inaccuracy, as to the house on the left of the road, while it really stands on the right; just as the words in Mrs. Howitt's letter slightly varied from those she had read in dream,—instructive inaccuracies these, not in the least invalidating the proofs which exist independent of them, but teaching us that, even through an agency such as we have been accustomed to call supernatural, truth may come to us, mingled with error, and that clairvoyance, even the most remarkable, is at best uncertain and fallible.

The next example—also of far-sight in dream—I obtained by personal interview with the gentleman who is the subject of it.

THE TWO FIELD-MICE.

In the winter of 1835–36, a schooner was frozen up in the upper part of the Bay of Fundy, close to Dorchester, which is nine miles from the river Pedeudiac. During the time of her detention she was intrusted to the care of a gentleman of the name of Clarke, who is at this time captain of the schooner Julia Hallock, trading between New York and St. Jago de Cuba.

Captain Clarke's paternal grandmother, Mrs. Ann Dawe Clarke, to whom he was much attached, was at that time living, and, so far as he knew, well. She was residing at Lyme-Regis, in the county of Dorset, England.

On the night of the 17th of February, 1836, Captain Clarke, then on board the schooner referred to, had a dream of so vivid a character that it produced a great impression upon him. He dreamed that, being at Lyme-Regis, he saw pass before him the funeral of his grandmother. He took note of the chief persons who composed the procession, observed who were the pall-bearers, who were the mourners, and in what order they walked, and distinguished who was the officiating pastor. He joined the procession as it approached the churchyard gate, and proceeded with it to the grave. He thought (in his dream) that the weather was stormy, and the ground wet, as after a heavy rain; and he noticed that the wind, being high, blew the pall partly off the coffin. The graveyard which they entered, the old Protestant one, in the center of the town, was the same in which, as Captain Clarke knew, their family burying-place was. He perfectly remembered its situation; but, to his surprise, the funeral procession did not proceed thither, but to another part of the churchyard, at some distance. There (still in his dream) he saw the open grave, partially filled with water, as from the rain; and, looking into it, he particularly noticed floating in the water two drowned field-mice. Afterward, as he thought, he conversed with his mother; and she told him that the morning had been so tempestuous that the funeral, originally appointed for ten o'clock, had been deferred till four. He remarked, in reply, that it was a fortunate circumstance; for, as he had just arrived in time to join the procession, had the funeral taken place in the forenoon he could not have attended it at all.

This dream made so deep an impression on Captain Clarke that in the morning he noted the date of it. Some time afterward there came the news of his grandmother's death, with the additional particular that she was buried on the same day on which he, being in North America, had dreamed of her funeral.

When, four years afterward, Captain Clarke visited Lyme-Regis, he found that every particular of his dream minutely corresponded with the reality. The pastor, the pall-bearers, the mourners, were the same persons he had seen. Yet this, we may suppose, he might naturally have anticipated. But the funeral *had* been appointed for ten o'clock in the morning, and, in consequence of the tempestuous weather and the heavy rain that was falling, it *had* been delayed until four in the afternoon. His mother, who attended the funeral, distinctly recollected that the high wind blew the pall partially off the coffin. In consequence of a wish expressed by the old lady shortly before her death, she was buried, not in the burying-place of the family, but at another spot, selected by herself; and to this spot Captain Clarke, without any indication from the family or otherwise, proceeded at once, as directly as if he had been present at the burial. Finally, on comparing notes with the old sexton, it appeared that the heavy rain of the morning had partially filled the grave, and that there were actually found in it two field-mice, drowned.

This last incident, even if there were no other, might suffice to preclude all idea of accidental coincidence.

The above was narrated to me by Captain Clarke himself,* with permission to use his name in attestation of its truth.†

---

* In New York, on July 28, 1859. The narrative is written out from notes taken on board his schooner.

† I originally intended to insert here a dream connected with a well-known incident in English history, and vouched for by Dr. Abercrombie in his "*Intellectual Powers,*" pp. 218, 219.

As there related, it is in substance to the effect that, eight days before the murder of Mr. Percival, Chancellor of the Exchequer, in the lobby of the English House of Commons, in 1812, a gentleman in Cornwall saw, in dream thrice repeated, every particular of the murder, even to the dress of the parties, and was told (still in dream) that it was the Chancellor who was shot; all which made so much impression on the dreamer that he was only deterred from giving notice to Mr. Percival by the assurances of his friends that, if he did so, he would be treated as a fanatic.

Dr. Carlyon, in his work already referred to, quotes and indorses the story, adding, "The dream in question occurred in Cornwall, to Mr. Williams, of Scorrier House, still alive, (February, 1836,) and now residing at Calstock, Devon, from whose lips I have more than once heard the relation."

There is, however, another and much more minute version of the story, given during Mr. Williams's life, in the (London) "Times" of August 16, 1828, and coming, as the editor states, from "a correspondent of un-

If, as to the faculty of farsight or natural clairvoyance in dream, evidently substantiated by the preceding examples, any should be tempted to regard it as a miraculous gift, they would do well to bear in mind the fact that, while in some of the examples of this faculty we find cases in which life and death are at stake, others, equally authentic, are to be found of the most trivial character.

Of the latter is the following example, for the accuracy of which Abercrombie vouches. "A lady in Edinburgh had sent her watch to be repaired. A long time elapsed without her being able to recover it; and, after many excuses, she began to suspect that something was wrong. She now dreamed that the watchmaker's boy, by whom the watch was sent, had dropped it in the street, and had injured it in such a manner that it could not be repaired. She went to the master, and, without any allusion to her dream, put the question to him directly, when he confessed that it was true."*

In this case, nothing can be more ridiculous than to imagine that there was miraculous intervention for the purpose of informing a lady why her watch was detained at the maker's; yet how extreme the improbability, also, that, among the ten thousand possible causes of that detention, chance should indicate to her, in dream, the very

---

questionable veracity," in which, while Mr. Scorrier's name and address are furnished, and all the particulars save one given by Dr. Abercrombie are strictly corroborated, that one fails. Dr. Abercrombie, who says he "derived the particulars from an eminent medical friend in England," mentions that the dream occurred *eight days before the murder;* while in the "Times" version it is expressly stated that it was "on the night of the 11th of May, 1812," *the same on which Mr. Percival was shot.*

Thus we are left in doubt whether this dream is of a prophetic or simply of a clairvoyant character. The one or the other it clearly is. But, in this uncertainty, after spending several days in collecting and collating the conflicting accounts, I omit all but this brief notice of the incident.

* Abercrombie's *"Intellectual Powers,"* p. 215.

one, though apparently among the most far-fetched and unlikely, that was found exactly to coincide with the fact as it occurred!

The attempt is futile to explain away even such a simple narrative as the foregoing, unless we impeach the good faith of the narrator; imagining, let us suppose, that he has willfully concealed some essential attendant circumstance, as, for instance, that the lady whose watch was injured had reason, from information obtained, to surmise that the boy might have dropped it. But, when Abercrombie vouches for the narrative as authentic, his voucher excludes, of course, suppositions which would deprive the anecdote of all value whatever, in the connection in which he publishes it.

In the three examples which follow, and which are of a different class from any of the preceding, we may go further yet, and assert that, unless the narrators directly lie, there are phenomena and laws connected with dreaming which have never yet been explained, and have scarcely been investigated.

The first was communicated to me in March, 1859, by Miss A. M. H——, the talented daughter of a gentleman well known in the literary circles of Great Britain. I give it in her words.

ONE DREAM THE COUNTERPART OF ANOTHER.

"We had a friend, S——, who some years ago was in a delicate state of health, believed to be consumptive. He lived several hundred miles from us, and, although our family were intimately acquainted with himself, we knew neither his home nor any of his family; our intercourse being chiefly by letters, received at intervals.

"One night, when there was no special cause for my mind reverting to our friend or to his state of health, I dreamed that I had to go to the town where he resided.

In my dream I seemed to arrive at a particular house, into which I entered, and went straight up-stairs into a darkened chamber. There, on his bed, I saw S—— lying as if about to die. I walked up to him; and, not mournfully, but as if filled with hopeful assurance, I took his hand and said, 'No, you are not going to die. Be comforted: you will live.' Even as I spoke I seemed to hear an exquisite strain of music sounding through the room.

"On awaking, so vivid were the impressions remaining that, unable to shake them off even the next day, I communicated them to my mother, and then wrote to S——, inquiring after his health, but giving him no clew to the cause of my anxiety.

"His reply informed us that he had been very ill,—indeed, supposed to be at the point of death,—and that my letter, which for several days he had been too ill to read, had been a great happiness to him.

"It was three years after this that my mother and I met S—— in London; and, the conversation turning on dreams, I said, 'By the way, I had a singular dream about you three years ago, when you were so ill:' and I related it. As I proceeded, I observed a remarkable expression spread over his face; and when I concluded he said, with much emotion, 'This is singular indeed; for I too had, a night or two before your letter arrived, a dream the very counterpart of yours. I seemed to myself on the point of death, and was taking final leave of my brother. "Is there any thing," he said, "I can do for you before you die?"—"Yes," I replied, in my dream; "two things. Send for my friend A. M. H——. I must see her before I depart."—"Impossible!" said my brother: "it would be an unheard-of thing: she would never come."—"She would," I insisted, in my dream, and added, "I would also hear my favorite sonata by Beethoven, ere I die."—"But these are trifles," exclaimed my brother, almost sternly. "Have you no desires more earnest at so solemn an hour?"—"No: to see my friend A. M. and to hear that sonata, that is all I wish." And, even as I spoke, in my dream I saw you enter. You walked up to the bed with a cheerful air; and, while the music I had longed for filled the room, you spoke to me encouragingly, saying I should not die.'"

Knowing the writer well, I can vouch for this narration; embodying, as it does, that rare and very remarkable phenomenon, two concurring and synchronous dreams.

The next example is adduced by Abercrombie[*] as having been mentioned by Mr. Joseph Taylor[†] for an undoubted fact. It occurred to the late Rev. Joseph Wilkins, afterward dissenting clergyman at Weymouth, in Dorsetshire, England, but then usher of a school in Devonshire, when he was twenty-three years of age; to wit, in the year 1754. Mr. Wilkins died November 22, 1800, in the seventieth year of his age. In the Obituary of the "Gentleman's Magazine" is a notice of his death, in which it is said of him, "For liberality of sentiment, generosity of disposition, and uniform integrity, he had few equals and hardly any superiors."[‡]

The original narrative was prepared and carefully preserved by himself in writing, and (the title only being added by me) is in these words:—

THE MOTHER AND SON.

" One night, soon after I was in bed, I fell asleep, and dreamed I was going to London. I thought it would not be much out of my way to go through Gloucestershire and call upon my friends there. Accord-

---

[*] " *Intellectual Powers,*" pp. 215, 216.
[†] He relates it in his work entitled " *Danger of Premature Interment.*"
[‡] " *Gentleman's Magazine*" for the year 1800, p. 1216.

ingly, I set out, but remembered nothing that happened by the way till I came to my father's house; when I went to the front door and tried to open it, but found it fast. Then I went to the back door, which I opened, and went in; but, finding all the family were in bed, I crossed the rooms only, went up-stairs, and entered the chamber where my father and mother were in bed. As I went by the side of the bed on which my father lay, I found him asleep, or thought he was so; then I went to the other side, and, having just turned the foot of the bed, I found my mother awake, to whom I said these words :—'Mother, I am going a long journey, and am come to bid you good-bye.' Upon which she answered, in a fright, 'Oh, dear son, thou art dead!' With this I awoke, and took no notice of it more than a common dream, except that it appeared to me very perfect. In a few days after, as soon as a letter could reach me, I received one by post from my father; upon the receipt of which I was a little surprised, and concluded something extraordinary must have happened, as it was but a short time before I had a letter from my friends, and all were well. Upon opening it I was more surprised still; for my father addressed me as though I was dead, desiring me, if alive, or whoever's hands the letter might fall into, to write immediately; but if the letter should find me living they concluded I should not live long, and gave this as the reason of their fears:—That on a certain night, naming it, after they were in bed, my father asleep and my mother awake, she heard somebody try to open the front door; but, finding it fast, he went to the back door, which he opened, came in, and came directly through the rooms up-stairs, and she perfectly knew it to be my step; but I came to her bedside, and spoke to her these words :—'Mother, I am going a long journey, and have come to bid you good-bye.' Upon which she answered me, in a fright, 'Oh, dear son, thou art dead!'—which were the circumstances and words of my dream. But she heard nothing more, and saw nothing more; neither did I in my dream. Upon this she awoke, and told my father what had passed; but he endeavored to appease her, persuading her it was only a dream. She insisted it was no dream, for that she was as perfectly awake as ever she was, and had not the least inclination to sleep since she was in bed. From these circumstances I am apt to think it was at the very same instant when my dream happened, though the distance between us was about one hundred miles; but of this I cannot speak positively. This occurred while I was at the academy at Ottery, Devon, in the year 1754; and at this moment every circumstance is fresh upon my mind. I have, since, had frequent opportunities of talking over the affair with my mother, and the whole was as fresh upon her mind as it was upon mine. I have often thought that her sensations, as to this matter, were stronger than mine. What may appear strange is, that I cannot remember any thing remarkable happening hereupon. This is only a plain, simple narrative of a matter of fact."

That nothing extraordinary occurred in the sequel—no sudden death, for example, of which the above might have been construed into a warning—is an instructive peculiarity in this case. Shall we say of it, as the superstitious usually say of such phenomena, that it was of a miraculous character? Then we have a miracle without a motive. This single incident, if we admit its authenticity, might alone suffice to disprove the common notions on this subject. And the total disconnection of the above facts from any alleged prediction or presentiment may stand as an additional voucher for their truth. There was nothing tending to mislead the imagination; no ground upon which any one would be tempted to erect a fanciful superstructure.

Nor does this narrative, inexplicable as the circumstances may appear, stand alone in its class. Another, remarkably well authenticated, is given, amid fifty other narratives of very apocryphal seeming, by Baxter, in his well-known "Certainty of the World of Spirits."* It is from a brother clergyman, residing in Kent. I transcribe it literally, adding the title only, as follows :—

THE MOTHER'S LONGING.

" REVEREND SIR :—

"Being informed that you are writing about witchcraft and apparitions, I take the liberty, though a stranger, to send you the following relation :—

"Mary, the wife of John Goffe, of Rochester, being afflicted with a long illness, removed to her father's house at West Malling, which is about nine miles distant from her own. There she died June the 4th, this present year, 1691.

"The day before her departure she grew very impatiently desirous to see her two children, whom she had left at home to the care of a nurse. She prayed her husband to hire a horse, for she must go home and die with the children. When they persuaded her to the contrary, telling her she was not fit to be taken out of her bed, nor able to sit on horseback, she intreated them, however, to try. 'If I cannot sit,' said she, 'I will lie all along upon the horse; for I must go to see my poor babes.' A minister who lives in the town was with her at ten o'clock that night, to whom she expressed good

---

* "*The Certainty of the World of Spirits,*" by Richard Baxter, London 1691, chap. vii. pp. 147 to 151.

hopes in the mercies of God, and a willingness to die: 'But,' said she, 'it is my misery that I cannot see my children.' Between one and two o'clock in the morning she fell into a trance. One widow Turner, who watched with her that night, says that her eyes were open and fixed and her jaw fallen. She put her hand upon her mouth and nostrils, but could perceive no breath. She thought her to be in a fit; and doubted whether she were dead or alive.

"The next morning this dying woman told her mother that she had been at home with her children. 'That is impossible,' said the mother; 'for you have been in bed all the while.' 'Yes,' replied the other, 'but I was with them last night when I was asleep.'

"The nurse at Rochester, widow Alexander by name, affirms, and says she will take her oath on't before a magistrate, and receive the sacrament upon it, that a little before two o'clock that morning she saw the likeness of the said Mary Goffe come out of the next chamber, (where the elder child lay in a bed by itself,) the door being left open, and stood by her bedside for about a quarter of an hour; the younger child was there lying by her. Her eyes moved and her mouth went; but she said nothing. The nurse, moreover, says that she was perfectly awake; it was then daylight, being one of the longest days in the year. She sate up in her bed and looked stedfastly upon the apparition. In that time she heard the bridge-clock strike two, and a while after said, 'In the name of the Father, Son, and Holy Ghost, what art thou?' Thereupon the appearance removed, and went away; she slipp'd on her cloaths and followed, but what became on't she cannot tell. Then, and not before, she began to be grievously affrighted, and went out of doors and walked upon the wharf (the house is just on the river-side) for some hours, only going in now and then to look to the children. At five-a-clock she went to a neighbor's house, and knocked at the door; but they would not rise. At six she went again; then they rose, and let her in. She related to them all that had pass'd: they would persuade her she was mistaken or dreamt. But she confidently affirmed, 'If ever I saw her in all my life, I saw her this night.'

"One of those to whom she made the relation (Mary, the wife of John Sweet) had a messenger came from Malling that forenoon, to let her know her neighbor Goffe was dying, and desired to speak with her. She went over, the same day, and found her just departing. The mother, among other discourse, related to her how much her daughter had long'd to see the children, and said she had seen them. This brought to Mrs. Sweet's mind what the nurse had told her that morning; for till then she had not thought to mention it, but disguised it, rather, as the woman's disturbed imagination.

"The substance of this I had related to me by John Carpenter, the father of the deceased, the next day after her burial. July the second, I fully discoursed the matter with the nurse and two neighbors to whose house she went that morning. Two days after, I had it from the mother, the minister that was with her in the evening, and the woman who sat up with her that last night. They all agree in the same story, and every one helps to strengthen the other's testimony. They appear to be sober, intelligent persons, far enough off from designing to impose a cheat upon the world, or to manage a lye; and what temptation they could lye under for so doing, I cannot conceive.

"Sir, that God would bless your pious endeavors for the conviction of Atheists and Sadduces, and the promoting of true religion and godliness, and that this narrative may conduce somewhat towards the further-

ing of that great work, is the hearty desire and prayer
of

"Your most faithful friend
"And humble servant,
"THO. TILSON, *Minister of Aylesford,*
nigh Maidstone, in Kent.
"AYLESFORD, July 6, 1691."

This story, simply and touchingly told, is a narrative of
events alleged to have occurred in the same year in which
Baxter's work was published,—to wit, in 1691; related
by a clergyman of the vicinity, writing of circumstances
all of which had transpired within five weeks of the
day on which he wrote, and most of which he had verified
within five days of the date of his letter,—namely, on
the 2d and 4th of July, 1691. The names and residences
of all the witnesses are given, and the exact time and
place of the occurrences to which they testify. It would
be difficult to find any narrative of that day better attested.

The exception which doubters will take to it is not,
probably, that the witnesses conspired to put forth a
falsehood, for that is incredible; but that the dying
mother, inspired with preternatural strength by the
earnest longing after her children, had actually arisen
during the night between the 3d and 4th of June, had
found her way from West Mulling to Rochester, entered
her dwelling and seen her children, and then returned,
before morning, to her father's house; that Mrs. Turner,
as sick-nurses will, had fallen asleep, and, even if she
did awake and miss her patient before her return, had
refrained from saying a word about it, lest she might
be taxed with neglect of duty. And, in support of such
a hypothesis, skepticism might quote this anecdote, related by Sir Walter Scott.*

---

* "*Letters on Demonology and Witchcraft,*" by Sir Walter Scott, Bart., 2d
ed., 1857, pp. 371 to 374.

A philosophical club at Plymouth were wont to hold their meetings, during the summer months, in a cave by the sea-shore, and at other times in a summer-house standing in the garden of a tavern, to the door of which garden some of the members, living adjacent, had private pass-keys. The members of the club presided alternately. On one occasion the president of the evening was ill,—reported to be on his death-bed; but, from respect, his usual chair was left vacant. Suddenly, while the members were conversing about him, the door opened, and the appearance of the president entered the room, wearing a white wrapper and night-cap, and presenting the aspect of death, took the vacant place, lifted an empty glass to his lips, bowed to the company, replaced his glass, and stalked out of the room. The appalled company, after talking over the matter, dispatched two of their number to ascertain the condition of their president. When they returned with the frightful intelligence that he had just expired, the members, fearing ridicule, agreed that they would remain silent on the subject.

Some years afterward, the old woman who had acted as sick-nurse to the deceased member, being on her death-bed, confessed to her physician, who happened to be one of the club, that, during her sleep, the patient, who had been delirious, awoke and left the apartment; that, on herself awaking, she hurried out of the house in search of him, met him returning, and replaced him in bed, where he immediately died. Fearing blame for her carelessness, she had refrained from saying any thing of the matter.

Scott, in quoting this and a few other simple explanations of what might seem extraordinary occurrences, remarks, that "to know what has been discovered in many cases, gives us the assurance of the ruling cause in all."* Nothing can be more illogical. It is a troublesome thing to get at the truth; but if we desire to get at it we must take the trouble. If it be a tedious process, it is the only safe one, to test each example by evidence sought and sifted (as the diplomatic phrase is) *ad hoc*. If, because we detect imposture in a single case, we slur over twenty others as equally unreliable, we are acting no whit more wisely than he who, having received in a certain town a bad dollar, presently concludes that none but counterfeits are to be met with there. It ought to make him more careful in examining the next coin he receives; nothing more. And so we, knowing that in some cases, as in this of the Plymouth club, appearances may deceive, should be upon our guard against such deceit,—not conclude that in every analogous example the same or similar explanation will serve.

Will it serve in the Mary Goffe case? The distance between her father's house and her own was nine miles. Three hours to go and three to return, six hours in all, —say from eleven till five o'clock,—would have been required to travel it by a person in good health, walking, without stopping, at an ordinary pace. One can believe, as in the Plymouth example, that a patient, in delirium, may, very shortly before his death, walk a few hundred yards. But is it credible that a dying woman, so weak that her friends considered her unfit to be taken out of her bed, should walk eighteen miles unaided and alone? The nurse declares that her patient fell into a trance between one and two o'clock, and that she put her hand upon her mouth and nostrils, but could perceive no breath. Suppose this a falsehood, invented to shelter negligence: can we imagine that, after a visit from a clergyman at ten, the nurse, attending a person

---

* *"Demonology and Witchcraft,"* p. 367.

hourly expected to die, should fall asleep before eleven o'clock, and not wake till after five, or that, if she did wake and find her patient gone, she would not alarm the house? But grant all these extreme improbabilities. Can we believe that the father and mother of a dying woman would both abandon her on the last night of her life for more than six hours? Or can we suppose, under such circumstances, that the patient could issue from her chamber and the house before eleven o'clock, and return to it after five, unseen by any one, either in going or returning?

Nor are these the only difficulties. Mrs. Goffe herself declared, next morning, that it was in dream only she had seen her children. And if this was not true, and if she actually walked to Rochester, is it credible that she would but look, in silence, for a few minutes, on her sleeping babes, and then, quitting them without even a word of farewell, recommence the weary way to her father's house? When she so earnestly begged her husband to hire a horse, what was the argument with which she urged her request? "She must go home, and die with the children."

I submit to the judgment of the reader these considerations. Let him give to them the weight to which he may deem them entitled. But if, finally, he incline to the theory of a nocturnal journey by the patient, then I beg of him to consider in what manner he will dispose of the parallel case,—that of the Rev. Mr. Wilkins, where the distance between mother and son was a hundred miles?

Abercrombie, admitting the facts of this latter case as Wilkins states them, merely says, "This singular dream must have originated in some strong mental impression which had been made on both individuals about the same time; and to have traced the source of it would have been a subject of great interest."

I cannot suppose that Abercrombie here means a mental impression *accidentally* made on mother and son at the same time. He was too good a logician not to know whither such a doctrine as that would lead. If we are to imagine all the details adduced, as the fruitless attempt to enter the front door, the entering by the back door, the going up-stairs and passing on to the paternal bedchamber, the exact terms of the question, the precise words of the reply, finally, the cessation of the dream or vision by mother and son at the very same point,—if, I say, we are to permit ourselves to interpret coincidences so numerous and minutely particular as these to be the mere effect of chance, where will our skepticism stop? Perhaps not until we shall have persuaded ourselves, also, that this world, with all it contains, is but the result of a fortuitous combination.

But if, as is doubtless the case, Dr. Abercrombie meant to intimate that this simultaneous impression on two distant minds must have occurred in accordance with some yet undiscovered psychological law, which it would be interesting to trace out, we may well agree with him in opinion.

It does not appear, however, that he regarded the incident in any other light than as an example of coinciding and synchronous dreams. Whether that be the true hypothesis may be questioned. In another chapter* will be adduced such evidence as I have obtained that the appearance of a living person at a greater or less distance from where that person actually is, and perhaps usually where the thoughts or affections of that person may be supposed, at the moment, to be concentrated, is a phenomenon of not infrequent occurrence. If it be admitted, it may furnish the true explanation

---

* See Book IV. chap. ii., on "*Apparitions of the Living.*"

of the Wilkins dream, the Goffe dream, and others similar in character.

The ingenious author of the "Philosophy of Mysterious Agents," who eschews every thing like Spiritualism, in dealing with the Wilkins narrative, of which he admits the authenticity, says, " It certainly shows a strange and hitherto unknown physical agent in or by which the brain may act even at a great distance, and produce physical results perfectly representing the cerebral action when the mind's controlling power is suspended."*

If this, as may happen, should seem to the reader somewhat obscure, let him, to aid his conceptions, take another paragraph. After copying the story itself, Mr. Rogers subjoins, " This is easily accounted for by the method we are considering this class of phenomena; and we can see no other in which there are not insuperable difficulties. In this case we have again the condition required for the play of mundane powers in reference to the brain; and that in which the brain, as a point, being irritated, may act, and by the mundane agency represent its action (as in this case) fifty miles or more distant."†

It does not strike me that by this method of Mr. Rogers the strange phenomenon we have been considering is, as he thinks, easily accounted for. How does he account for it? The doctrine of chance, he sees, is quite untenable. The doctrine of Spiritualism he repudiates. To avoid both, he suggests that the brain of the son, in Devonshire, being in activity during the suspended volition incident to sleep, represented its action on the brain of the mother, a hundred miles off, in

* *"Philosophy of Mysterious Agents, Human and Mundane,"* by E. C. Rogers, Boston, 1853, p. 283.
† *Work cited,* pp. 284, 285.

Gloucestershire; and that this represented action was due to a mundane agency strange and unknown.

To say that the two minds were, in some mode or other, placed in relation, is only an admission that the coincidence of sensations and ideas in both was not fortuitous. If, as we may freely further admit, the agency be, as Mr. Rogers alleges, strange and unknown, why assume it to be physical? And by such assumption do we account for the phenomenon,—not to say easily, but at all? Have we done more than employ vague words?—and words, vague as they are, which we do not seem justified in employing? What do we know about a brain, irritated, acting physically at a hundred miles' distance? What do we mean by such a brain *representing its action*, at that distance, on another? What sort of mundane agency can we imagine as the instrument of such action? And if we are to esteem a mere physical agent capable of thus connecting, without regard to distance, mind with mind, what need of any hypothetical soul or spirit to account for the entire wondrous range of mental phenomena?

Here again it behooves us to ask whither, in an attempt to escape the hypothesis of spiritual agency, our steps are invited? To the confines, it would seem, of materialism.

As the class of phenomena we have been here examining will usually be regarded as among the least credible of those connected with the subject of dreaming, I may state that the above are not the only examples on record. Kerner, in his "Seeress of Prevorst," furnishes one, attested by himself and by a physician attending the seeress's father.* Sinclair records another;† but

---

* *"Die Seherin von Prevorst,"* by Justinus Kerner, 4th edition, Stuttgart, 1846, pp. 132 to 134.

† In his *"Satan's Invisible World Discovered,"* Edinburgh, 1789. It is

how good the authority is in this last case I am not able to say.

An important inquiry remains unbroached. Are there any reliable cases presenting, or seeming to present, evidence that the faculty of prescience in dreams is an actual phenomenon, and that this faculty is sometimes enjoyed, as clairvoyance is said to be, specially by certain persons? Are there—as the phrase has been used in regard to the alleged second-sight of the Scottish Highlands—*seers*, thus habitually gifted?

Distinguished men have asserted that there are; Goethe, for example, in regard to his maternal grandfather. I translate from his Autobiography.

THE GRANDFATHER OF GOETHE.

"But what still increased the veneration with which we regarded this excellent old man was the conviction that he possessed the gift of prophecy, especially in regard to matters that concerned him and his. It is true that he confided the full knowledge and particulars of this faculty to no one except our grandmother; yet we children knew well enough that he was often informed, in remarkable dreams, of things that were to happen. For example, he assured his wife, at a time when he was still one of the youngest magistrates, that at the very next vacancy he would be appointed to a seat on the board of aldermen. And when, very soon after, one of the aldermen was struck with a fatal stroke of apoplexy, he ordered that, on the day when the choice was to be made by lot, the house should be arranged and every thing prepared to receive the guests coming to congratulate him on his elevation. And, sure enough, it was for him that was drawn the golden ball which decides the

---

the story of Sir George Horton, who is stated to have dreamed that he interfered to prevent his two sons fighting a duel, and actually to have appeared to them, and prevented it, sixty miles off, at the same time.

choice of aldermen in Frankfort. The dream which
foreshadowed to him this event he confided to his wife,
as follows. He found himself in session with his col-
leagues, and every thing was going on as usual, when
an alderman (the same who afterward died) descended
from his seat, came to my grandfather, politely begged
him to take his place, and then left the chamber. Something similar happened on occasion of the provost's
death. It was usual in such case to make great haste
to fill the vacancy, seeing that there was always ground
to fear that the emperor, who used to nominate the
provost, would some day or other re-assert his ancient
privilege. On this particular occasion the sheriff received orders at midnight to call an extra session for
next morning. When, in his rounds, this officer reached
my grandfather's house, he begged for another bit of
candle, to replace that which had just burned down in
his lantern. 'Give him a whole candle,' said my grandfather to the women: 'it is for me he is taking all this
trouble.' The event justified his words. He was actually chosen provost. And it is worthy of notice that,
the person who drew in his stead having the third and
last chance, the two silver balls were drawn first, and
thus the golden one remained for him at the bottom of
the bag.

"His dreams were matter-of-fact, simple, and without
a trace of the fantastic or the superstitious, so far, at
least, as they ever became known to us. I recollect,
too, that when, as a boy, I used to look over his books and
papers, I often found, mixed up with memoranda about
gardening, such sentences as these:—'Last night * * *
came to me and told me * * *,'—the name and the circumstance being written in cipher. Or, again, it ran
thus:—'Last night I saw * * *,'—the rest in characters
unintelligible to me. It is further remarkable, in this
connection, that certain persons who had never pos-

sessed any extraordinary power sometimes acquired it, for the time-being, when they remained near him; for example, the faculty of presentiment, by visible signs, in cases of sickness or death occurring at the time, but at a distance. Yet none either of his children or of his grandchildren inherited this peculiarity."*

The particular examples here cited may be explained away; but it is evident that Goethe, who had the best means of knowing, regarded the proofs that his grandfather really was endowed with this prophetic instinct to be conclusive.

Macario mentions a similar case, the evidence for which seems unquestionable. I translate from his work on Sleep.

THE VISIT FORETOLD.

"Here is a fact which occurred in my own family, and for the authenticity of which I vouch. Madame Macario set out, on the 6th of July, 1854, for Bourbon l'Archambault, for the benefit of the waters there, in a rheumatic affection. One of her cousins, Monsieur O——, who inhabits Moulins, and who habitually dreams of any thing extraordinary that is to happen to him, had, the night before my wife set out, the following dream. He thought he saw Madame Macario, accompanied by her little daughter, take the railroad-cars, to commence her journey to the Bourbon baths. When he awoke, he bade his wife prepare to receive two cousins with whom she was yet unacquainted. They would arrive, he told her, that day at Moulins, and would set out in the evening for Bourbon. 'They will surely not fail,' he added, 'to pay us a visit.' In effect, my wife and daughter did arrive at Moulins; but, as the

---

* "*Aus meinem Leben,*" by J. W. von Goethe, Stuttgart, 1853, vol. i. pp. 41 to 43.

weather was very bad, the rain falling in torrents, they stopped at the house of a friend near the railroad-station, and, their time being short, did not visit their cousin, who lived in a distant quarter of the town. He, however, was not discouraged. 'Perhaps it may be to-morrow,' he said. But the next day came, and no one appeared. Being thoroughly persuaded, nevertheless, on account of his experience in finding such dreams come true, that his cousins had arrived, he went to the office of the diligence that runs from Moulins to Bourbon, to inquire if a lady, accompanied by her daughter, (describing them,) had not set out the evening before for Bourbon. They replied in the affirmative. He then asked where that lady had put up at Moulins, went to the house, and there ascertained that all the particulars of his dream were exactly true. In conclusion, I may be allowed to remark that Monsieur O—— had no knowledge whatever of the illness nor of the projected journey of Madame Macario, whom he had not seen for several years."*

The remarkable feature in the above is the confidence of Monsieur O—— in the presage of his dream, indicating that he had good reason to trust in similar intima-

---

* *"Du Sommeil, des Rêves, et du Somnambulisme,"* par M. Macario, p. 82.

The incident reminds one of Scott's lines, in which, in the "Lady of the Lake," Ellen addresses Fitz-James:—

> ——As far as yesternight
> Old Allan-Bane foretold your plight;
> A gray-haired sire, whose look intent
> Was on the visioned future bent.
> He saw your steed, a dappled gray,
> Lie dead beneath the birchen way;
> Painted exact your form and mien,
> Your hunting-suit of Lincoln green
>   *   *   *   *   *
> And bade that all should ready be
> To grace a guest of fair degree.

tions. For the rest, it is difficult to call in question the truth or the accuracy of an observation as to which the evidence is so direct and the authority so respectable.

Considering the extraordinary character of this alleged faculty of foresight, or prophetic instinct, in dreams, I esteem myself fortunate in being able to adduce several other well-authenticated narratives directly bearing upon it. It does not appear, however, that in these cases, as in the preceding, the dreamers were habitual seers.

In the first, a highly improbable event was fore-shadowed, with distinctness, a year before it occurred. I had the narrative in writing from a lady, whose name, if it were proper for me to give it, would be to the public an all-sufficient voucher for the truth of the story.

THE INDIAN MUTINY.

"Mrs. Torrens, the widow of General Torrens, now residing at Southsea, near Portsmouth, about a year previous to the Indian mutiny dreamed that she saw her daughter, Mrs. Hayes, and that daughter's husband, Captain Hayes, attacked by sepoys; and a frightful murderous struggle ensued, in which Captain Hayes was killed.

"She wrote instantly to entreat that her daughter and the children would presently come home; and, in consequence of her extreme importunity, her grand-children arrived by the following ship. This was before an idea was entertained of the mutiny. I have seen these children often, in safety, at Southsea. Mrs. Hayes remained with her husband, and suffered the whole horrors of the siege at Lucknow, where Captain Hayes fell by the hands of sepoys,—who first put out his eyes, and then killed him."

I shall now present an anecdote, as directly authenti-cated as either of the foregoing, which I find in the Appendex to Dr. Binns' "Anatomy of Sleep."* It was communicated to the author by the Hon. Mr. Talbot, father of the present Countess of Shrewsbury, and is given in his own words, and under his own signature, (the title only added by me,) as follows:—

BELL AND STEPHENSON.

"In the year 1768, my father, Matthew Talbot, of Castle Talbot, county Wexford, was much surprised at the recurrence of a dream three several times during the same night, which caused him to repeat the whole circumstance to his lady the next morning. He dreamed that he had arisen as usual, and descended to his library, the morning being hazy. He then seated himself at his secretoire to write; when, happening to look up a long avenue of trees opposite the window, he perceived a man in a blue jacket, mounted on a white horse, coming toward the house. My father arose, and opened the window: the man, advancing, presented him with a roll of papers, and told him they were invoices of a vessel that had been wrecked and had drifted in during the night on his son-in-law's (Lord Mount Morris's) estate, hard by, and signed '*Bell and Stephenson.*'

"My father's attention was called to the dream only from its frequent recurrence; but when he found himself seated at his desk on the misty morning, and beheld the identical person whom he had seen in his dream, in the blue coat, riding on a gray horse, he felt surprised, and, opening the window, waited the man's approach He immediately rode up, and, drawing from his pocket a packet of papers, gave them to my father, stating that they were invoices belonging to an American vessel which had been wrecked and drifted upon his lordship's estate; that there was no person on board to lay claim

* "*The Anatomy of Sleep*," by Edward Binns, M.D., 2d ed. London, 1845, pp. 459, 460.

to the wreck; but that the invoices were signed '*Stephenson and Bell.*'

"I assure you, my dear sir, that the above actually occurred, and is most faithfully given; but it is not more extraordinary than other examples of the prophetic powers of the mind or soul during sleep, which I have frequently heard related.

"Yours, most faithfully,

"WILLIAM TALBOT.

"ALTON TOWERS, October 23, 1842."

In the above we find the same strange element of slight inaccuracy mixed with marvelous coincidence of detail already several times noticed. The man with his blue coat; the white or gray horse; the vessel wrecked on Lord Mount Morris's estate; the roll of invoices presented,—all exhibit complete correspondence between the foreshadowing dream and the actual occurrences. The names on the invoices, too, correspond; but the order in which they stand is reversed: in the dream, "Bell and Stephenson;" on the invoices themselves, "Stephenson and Bell."

Lest I should weary the reader by too much extending this chapter, and by too great an accumulation of examples, which might (as to many of the points noticed) be multiplied without limit, while perhaps those cited may suffice as a fair specimen of the whole, I shall adduce but one more,—an example quite as remarkable as any of the preceding, of prevision in dream; a narrative which was verified by one of the most accredited writers on intellectual philosophy, (for such Dr. Abercrombie must be admitted to be,) and for which, in addition, I have obtained an important voucher. Dr. Abercrombie, after declaring that he is "enabled to give it as perfectly authentic," relates it (without the title here given) in these words:—

THE NEGRO SERVANT.

"A lady dreamed that an aged female relative had been murdered by a black servant; and the dream occurred more than once.* She was then so much impressed by it that she went to the house of the lady to whom it related, and prevailed upon a gentleman to watch in an adjoining room during the following night. About three o'clock in the morning, the gentleman, hearing footsteps on the stairs, left his place of concealment, and met the servant carrying up a quantity of coals. Being questioned as to where he was going, he replied, in a confused and hurried manner, that he was going to mend his mistress's fire; which, at three o'clock in the morning, in the middle of summer, was evidently impossible; and, on further investigation, a strong knife was found concealed beneath the coals."†

This narrative, remarkable as it is, is not given in sufficient detail. It does not intimate whether the lady who dreamed knew or not, at the time, that her aged relative had a negro servant. Nor does it say any thing of the subsequent conduct and fate of that servant. Nor does it furnish the names of the parties. I am, fortunately, enabled to supply these deficiencies.

While in Edinburgh, in October, 1858, I had occasion to submit this chapter to a lady,—the daughter of a distinguished statesman, and herself well known by

---

* It is worthy of attention that many of these remarkable dreams occur more than once, as if (one might suppose) to produce on the dreamer the deeper impression. In the preceding dream by Mr. Talbot, in that which disclosed the death of Percival, in Mrs. Griffith's warning dream, in Alderman Clay's dream, and others, the vision was thrice repeated.

† "Intellectual Powers," p. 214.

numerous and successful works,—who, in returning it to me, kindly appended to the above narrative the following note :—

"This lady was Mrs. Rutherford, of Egerton, grand-aunt of Sir Walter Scott; and I have myself heard the story from the family. The lady who dreamed was the daughter of Mr. Rutherford, then absent from home. On her return, she was astonished, on entering her mother's house, to meet the very black servant whom she had seen in her dream, as he had been engaged during her absence. This man was, long afterward, hung for murder; and, before his execution, he confessed that he had intended to assassinate Mrs. Rutherford."

The story, with this attesting voucher,—giving the names of the persons referred to, and supplying particulars which greatly add to the value of the illustration,—is, I think, the very strongest example of prevision in dream I ever met with. Let us briefly scrutinize it.

In the first place, the dream indicated two particulars: the one, that the dreamer's mother would be murdered; the other, that the murder would be committed by a negro. Had the daughter known that her mother had a black servant, it would not be proper to regard these as separate contingencies: indeed, something in the man's manner might be imagined to have created suspicion, and so given shape to the dream. But the daughter *did not know*, when she dreamed, *that her mother had a negro servant*. She was astonished to meet him, on her return home. This is one of the strongest points in the case; for it precludes all argument that the negro's concern in the matter was naturally suggested to the dreamer.

Here, then, is the indication in dream of two independent specifications, correctly to have determined either of which would have been, if an accident, one of which the mathematical expectation is exceedingly small. In the quiet of domestic life, in a civilized country and a respectable rank, a deliberate murder does not occur to one out of millions of persons. There were millions to one, then, against the fortuitous predicting, in the case of a particular individual, of that single event. So, again, in regard to the other specification. Negroes are rare in Scotland. Had the dream merely been that a negro would commit a murder in Edinburgh, without designating the murdered person, how difficult to imagine, in case the event, occurring within a few days, had justified the prediction, that such fulfillment was purely accidental! But when there is question of the double event, the mathematical expectation diminishes till, in practice, it may be regarded as inappreciable. The chances against that double event, as a purely fortuitous occurrence, are such as we constantly act upon in daily life with the same assurance as upon certainty itself.

It is true that, with that inexplicable dimness of vision which seems so often to characterize similar phenomena, the coming event is indicated only, not distinctly foretold. The daughter's dream was that her mother *had been* murdered; and this had not taken place. The effect upon her mind, however, aided by the repetition of her dream, was such as to cause her to take precautions against such a contingency in the future; and it so happened that on the very night the precaution was taken the attempt was made. Here is a third coincidence.

Was this all accident? Was there no warning given? Was there no intention, by acting in dream on the daughter's mind, to save the mother's life? If we answer these questions in the negative, are we not discarding the clearest rules of evidence which, at the bidding of reason, we have adopted for the government of daily life?

But if, on the other hand, we admit that there *was* a warning,—that there *was* an intention,—then, who gave that warning? And what intelligence was it that intended?

It may be regarded as a mere cutting of the Gordian knot to assume the theory of spiritual guardianship.* Yet, if that theory be rejected, have we any other with which to supply its place?

But, without touching further for the present on this latter hypothesis, let us here pause for a moment to reflect whither the actual evidence at which we have arrived—culled, surely, from no suspicious source—is leading us on? If we assent to it,—if, with Abercrombie and the indorser of his narrative touching Mrs. Rutherford's negro servant, we feel compelled to admit that narrative as a fact,—shall we ignore the legitimate, the unavoidable, consequences? Shall we continue, with Macnish, to declare that the belief in the occasional power of dreams to give us an insight into futurity is "an opinion so singularly unphilosophical" as to be unworthy of notice? Shall we put aside, unexamined, with contempt or derision, instead of scrutinizing with patient care, the pretensions of certain observers as to the higher phenomena said to characterize some states of somnambulism,—as clearsight, farsight, and this very faculty of prevision? If we are to speak of the singularly unphilosophical, such a proceeding as this would surely supply a remarkable example of it.

And is there not abundant justification for the remark heretofore made, that it behooves us, if we would obtain a comprehensive view of this subject, to

---

* See, in this connection, the narratives entitled "*The Rejected Suitor*" and "*How Senator Linn's Life was Saved:*" both in Book V.

study all the various hypnotic states in their connection with each other? Before we undertake the wonders of mesmerism, let us dispose of the greater wonders of sleep.

Finally, that such inquiry should be slighted is the less defensible, seeing that it occurs in Christian countries, where the Bible is read and its teachings venerated. But if there be one doctrine there taught plainly, unequivocally, by direct allegation and by numerous examples, in the Old Testament as in the New, it is the same which has prevailed, as Cicero reminds us,* in every nation, whether polished and learned, or barbarous and unlettered; the doctrine, namely, that in the visions of the night men occasionally receive more than is taught them throughout all the waking vigilance of the day.

The illustrations of such a doctrine are scattered all over the Bible. The Old Testament especially is full of them: witness the dreams of Abimelech, of Pharaoh, of Saul, of Solomon, of Nebuchadnezzar; and, again, of Jacob, of Laban, of Daniel. But, passing by the Old to the dreams of the New Testament, we find that upon certain of these repose, in a measure, some of the very articles of faith cardinal to the creed of the orthodox church, whether Protestant or Catholic. Such are the dreams of the Wise Men of the East, of Joseph, of the wife of Pilate.

It is very true, and should be here taken into account, that most writers who deny to dreams any extraordinary or prophetic character make exception, directly or by implication, of those recorded in Scripture. But Scripture itself nowhere authorizes any such distinction. Elihu announces a general truth in general terms:—"In slumberings upon the bed, God

* *"De Divinatione,"* lib. i. §§ 1, 2, and 3.

openeth the ears of men and sealeth their instruction."
Shall we limit this to the men of any particular age?
By what warrant? By a similar license, can we not
explain away any text whatever? that, for instance,
with which Elihu closes his eloquent remonstrance:—
"God respecteth not any that are wise of heart."
Many will be found disregarding, in practice, the im-
plied warning against presumptuous self-sufficiency, but
few bold enough to allege that, though the observation
applied to the self-wise in the times of Job, it is antiquated and inapplicable, in these latter days, to ourselves.

If we would not be found thus bold in casuistry,—if,
in connection with the phenomena here briefly and imperfectly examined, we accept and take home in our
own case the lesson embodied in Elihu's words,—we may
be induced to conclude that it behooves us to devote more
time and attention to an important and neglected subject* than men have hitherto bestowed upon it, before
authoritatively pronouncing, as to all modern dreams
whatever, that they are the mere purposeless wanderings
of a vagrant imagination; that they never exhibit an
intelligence which exceeds that of the waking sense;
that never, under any circumstances, do they disclose
the distant or foreshadow the future; that never, in
any case, do they warn or avert: in a word, that all
visions of the night, without exception, are utterly
inconsequent, fantastic, and unreliable.

---

* Abercrombie concludes his chapter on Dreaming as follows:—"The
slight outline which has now been given of dreaming may serve to show
that the subject is not only curious, but important. It appears to be
worthy of careful investigation; and there is much reason to believe that
an extensive collection of authentic facts, carefully analyzed, would unfold
principles of very great interest in reference to the philosophy of the
mental powers."—"*Intellectual Powers,*" p. 224.

O   18*

BOOK III.

DISTURBANCES POPULARLY TERMED HAUNTINGS.

CHAPTER I.

GENERAL CHARACTER OF THE PHENOMENA.

"For this is not a matter of to-day
Or yesterday, but hath been from all time;
And none can tell us whence it came, or how."

SOPHOCLES.

THAT extraordinary and influential movement, commonly denominated spiritual, which has overrun these United States, and has spread hence, to a greater or less extent, over every country of Europe, had its origin in a phenomenon, or alleged phenomenon, of the character which has usually been termed a haunted house.

In a work like the present, then, it is fitting that this class of phenomena, slighted and derided by modern Sadducism though they be, should have place as worthy of serious examination.

And in prosecuting such an examination, by citing the best-attested examples, the fair question is not, whether in these each minute particular is critically exact;—for what history, ancient or modern, would endure such a test?—but whether, in a general way, the narratives bear the impress of truth; whether there be sufficient evidence to indicate that they are based on a substantial reality. In such an inquiry, let us take with us two considerations: remembering, on the one hand,

210

that, when the passions of wonder and fear are strongly excited, men's imaginations are prone to exaggerate; and, on the other, that, as elsewhere set forth,* there are no *collective* hallucinations.

The fair question is, then, whether, even if this haunting of houses be often a mere popular superstition, there be yet no actual truth, no genuine phenomena, underlying it.

In winnowing, from out a large apocryphal mass, the comparatively few stories of this class which come down to us in authentic form, vouched for by respectable cotemporary authority, sustained by specifications of time and place and person, backed sometimes by judicial oaths, one is forcibly struck by the observation that, in thus making the selection, we find thrown out all stories of the ghostly school of horror, all skeleton specters with the worms creeping in and out, all demons with orthodox horns and tail, all midnight lights burning blue, with other similar embellishments; and there remain a comparatively sober and prosaic set of wonders,—inexplicable, indeed, by any known physical agency, but shorn of that gaudy supernaturalism in which Anne Radcliffe delighted, and which Horace Walpole scorned not to employ.

In its place, however, we find an element which by some may be considered quite as startling and improbable. I allude to the mischievous, boisterous, and freakish aspect which these disturbances occasionally assume. So accustomed are we to regard all spiritual visitations, if such there be, as not serious and important only, but of a solemn and reverential character, that our natural or acquired repugnance to admit the reality of any phenomena not explicable by mundane agency is greatly

---

* See next chapter, where the distinction is made between *illusion* and *hallucination ;* the one based on a reality, the other a mere disease of the senses.

increased when we discover in them more whim and triviality.

It is very certain that, if disturbances of the character alluded to be the work of disembodied spirits, it appears to be of spirits of a comparatively inferior order; as imps, we might say, of frolic and misrule; not wicked, it would seem, or, if wicked, restrained from inflicting serious injury, but, as it were, tricksy elves, sprites full of pranks and levities,—a sort of *Pucks*,—"esprits espiègles," as the French phrase it; or as the Germans, framing an epithet expressly for this supposed class of spirits, have expressed it, *poltergeister*.

If it may be plausibly argued that we cannot reasonably imagine spirits revisiting the scenes of their former existence with no higher aim, for no nobler purpose, than these narratives disclose, it must be conceded also, for the very same reason, that men were not likely to invent stories of such a character with no actual foundation whereupon to build. Imagination, once at work, would not restrict itself to knockings, and scrapings, and jerking furniture about, and teasing children, and similar petty annoyances. It would conjure up something more impressive and mysterious.

But my business here is with facts, not theories; with what we find, not with what, according to our present notions, we might expect to find. How much is there in nature, which, if we sat down beforehand to conjecture probabilities, would directly belie our anticipations!

And in making choice of facts, or what purport to be so, I shall not go back further than two centuries.*

---

* Those who are disposed to amuse themselves (for, in truth, it amounts to little more than amusement) may find in various ancient writers narratives of haunted houses, apparently as well attested as any other portion of the history of the time. Pliny the Younger has one (*Plin. Junior, Epist. ad Suram.* lib. vii. cap. 27) which he relates as having occurred to the philosopher Athenodorus. The skeptical Lucian (in *Philo-pseud.* p. 840) relates another of a man named Arignotes. In later days, Antonio

Until printing became a common art, and books were freely read beyond the limits of a learned and restricted circle, a narrative of questionable events could not obtain that extended circulation which would expose it to general criticism, afford fair chance for refutation, and thus give to future ages some guarantee against the frequent errors of an *ex-parte* statement.

Torquemada (in his "*Flores Curiosas,*" Salamanca, 1570) has the story of a certain Vasquez de Ayola. In all these three cases a specter is alleged to have disappeared on a spot where, on digging, a skeleton was found. Alexander ab Alexandro, a learned Neapolitan lawyer of the fifteenth century, states, as a fact of common notoriety, that in Rome there are a number of houses so much out of repute as being haunted that no one will venture to inhabit them; and he adds, that, desiring to test the truth of what was said in regard to one of these houses, he, along with a friend named Tuba and others, spent a night there, when they were terrified by the appearance of a phantom and by the most frightful noises and disturbances. —*Alexander ab Alexandro,* lib. v. cap. 23.

A hundred similar cases might be adduced, especially from the writings of the ancient fathers, as St. Augustin, St. Germain, St. Gregory, and others.

But no reliable inference can be drawn from these vague old stories, except the universal prevalence, in all ages, of the same idea.

CHAPTER II.

NARRATIVES.

"I have no humor nor delight in telling stories, and do not publish these for the gratification of those that have; but I record them as arguments for the confirmation of a truth, which hath indeed been attested by multitudes of the like evidences in all places and times."—REV. JOSEPH GLANVIL: *Pref. to his Sadducismus Triumphatus.*

THE first narrative I select was the object of interest and controversy all over England for twenty years and more, and was published, almost at the time of the alleged occurrences, by a man of character and station.

THE GLANVIL NARRATIVE.

Disturbances at Mr. Mompesson's house at Tedworth.

1661 to 1663.

The Rev. Joseph Glanvil, chaplain-in-ordinary to Charles II., was a man well and favorably known in his day, as much by various theological works as by his defense of the Baconian philosophy, and as the champion, against certain detractors, of the Royal Society, of which he was a member.

In the year 1666 he published his "*Sadducismus Triumphatus,*" in which, to sustain the popular opinions of that age on the subject of witches and apparitions, he includes what he calls a "choice collection of modern relations." Most of these are from hearsay, some based on the confessions of the accused and other evidences now admitted to be untrustworthy; but the first and principal relation, entitled by Glanvil "The Dæmon of Tedworth," is of a different character, being a narrative of events occurring, at intervals throughout two entire

214

years, in the house of a gentleman of character and standing, Mr. John Mompesson, of Tedworth, in the county of Wilts; a portion of which events were witnessed by Glanvil himself.

It appears that in March, 1661, Mr. Mompesson, in his magisterial capacity, had caused to be arrested a vagrant drummer, who had been annoying the country by noisy demands for charity, and that he had caused his drum to be taken from him and left in the bailiff's hands. This fact Mr. Mompesson imagined to be connected with the disturbances that followed, and of which the chief details are here given, quoted literally from Glanvil's work.

"About the middle of April following, (that is, in 1661,) when Mr. Mompesson was preparing for a journey to London, the bailiff sent the drum to his house. When he was returned from that journey, his wife told him that they had been much affrighted in the night by thieves, and that the house had like to have been broken up. And he had not been at home above three nights when the same noise was heard that had disturbed the family in his absence. It was a very great knocking at his doors and the outsides of his house. Hereupon he got up and went about the house with a brace of pistols in his hands. He opened the door where the great knocking was, and then he heard the noise at another door. He opened that also, and went out round his house, but could discover nothing, only he still heard a strange noise and hollow sound. When he got back to bed, the noise was a thumping and drumming on the top of his house, which continued a good space, and then by degrees went off into the air.

"After this, the noise of thumping and drumming was very frequent, usually five nights together, and then it would intermit three. It was on the outsides of the house, which was most of it of board. It constantly came as they were going to sleep, whether early or late. After a month's disturbance without, it came into the room where the drum lay, four or five nights in seven, within half an hour after they were in bed, continuing almost two. The sign of it, just before it came, was an hurling in the air over the house; and at its going off, the beating of a drum like that at the breaking up of a guard. It continued in this room for the space of two months, which time Mr. Mompesson himself lay there to observe it."*

During Mrs. Mompesson's confinement, and for three weeks afterward, it intermitted; but "after this civil cessation," says Glanvil, "it returned in a ruder manner than before, and followed and vext the youngest children, beating their bedsteads with that violence, that all present expected when they would fall to pieces. In laying hands on them, one should feel no blows, but might perceive them to shake exceedingly. For an hour together it would beat 'Round-Heads and Cuckolds,' the 'Tat-too,' and several other points of war, as well as any drummer. After this, they would hear a scratching under the children's bed, as if by something that had iron talons. It would lift the children up in their beds, follow them from one room to another, and for a while haunted none particularly but them."

The next portion of the recital is still more marvelous; and Glanvil states that the occurrences took place in the presence of a minister of the gospel, Mr. Cragg, and of many neighbors who had come to the house on a visit.

"The minister went to prayers with them, kneeling at the children's bedside, where it was then very troublesome and loud. During prayer-time it withdrew into

* "Sadducismus Triumphatus; or, Full and Plain Evidence concerning Witches and Apparitions," by Joseph Glanvil, late Chaplain-in-ordinary to His Majesty, and Fellow of the Royal Society, 3d ed., London, 1689, pp. 322–323.

the cock-loft, but returned as soon as prayers were done; and then, in sight of the company, the chairs walkt about the room of themselves, the children's shoes were hurled over their heads, and every loose thing moved about the chamber. At the same time a bed-staff was thrown at the minister, but so favorably, that a lock of wool could not have fallen more softly; and it was observed, that it stopt just where it lighted, without rolling or moving from the place." (p. 324.)

However whimsical and unlikely all this may appear, we shall find it paralleled in modern examples occurring both in Europe and America.

The next extract introduces a new feature, well deserving our attention. It is the earliest indication I have found, of that responding of the sounds, with apparent intelligence, which has expanded in these United States to such vast proportions.

"Mr. Mompesson perceiving that it so much persecuted the little children, he lodged them at a neighbor's house, taking his eldest daughter, who was about ten years of age, into his own chamber, where it had not been a month before. As soon as she was in bed, the disturbance began there again, continuing three weeks, drumming and making other noises; and *it was observed that it would exactly answer in drumming any thing that was beaten or called for.*" (p. 324.)

Here is another extract, confirming similar observations touching the conduct of animals during like disturbances elsewhere.

"It was noted that when the noise was loudest, and came with the most sudden and surprising violence, no dog about the house would move, though the knocking was oft so boisterous and rude, that it hath been heard at a considerable distance in the fields, and awakened the neighbors in the village, none of which live very near this." (p. 324.)

19

The disturbances continued *throughout two years*, some of them being recorded (p. 332) as having taken place in the month of April, 1663. Mr. Mompesson and his friends ascribed them to the malice of the drummer, in league with the Evil One. And in this they were confirmed by the following incidents, occurring in the month of January, 1662. Those who have any experience in similar communications of our day know well how little confidence ought to be placed in such, when uncorroborated by other evidence, except as an indication of some occult intelligence.

"During the time of the knocking when many were present, a gentleman of the company said, 'Satan, if the drummer set thee to work, give three knocks and no more;' which it did very distinctly, and stopt. Then the gentleman knockt, to see if it would answer him as it was wont; but it did not. For farther trial, he bid it, for confirmation, if it were the drummer, to give five knocks and no more that night, which it did, and left the house quiet all the night after. This was done in the presence of Sir Thomas Chamberlain, of Oxford, and divers others." (p. 326.)

So far the narrative, as derived by our author from Mr. Mompesson and others; but Mr. Glanvil himself visited the scene of the disturbance in January, 1662, and gives us the result of his personal observations, as follows:—

"About this time I went to the house, on purpose to inquire the truth of those passages, of which there was so loud a report. It had ceased from its drumming and ruder noises before I came thither; but most of the more remarkable circumstances before related were confirmed to me there, by several of the neighbors together, who had been present at them. At this time it used to haunt the children, and that as soon as they were laid. They went to bed that night I was there, about eight of the clock, when a maid-servant, coming down from them, told us it was come. The neighbors that were there, and two ministers who had seen and heard divers times, went away; but Mr. Mompesson and I, and a gentleman that came with me, went up. I heard a strange scratching as we went up the stairs, and when we came into the room, I perceived it was just behind the bolster of the children's bed, and seemed to be against the tick. It was loud scratching, as one with long nails could make upon a bolster. There were two little modest girls in the bed, between seven and eleven years old, as I guest. I saw their hands out of the cloaths, and they could not contribute to the noise that was behind their heads. They had been used to it, and had still somebody or other in the chamber with them, and therefore seemed not to be much affrighted. I, standing at the bed's head, thrust my hand behind the bolster, directing it to the place whence the noise seemed to come. Whereupon the noise ceased there, and was heard in another part of the bed. But when I had taken out my hand it returned, and was heard in the same place as before. I had been told that it would imitate noises, and made trial by scratching several times upon the sheet, as 5, and 7, and 10, which it followed and still stopped at my number. I searched under and behind the bed, turned up the clothes to the bed-cords, graspt the bolster, sounded the wall behind, and made all the search that possibly I could, to find if there were any trick, contrivance, or common cause of it: the like did my friend; but we could discover nothing. So that I was then verily persuaded, and am so still, that the noise was made by some dæmon or spirit. After it had scratched about half an hour or more, it went into the midst of the bed, under the children, and there seemed to pant, like a dog out of breath, very loudly. I put my hand upon the place, and felt the bed bearing up against it, as if something within had thrust it up. I grasped the feathers to feel if any living thing were in it. I looked under, and everywhere about, to see if there were any dog or cat, or any such creature, in the room, and so we all did, but found nothing. The motion it caused by this panting was so strong, that it shook the rooms and windows very sensibly. It continued more than half an hour, while my friend and I staid in the room; and as long after, as we were told.

"It will, I know, be said, by some, that my friend and I were under some affright, and so fancied noises and sights that were not. This is the eternal evasion. But if it be possible to know how a man is affected when in fear, and when unconcerned, I certainly know, for mine own part, that during the whole time of my being in the room, and in the house, I was under no more affrightment, than I am while I write this relation. And if I know that I am now awake, and that I see the objects that are before me, I know that I heard and saw the particulars that I have told." (pp. 328 to 330.)

Mr. Glanvil concludes the relation, the repetitions and less interesting portions of which, for brevity's sake, I have omitted, as follows:—

"Thus I have written the sum of Mr. Mompesson's disturbance, which I had partly from his own mouth related before divers, who had been witnesses of all, and confirmed his relation; and partly from his own letters, from which the order and series of things is taken. The same particulars he writ also to Dr. Creed, then Doctor of the chair in Oxford." (p. 334.)

It remains to be stated that, some time after the drummer's first commitment, Mr. Mompesson had him again taken up for felony, (under the statute of I. James, chap. 12,) for the supposed witchcraft about his house. The grand jury found a true bill; but, to the honor of the petty jury be it said, the man was acquitted, his connection with the disturbances not being proved. The reality of the disturbances was sworn to by various witnesses. To this fact Mr. Mompesson alludes in a letter written by him to a Mr. James Collins, dated Tedworth, August 8, 1674, and published entire in Glanvil's book. I quote from that letter:—

"The evidence upon oath were myself, Mr. William Maton, one Mr. Walter Dowse,—all yet living, and, I think, of as good repute as any this country has in it,— and one Mr. Joseph Cragg, then minister of the place, but since dead. We all deposed several things that we conceived impossible to be done by any natural agents, as the motion of chairs, stools, and bed-staves, nobody being near them, the beating of drums in the air over the house in clear nights, and nothing visible, the shaking of the floor and strongest parts of the house in still and calm nights, with several other things of the like nature."*

In another letter, addressed by Mr. Mompesson to Mr. Glanvil himself, under date November 8, 1672, he says,—

"Meeting with Dr. Pierce accidentally at Sir Robert Button's, he acquainted me of something that passed between my Lord of R—— and yourself about my troubles, &c.; to which (having but little leisure) I do give you this account: That I have been very often of late asked the question, 'Whether I have not confessed to his majesty, or any other, a cheat discovered about that affair.' To which I gave, and shall to my dying day give, the same answer: That I must belie myself, and perjure myself also, to acknowledge a cheat in a thing where I am sure there neither was or could be any, as I, the minister of the place, and two other honest gentlemen deposed at the assizes upon my impleading the drummer. If the world

---

* Mompesson's letter to Collins, given entire in the preface to the second part of Glanvil's "*Sadducismus Triumphatus*," 3d ed., 1689. It does not appear in the 1st edition, not having been then written.

will not believe it, it shall be indifferent to me, praying God to keep me from the same or the like affliction."*

Such is a compendium of the essential facts in this case, literally extracted from Glanvil's work, to which for a more detailed account the curious reader is referred.

In connection with the above narrative, it is chiefly to be noted,—

That the disturbances continued for two entire years, namely, from April, 1661, until April, 1663; and that Mr. Mompesson took up his quarters for the night, for two months at a time, in a particular chamber, expressly for the purpose of observing them.

That the sounds produced were so loud as to awaken the neighbors in the adjoining village, at a considerable distance from Mr. Mompesson's house.

That the motion in the children's bed, in Mr. Glanvil's presence, was so great as sensibly to shake the doors and windows of the house.

That the facts, collected by Glanvil at the time they occurred, were published by him four years afterward, to wit, in 1666; and that the more important of these facts were sworn to in a court of justice.

That ten years after these occurrences took place, and when it was reported that Mr. Mompesson had admitted the discovery of a trick, that gentleman explicitly denied that he had ever discovered any natural cause for the phenomena, and in the most solemn manner indorsed his former declarations to Mr. Glanvil.

---

* The letter is given entire in the preface to Glanvil's work, 3d edition.

It is remarkable how unscrupulously some men who ought to know better deny, without any foundation, the truth of some unwelcome fact. In the "*Philosophy of Mystery*," by Walter Cooper Dendy, Fellow and Honorary Secretary to the Medical Society of London, the author, speaking of the "mystery of the Demon of Tedworth," says, "This also was the source of extreme wonder until the drummer was tried and convicted and Mr. Mompesson confessed that the mystery was the effect of contrivance." — Chapter "*Illustration of Mysterious Sounds*," pp. 149, 150.

When to these considerations are added the following remarks of Mr. Glanvil regarding the character of Mr. Mompesson and the chances of imposture under the circumstances, the reader has before him all the materials for judging in this case.

"Mr. Mompesson is a gentleman of whose truth in this account I have not the least ground of suspicion, he being neither vain nor credulous, but a discreet, sagacious, and manly person. Now, the credit of matters of fact depends much upon the relators, who, if they cannot be deceived themselves nor supposed anyways interested to impose upon others, ought to be credited. For upon these circumstances all human faith is grounded, and matter of fact is not capable of any proof besides but that of immediate sensible evidence. Now, this gentleman cannot be thought ignorant whether that he relates be true or no,—the scene of all being his own house, himself the witness, and that not of a circumstance or two, but of an hundred, nor of once or twice only, but for the space of some years, during which he was a concerned and inquisitive observer. So that it cannot with any show of reason be supposed that any of his servants abused him, since in all that time he must needs have detected the deceit. And what interest could any of his family have had (if it had been possible to have managed without discovery) to continue so long, so troublesome, and so injurious an imposture? Nor can it with any whit of more probability be imagined that his own melancholy deluded him, since (besides that he is no crazy nor imaginative person) that humor could not have been so lasting and pertinacious. Or, if it were so in him, can we think he affected his whole family and those multitudes of neighbors and others who had so often been witnesses of those passages? Such supposals are wild, and not like to tempt any but those whose wills are their reasons. So that, upon the whole, the principal relator, Mr. Mompesson himself, knew whether what he reports was true or not, whether those things acted in his house were contrived cheats or extraordinary realities. And, if so, what interest could he serve in carrying on or conniving at a juggling design and imposture?

"He suffered by it in his name, in his estate, in all his affairs, and in the general peace of his family. The unbelievers in the matter of spirits and witches took him for an impostor. Many others judged the permission of such an extraordinary evil to be the judgment of God upon him for some notorious wickedness or impiety. Thus his name was continually exposed to censure, and his estate suffered by the concourse of people from all parts to his house; by the diversion it gave him from his affairs; by the discouragement of servants, by reason of which he could hardly get any to live with him. To which I add, the continual hurry that his family was in, the affrights, and the watchings and disturbance of his whole house, (in which himself must needs be the most concerned.) I say, if these things are considered, there will be little reason to think he would have any interest to put a cheat upon the world in which he would most of all have injured and abused himself."*

Leaving this case in the reader's hands, I pass to another, occurring in the eighteenth century.

THE WESLEY NARRATIVE.

Disturbances in Mr. Wesley's parsonage at Epworth.

1716 and 1717.

In the year 1716, the Rev. Samuel Wesley, father of the celebrated John Wesley the founder of Methodism, was rector of Epworth, in the county of Lincoln, England. In his parsonage-house, the same in which John was born, there occurred, throughout the months of

---

* *"Sadducismus Triumphatus,"* pp. 334 to 336.

December, 1716, and of January, 1717, sundry disturbances, of which Mr. Samuel Wesley kept a detailed journal. The particulars are further preserved in twelve letters written on the subject, at the time, to and from various members of the family. In addition to this, Mr. John Wesley himself went down to Epworth in the year 1720, inquired carefully into the particulars, received statements in writing from each member of the family touching what they had seen and heard, and compiled from these a narrative which he published in the "Arminian Magazine."

The original documents were preserved in the family, came into the hands of Mrs. Earle, grand-daughter of Mr. Samuel Wesley, (the eldest brother of John,) were intrusted by her to a Mr. Babcock, and by him given to the well-known Dr. Joseph Priestley, by whom the whole were first published in 1791.*

They have been reprinted by Dr. Adam Clarke, in his "Memoirs of the Wesley Family."† They cover forty-six pages of that work; and, as they contain numerous repetitions, I content myself with transcribing a portion only, commencing with the narrative drawn up by Mr. John Wesley, to which I have already referred.

NARRATIVE.

"On December 2, 1716, while Robert Brown, my father's servant, was sitting with one of the maids, a little before ten at night, in the dining-room, which opened into the garden, they both heard one knocking at the door. Robert rose and opened it, but could see

---

* "*Original Letters by the Rev. John Wesley and his Friends, illustrative of his Early History,*" with other Curious Papers, communicated by the late Rev. S. Babcock. To which is prefixed An Address to the Methodists, by Joseph Priestley, LL.D., F.R.S., &c., London, 1791: an octavo volume of 170 pages. This pamphlet is scarce.

† "*Memoirs of the Wesley Family,*" collected principally from original documents. By Adam Clarke, LL.D., F.A.S., 2d ed., London, 1843.

P

nobody. Quickly it knocked again, and groaned. 'It is Mr. Turpine,' said Robert: 'he has the stone, and uses to groan so.' He opened the door again twice or thrice, the knocking being twice or thrice repeated; but, still seeing nothing, and being a little startled, they rose up and went to bed. When Robert came to the top of the garret stairs, he saw a handmill which was at a little distance whirled about very swiftly. When he related this he said, 'Nought vexed me but that it was empty. I thought if it had but been full of malt he might have ground his heart out for me.' When he was in bed, he heard as it were the gobbling of a turkey-cock close to the bedside, and soon after the sound of one stumbling over his shoes and boots; but there was none there: he had left them below. The next day, he and the maid related these things to the other maid, who laughed heartily, and said, 'What a couple of fools are you! I defy any thing to fright me.' After churning in the evening, she put the butter in the tray, and had no sooner carried it into the dairy than she heard a knocking on the shelf where several puncheons of milk stood, first above the shelf, then below. She took the candle, and searched both above and below, but, being able to find nothing, threw down butter, tray, and all, and ran away for life. The next evening, between five and six o'clock, my sister Molly, then about twenty years of age, sitting in the dining-room reading, heard as if it were the door that led into the hall open, and a person walking in that seemed to have on a silk night-gown, rustling and trailing along. It seemed to walk round her, then to the door, then round again; but she could see nothing. She thought, 'It signifies nothing to run away; for, whatever it is, it can run faster than me.' So she rose, put her book under her arm, and walked slowly away. After supper, she was sitting with my sister Sukey (about a year older than her) in one of the chambers, and telling her what had happened. She made quite light of it, telling her, 'I wonder you are so easily frighted: I would fain see what would fright me.' Presently a knocking began under the table. She took the candle and looked, but could find nothing. Then the iron casement began to clatter, and the lid of a warming-pan. Next the latch of the door moved up and down without ceasing. She started up, leaped into the bed without undressing, pulled the bed-clothes over her head, and never ventured to look up until next morning.

"A night or two after, my sister Hetty (a year younger than my sister Molly) was waiting as usual, between nine and ten, to take away my father's candle, when she heard one coming down the garret stairs, walking slowly by her, then going down the best stairs, then up the back stairs, and up the garret stairs; and at every step it seemed the house shook from top to bottom. Just then my father knocked. She went in, took his candle, and got to bed as fast as possible. In the morning she told this to my eldest sister, who told her, 'You know I believe none of these things: pray let me take away the candle to-night, and I will find out the trick.' She accordingly took my sister Hetty's place, and had no sooner taken away the candle than she heard a noise below. She hastened downstairs to the hall, where the noise was, but it was then in the kitchen. She ran into the kitchen, where it was drumming on the inside of the screen. When she went round, it was drumming on the outside, and so always on the side opposite to her. Then she heard a knocking at the back kitchen door. She ran to it, unlocked it softly, and, when the knocking was repeated, suddenly opened it; but nothing was to be seen. As soon as she had shut it, the knocking began again.

She opened it again, but could see nothing. When she went to shut the door, it was violently thrust against her; but she set her knee and her shoulder to the door, forced it to, and turned the key. Then the knocking began again; but she let it go on, and went up to bed. However, from that time she was thoroughly convinced that there was no imposture in the affair.

"The next morning, my sister telling my mother what had happened, she said, 'If I hear any thing myself, I shall know how to judge.' Soon after she begged her to come into the nursery. She did, and heard, in the corner of the room, as it were the violent rocking of a cradle; but no cradle had been there for some years. She was convinced it was preternatural, and earnestly prayed it might not disturb her in her own chamber at the hours of retirement; and it never did. She now thought it was proper to tell my father. But he was extremely angry, and said, 'Sukey, I am ashamed of you. These boys and girls frighten one another; but you are a woman of sense, and should know better. Let me hear of it no more.'

"At six in the evening he had family prayers as usual. When he began the prayer for the king, a knocking began all round the room, and a thundering knock attended the *Amen*. The same was heard from this time every morning and evening while the prayer for the king was repeated   As both my father and mother are now at rest, and incapable of being pained thereby, I think it my duty to furnish the serious reader with a key to this circumstance.

"The year before King William died, my father observed my mother did not say amen to the prayer for the king. She said she could not, for she did not believe the Prince of Orange was king. He vowed he would never cohabit with her until she did. He then took his horse and rode away; nor did she hear any thing of him for a twelve-month. He then came back, and lived with her as before. But I fear his vow was not forgotten before God.

"Being informed that Mr. Hoole, the vicar of Haxey, (an eminently pious and sensible man,) could give me some further information, I walked over to him. He said, 'Robert Brown came over to me, and told me your father desired my company. When I came, he gave me an account of all that had happened, particularly the knocking during family prayer. But that evening (to my great satisfaction) we had no knocking at all. But between nine and ten a servant came in, and said, "Old Jeffrey is coming, (that was the name of one that died in the house,) for I hear the signal." This they informed me was heard every night about a quarter before ten. It was toward the top of the house, on the outside, at the northeast corner, resembling the loud creaking of a saw, or rather that of a windmill when the body of it is turned about in order to shift the sails to the wind. We then heard a knocking over our heads; and Mr. Wesley, catching up a candle, said, "Come, sir, now you shall hear for yourself." We went up-stairs; he with much hope, and I (to say the truth) with much fear. When we came into the nursery, it was knocking in the next room; when we went there, it was knocking in the nursery. And there it continued to knock, though we came in, particularly at the head of the bed (which was of wood) in which Miss Hetty and two of her younger sisters lay. Mr. Wesley observing that they were much affected,—though asleep, sweating, and trembling exceedingly,—was very angry, and, pulling out a pistol, was going to fire at the place from whence the sound came. But I snatched him by the arm, and said, "Sir, you are convinced this is something preternatural. If so, you cannot hurt it; but you give it power to hurt you." He then went

20

close to the place, and said, sternly, "Thou deaf and dumb devil! why dost thou fright these children, that cannot answer for themselves? Come to me, in my study, that am a man!" Instantly, it knocked his knock (the particular knock which he always used at the gate) as if it would shiver the board to pieces; and we heard nothing more that night.'

"Till this time my father had never heard the least disturbance in his study. But the next evening, as he attempted to go into his study, (of which none had the key but himself,) when he opened the door, it was thrust back with such violence as had like to have thrown him down. However, he thrust the door open, and went in. Presently there was a knocking, first on one side, then on the other, and, after a time, in the next room, wherein my sister Nancy was. He went into that room, and, the noise continuing, adjured it to speak, but in vain. He then said, 'These spirits love darkness: put out the candle, and perhaps it will speak.' She did so, and he repeated his adjuration; but still there was only knocking, and no articulate sound. Upon this he said, 'Nancy, two Christians are an overmatch for the devil. Go all of you down-stairs: it may be when I am alone he will have courage to speak.' When she was gone, a thought came in his head, and he said, 'If thou art the spirit of my son Samuel, I pray knock three knocks, and no more.' Immediately all was silence, and there was no more knocking at all that night. I asked my sister Nancy (then fifteen years old) whether she was not afraid when my father used that adjuration. She answered she was sadly afraid it would speak when she put out the candle: but she was not at all afraid in the day-time, when it walked after her, only she thought when she was about her work he might have done it for her, and saved her the trouble.

"By this time all my sisters were so accustomed to

these noises that they gave them little disturbance. A gentle tapping at their bed-head usually began between nine and ten at night. They then commonly said to each other, 'Jeffrey is coming: it is time to go to sleep.' And if they heard a noise in the day, and said to my youngest sister, 'Hark, Kezzy, Jeffrey is knocking above,' she would run up-stairs and pursue it from room to room, saying she desired no better diversion.

" A few nights after, my father and mother had just gone to bed, and the candle was not taken away, when they heard three blows, and a second and a third three, as it were with a large oaken staff, struck upon a chest which stood by the bedside. My father immediately arose, put on his night-gown, and, hearing great noises below, took the candle and went down ; my mother walked by his side. As they went down the broad stairs, they heard as if a vessel full of silver was poured upon my mother's breast and ran jingling down to her feet. Quickly after, there was a sound as if a large iron bell was thrown among many bottles under the stairs ; but nothing was hurt. Soon after, our large mastiff dog came, and ran to shelter himself between them. While the disturbances continued he used to bark and leap, and snap on one side and the other, and that frequently before any person in the room heard any noise at all. But after two or three days he used to tremble, and creep away before the noise began. And by this the family knew it was at hand; nor did the observation ever fail.

" A little before my father and mother came into the hall, it seemed as if a very large coal was violently thrown upon the floor and dashed all in pieces; but nothing was seen. My father then cried out, 'Sukey, do you not hear? all the pewter is thrown about the kitchen.' But when they looked, all the pewter stood in its place   There then was a loud knocking at the back door. My father opened it, but saw nothing. It was then at the fore door. He opened that, but it was still lost labor. After opening first the one, then the other, several times, he turned and went up to bed. But the noises were so violent over the house that he could not sleep till four in the morning.

"Several gentlemen and clergymen now earnestly advised my father to quit the house. But he constantly answered, 'No: let the devil flee from me; I will never flee from the devil.' But he wrote to my eldest brother, at London, to come down. He was preparing so to do, when another letter came informing him the disturbances were over, after they had continued (the latter part of the time day and night) from the 2d of December to the end of January."*

The journal of Mr. Wesley, Sen., (p. 247,) fully corroborates his son's narrative, adding some further particulars. He notices that, on the 23d December, in the nursery, when his daughter Emily knocked, it answered her. On another occasion, he says, "I went down-stairs, and knocked with my stick against the joists of the kitchen. It answered me as often and as loud as I knocked; but then I knocked as I usually do at my door,—1,—2, 3, 4, 5, 6,—7; but this puzzled it, and it did not answer, or not in the same method, though the children heard it do the same exactly twice or thrice after." This corresponds with what Mr. Hoole said about "its knocking Mr. Wesley's knock."

On the 25th of December, he says, " The noises were so violent it was vain to think of sleep while they continued." So, again, on December 27, he adds, "They were so boisterous that I did not care to leave my family,"—as he wished to do, to pay a visit to a friend, Mr. Downs.

---

* *"Memoirs of the Wesley Family,"* vol. i. pp. 253 to 260.

He says, also, "I have been thrice pushed by an invisible power, once against the corner of my desk in the study, a second time against the door of the matted chamber, a third time against the right side of the frame of my study door, as I was going in."

As to the dog, under date December 25, his record is, "Our mastiff came whining to us, as he did always after the first night of its coming; for then he barked violently at it, but was silent afterwards, and seemed more afraid than any of the children."

The letters corroborating the various details are too long and numerous to be here transcribed. I extract, as a specimen, from one written by Emily Wesley (afterward Mrs. Harper) to her brother Samuel. She says,—

"I thank you for your last, and shall give you what satisfaction is in my power concerning what has happened in our family. I am so far from being superstitious, that I was too much inclined to infidelity: so that I heartily rejoice at having such an opportunity of convincing myself, past doubt or scruple, of the existence of some beings besides those we see. A whole month was sufficient to convince anybody of the reality of the thing, and to try all ways of discovering any trick, had it been possible for any such to have been used. I shall only tell you what I myself heard, and leave the rest to others.

"My sisters in the paper chamber had heard noises, and told me of them; but I did not much believe till one night, about a week after the first groans were heard, which was the beginning. Just after the clock had struck ten, I went down-stairs to lock the doors, which I always do. Scarce had I got up the best stairs, when I heard a noise like a person throwing down a vast coal in the middle of the fore kitchen, and all the splinters seemed to fly about from it. I was not much frighted, but went to my sister Sukey, and we together went all over the low rooms; but there was nothing out of order.

" Our dog was fast asleep, and our only cat in the other end of the house. No sooner was I got up-stairs and undressing for bed, but I heard a noise among many bottles that stand under the best stairs, just like the throwing of a great stone among them which had broken them all to pieces. This made me hasten to bed. But my sister Hetty, who sits always to wait on my father going to bed, was still sitting on the lowest step on the garret stairs, the door being shut at her back, when, soon after, there came down the stairs behind her something like a man in a loose night-gown trailing after him, which made her fly rather than run to me in the nursery.

" All this time we never told my father of it; but soon we did. He smiled, and gave no answer, but was more careful than usual from that time to see us in bed, imagining it to be some of us young women that sat up late and made a noise. His incredulity, and especially his imputing it to us or our lovers, made me, I own, desirous of its continuance till he was convinced. As for my mother, she firmly believed it to be rats, and sent for a horn to blow them away. I laughed to think how wisely they were employed who were striving half a day to fright away Jeffrey (for that name I gave it) with a horn.

" But, whatever it was, I perceived it could be made angry; for from that time it was so outrageous, there was no quiet for us after ten at night. I heard frequently, between ten and eleven, something like the quick winding-up of a jack at the corner of the room by my bed's head, just like the running of the wheels and the creaking of the iron-work. This was the common signal of its coming. Then it would knock on the floor three times, then at my sister's bed's head, in the same room, almost always three together, and then stay. The sound was hollow and loud, so as none of us could ever imitate.

"It would answer to my mother if she stamped on the floor and bid it. It would knock when I was putting the children to bed, just under me, where I sat. One time little Kezzy, pretending to scare Polly, as I was undressing them, stamped with her foot on the floor; and immediately it answered with three knocks, just in the same place. It was more loud and fierce if any one said it was rats, or any thing natural.

"I could tell you abundance more of it, but the rest will write, and therefore it would be needless. I was not much frighted at first, and very little at last; but it was never near me, except two or three times, and never followed me, as it did my sister Hetty. I have been with her when it has knocked under her; and when she has removed it has followed, and still kept just under her feet, which was enough to terrify a stouter person." (pp. 270 to 272.)

Under date January 19, 1717, Mr. Samuel Wesley, Jr., wrote to his mother, propounding certain questions, to which she most satisfactorily replied, adding, "But, withal, I desire that my answers may satisfy none but yourself; for I would not have the matter imparted to any."

From a memorandum of Mr. John Wesley, detailing the "general circumstances, of which most if not all the family were frequent witnesses," I extract as follows:—

"Before it came into any room, the latches were frequently lifted up, the windows clattered, and whatever iron or brass was about the chamber rung and jarred exceedingly.

"When it was in any room, let them make what noise they would, as they sometimes did on purpose, its dead, hollow note would be clearly heard above them all.

"The sound very often seemed in the air in the middle of a room; nor could they ever make any such themselves, by any contrivance.

"It never came by day till my mother ordered the horn to be blown. After that time scarce any one could go from one room into another but the latch of the room they went to was lifted up before they touched it.

"It never came into my father's study till he talked to it sharply, called it deaf and dumb devil, and bid it cease to disturb the innocent children and come to him in his study if it had any thing to say to him.

"From the time of my mother's desiring it not to disturb her from five to six, it was never heard in her chamber from five till she came down-stairs, nor at any other time when she was employed in devotion." (pp. 284, 285.)

It remains to be stated that one member, at least, of the family, Emily Wesley, a portion of whose letter on the subject has already been given, conceived herself to have been followed by the Epworth spirit through life. Dr. Clarke states that he possesses an original letter from that lady to her brother John, dated February 16, 1750,—that is, thirty-four years after the preceding events happened,—from which letter he publishes the following extract:—

"I want sadly to see you, and talk some hours with you, as in times past. One doctrine of yours and of many more,—namely, no happiness can be found in any or all things in the world: that, as I have sixteen years of my own experience which lie flatly against it, I want to talk with you about it. Another thing is, that wonderful thing called by us Jeffrey. You won't laugh at me for being superstitious if I tell you how certainly that *something* calls on me against any extraordinary new affliction; but so little is known of the invisible world that I, at least, am not able to judge whether it be a friendly or an evil spirit."*

As to the causes of these disturbances, Dr. Clarke has the following:—"For a considerable time all the family believed it to be a trick; but at last they were all satisfied it was something supernatural.". . . "Mr. John Wesley believed that it was a messenger of Satan sent to buffet his father for his rash promise of leaving his family, and very improper conduct to his wife, in consequence of her scruple to pray for the Prince of Orange as King of England." . . . "With others the house was considered as haunted." . . . "Dr. Priestley thinks the whole trick and imposture. It must be, on his system of materialism; but this does not solve the difficulty; it only cuts the knot." . . . "Mrs. Wesley's opinion was different from all the rest, and was probably the most correct: she supposed that 'these noises and disturbances portended the death of her brother, then abroad in the East India Company's service.' This gentleman, who had acquired a large fortune, suddenly disappeared, and was never heard of more,—at least, as far as I can find from the remaining branches of the family, or from any of the family documents." (pp. 287 to 289.)

These disturbances, though not so persistent as those of Tedworth, extended through two entire months,—a period sufficient, it would seem, for a family so strong-minded and stout-hearted as the Wesleys to detect any imposture. And, unless we are to suspect Emily Wesley of a superstition which her letters are very far from indicating, phenomena of a somewhat similar character accompanied her through a long lifetime.

Dr. Priestley, with all his skeptical leanings, speaking

---

* "*Memoirs of the Wesley Family*," vol. i. p. 286.

of the Epworth narrative, is fain to admit that "it is perhaps the best-authenticated and the best-told story of the kind that is anywhere extant."* He enters, however, into an argument to prove that there could be nothing supernatural in it; for which his chief reason is, that he could see no good to be answered by it. His conclusion is, "What appears most probable at this distance of time, in the present case, is, that it was a trick of the servants, assisted by some of the neighbors; and that nothing was meant by it besides puzzling the family and amusing themselves;" a supposition which Dr. Clarke rejects. He says, expressly, "The accounts given of these disturbances are so circumstantial and authentic as to entitle them to the most implicit credit. The eye and ear witnesses were persons of strong understandings and well-cultivated minds, untinctured by superstition, and in some instances rather skeptically inclined." And he adds, "Nothing apparently preternatural can lie further beyond the verge of imposture than these accounts; and the circumstantial statements contained in them force conviction of their truth on the minds of the incredulous."†

Southey, in his Life of Wesley, gives the account of these disturbances; and this is his comment upon it:—

"An author who, in this age, relates such a story and treats it as not utterly incredible and absurd, must expect to be ridiculed; but the testimony upon which it rests is far too strong to be set aside because of the strangeness of the relation." . . . "Such things may be preternatural, and yet not miraculous; they may not be in the ordinary course of nature, and yet imply no alteration of its laws. And with regard to the good end which they may be supposed to answer, it would be

* Dr. Priestley's pamphlet already cited, preface, p. xi.
† "*Memoirs of the Wesley Family*," vol. i. pp. 245, 246.

end sufficient if sometimes one of those unhappy persons who, looking through the dim glass of infidelity, see nothing beyond this life and the narrow sphere of mortal existence, should, from the well-established truth of one such story, (trifling and objectless as it might otherwise appear,) be led to a conclusion that there are more things in heaven and earth than are dreamed of in his philosophy."

Coleridge's opinion was very different. In his copy of Southey's work, which he left to Southey, he wrote, against the story of the Wesley disturbances, the following note:—"All these stories, and I could produce fifty, at least, equally well authenticated, and, as far as the veracity of the narrators and the single fact of their having seen and heard such and such sights or sounds, above all rational skepticism, are as much like one another as the symptoms of the same disease in different patients. And this, indeed, I take to be the true and only solution; a contagious nervous disease, the acme or intensest form of which is catalepsy.—S. T. C."*

It is an odd reason to allege *against* the credibility of such narratives that they are very numerous, and that in their general character they all agree. Nor is the short-cut by which the poet reaches an explanation of the phenomena less remarkable. Wesley and his family, he admits, *did* see and hear what they allege they did; but they were all cataleptics. What! the mastiff also?

It is not my purpose, however, here to comment on these conflicting opinions, but only to submit them. They all come from men of high character and standing.

I pass by various records of disturbances similar to the above, described as occurring in England and else-

* "*The Asylum Journal of Mental Science*" (published by an Association of Medical Officers of Asylums and Hospitals for the Insane) for April, 1858, London, p. 395.

where throughout the eighteenth century, because in the details given there is little beyond what is to be found in the foregoing, and because, as none of them are vouched for by names of such weight as those which attest the preceding examples, they will surely not be received if the others be rejected. Some of these are noticed in the journals of the day : for example, one recently disinterred from the columns of the " New York Packet," and which appeared in its issue of March 10, 1789. It is in the shape of a communication to the editor, dated Fishkill, March 3, 1789. The correspondent says,—

"Were I to relate the many extraordinary, though not less true, accounts I have heard concerning that unfortunate girl at New Havensack, your belief might perhaps be staggered and your patience tired. I shall therefore only inform you of what I have been eye-witness to. Last afternoon my wife and myself went to Dr. Thorn's; and, after sitting for some time, we heard a knocking under the feet of a young woman that lives in the family. I asked the doctor what occasioned the noise. He could not tell, but replied that he, together with several others, had examined the house, but were unable to discover the cause. I then took a candle and went with the girl into the cellar. There the knocking also continued; but, as we were ascending the stairs to return, I heard a prodigious rapping on each side, which alarmed me very much. I stood still some time, looking around with amazement, when I beheld some lumber which lay at the head of the stairs shake considerably.

"About eight or ten days after, we visited the girl again. The knocking still continued, but was much louder. Our curiosity induced us to pay the third visit, when the phenomena were still more alarming. I then saw the chairs move; a large dining-table was thrown against me; and a small stand, on which stood a candle, was tossed up and thrown in my wife's lap; after which we left the house, much surprised at what we had seen."

Others were published in pamphlets at the time; as, the disturbances in Mrs. Golding's dwelling and elsewhere at Stockwell, occurring on the 6th and 7th of January, 1772, chiefly marked by the moving about and destruction of furniture in various houses, but always in the presence of Mrs. Golding and her maid. The pamphlet is reprinted in a modern publication.*

This case, however, with several others, including that of the "electric girl" reported by Arago, seems to belong to a different class from those I am now relating; since in the latter the occult agency appears to have attached itself to persons and to have exhibited no intelligence.

Two other examples, of somewhat later date, and in which the annoyances suffered seem partly of a local, partly of a personal, character, will be found in that magazine, of which John Wesley was for many years the editor. They are probably from his pen.†

I pass on to an example occurring at the commencement of the present century on the continent of Europe.

---

* By Mrs. Crowe, in her "*Night Side of Nature,*" pp. 412 to 422. The pamphlet is entitled "An authentic, candid, and circumstantial narrative of the astonishing transactions at Stockwell, in the county of Surrey, on Monday and Tuesday, the 6th and 7th January, 1772, containing a series of the most surprising and unaccountable events that ever happened, which continued, from first to last, upwards of twenty hours, and at different places. Published with the consent and approbation of the family and other parties concerned, to authenticate which the original copy is signed by them."

† For the first, occurring to two sisters named Dixon, see the "*Arminian Magazine*" for the year 1786, pp. 660, 662. The disturbances commenced in 1779, and are said to have continued upward of six years. The second is given in the same magazine for 1787; commencing about a week before Christmas in the year 1780.

THE CASTLE OF SLAWENSIK.

Disturbances in Upper Silesia,

1806-07.

In the month of November, 1806, Councilor Hahn, attached to the court of the then reigning Prince of Hohenlohe Neuenstein-Ingelfingen, received orders from that prince to proceed to one of his castles in Upper Silesia, called Slawensik, there to await his orders. Hahn was accompanied by a certain Charles Kern, cornet in a hussar regiment, who had been taken prisoner by the French in a recent campaign against the Prussians, and had just returned on parole.

Both Hahn and Kern were in good health, and were men free from all taint of superstition. Hahn had been a student of philosophy under Fichte, was an admirer of Kant's doctrines, and at that time a confirmed materialist.

Having been intimate friends in youth, they occupied at Slawensik the same chamber. It was a corner room on the first floor, the windows looking out on the north and east. On the right, as one entered this room, was a glass door, opening through a wainscot partition into another room, in which household utensils were kept. This door was always kept locked. Neither in this latter room nor in that occupied by the two friends was there any opening communicating from without, except the windows. No one at that time resided in the castle besides Hahn and Kern, except Hahn's servant and two of the prince's coachmen.

It was under these circumstances and in this locality that the following disturbances occurred. They were written out by Hahn in November, 1808; and in 1828 the manuscript was communicated by the writer to Dr. Kerner, the author of the "Seeress of Prevorst," and by him first published as confirmatory of somewhat similar phenomena witnessed by himself in the case of the seeress. I translate the chief part of Hahn's narrative, omitting some portions in which he relates what others had reported to him; premising that it is written in the third person.

"On the third evening after their arrival in the castle, the two friends were sitting reading at a table in the middle of the room. About nine o'clock their occupation was interrupted by the frequent falling of small bits of lime over the room. They examined the ceiling, but could perceive no signs of their having fallen thence. As they were conversing of this, still larger pieces of lime fell around them. This lime was cold to the touch, as if detached from an outside wall.

"They finally set it down to the account of the old walls of the castle, and went to bed and to sleep. The next morning they were astonished at the quantity of lime that covered the floor, the more so as they could not perceive on walls or ceiling the slightest appearance of injury. By evening, however, the incident was forgotten, until not only the same phenomenon recurred, but bits of lime were thrown about the room, several of which struck Hahn. At the same time loud knockings, like the reports of distant artillery, were heard, sometimes as if on the floor, sometimes as if on the ceiling. Again the friends went to bed; but the loudness of the knocks prevented their sleeping. Kern accused Hahn of causing the knockings by striking on the boards that formed the under portion of his bedstead, and was not convinced of the contrary till he had taken the light and examined for himself. Then Hahn conceived a similar suspicion of Kern. The dispute was settled by both rising and standing close together, during which time the knockings continued as before. Next evening, besides the throwing of lime and the knockings, they heard another sound, resembling the distant beating of a drum.

"Thereupon they requested of a lady who had charge of the castle, Madame Knittel, the keys of the rooms above and below them; which she immediately sent them by her son. Hahn remained in the chamber below, while Kern and young Knittel went to examine the apartments in question. Above they found an empty room, below a kitchen. They knocked; but the sounds were entirely different from those that they had heard, and which Hahn at that very time continued to hear, in the room below. When they returned from their search, Hahn said, jestingly, 'The place is haunted.' They again went to bed, leaving the candles burning; but things became still more serious, for they distinctly heard a sound as if some one with loose slippers on were walking across the room; and this was accompanied also with a noise as of a walking-stick on which some one was leaning, striking the floor step by step; the person seeming, as far as one could judge by the sound, to be walking up and down the room. Hahn jested at this, Kern laughed, and both went to sleep, still not seriously disposed to ascribe these strange phenomena to any supernatural source.

"Next evening, however, it seemed impossible to ascribe the occurrences to any natural cause. The agency, whatever it was, began to throw various articles about the room; knives, forks, brushes, caps, slippers, padlocks, a funnel, snuffers, soap, in short, whatever was loose about the apartment. Even candlesticks flew about, first from one corner, then from another. If the things had been left lying as they fell, the whole room would have been strewed in utter confusion. At the same time, there fell, at intervals, more lime; but the knockings were discontinued. Then the friends called up the two coachmen and Hahn's servant, besides young

Knittel, the watchman of the castle, and others; all of whom were witnesses of these disturbances."

This continued for several nights; but all was usually quiet by morning,—sometimes by one o'clock at night. Hahn continues:—

"From the table, under their very eyes, snuffers and knives would occasionally rise, remain some time in the air, and then fall to the floor. In this way a large pair of scissors belonging to Hahn fell between him and one of the coachmen, and remained sticking in the floor.

"For a few nights it intermitted, then recommenced as before. After it had continued about three weeks, (during all which time Hahn persisted in remaining in the same apartment,) tired out, at length, with the noises which continually broke their rest, the two friends resolved to have their beds removed into the corner room above, so as to obtain, if possible, a quiet night's sleep. But the change was unavailing. The same loud knockings followed them; and they even remarked that articles were flung about the room which they were quite certain they had left in the chamber below. 'Let them fling as they will,' exclaimed Hahn: 'I must have sleep!' Kern, half undressed, paced the room in deep thought. Suddenly he stopped before a mirror, into which he chanced to look. After gazing upon it for some ten minutes, he began to tremble, turned deadly pale, and moved away. Hahn, thinking that he had been suddenly taken ill from the cold, hastened to him and threw a cloak over his shoulders. Then Kern, naturally a fearless man, took courage, and related to his friend, though still with quivering lips, that he had seen in the mirror the appearance of a female figure, in white, looking at him, and apparently before him, for he could see the reflection of himself behind it. It was some time before he could persuade himself that he really saw this figure; and for that reason he remained so long before the glass.   Willingly would he have believed that it was a mere trick of his imagination; but as the figure looked at him full in the face, and he could perceive its eyes move, a shudder passed over him, and he turned away. Hahn instantly went to the mirror and called upon the image to show itself to him; but, though he remained a quarter of an hour before it, and often repeated his invocation, he saw nothing.   Kern told him that the figure exhibited old but not disagreeable features, very pale but tranquil-looking; and that its head was covered with white drapery, so that the face only appeared. . . .

"By this time a month had passed; the story of these disturbances had spread over the neighborhood, and had been received by many with incredulity; among the rest, by two Bavarian officers of dragoons, named Cornet and Magerle.   The latter proffered to remain alone in the room; so the others left him there about twilight.   But they had been but a short time in the opposite room, when they heard Magerle swearing loudly, and also sounds as of saber-blows on tables and chairs.   So, for the sake of the furniture at least, they judged it prudent to look in upon Magerle.   When they asked him what was the matter, he replied, in a fury, 'As soon as you left, the cursed thing began pelting me with lime and other things.   I looked everywhere, but could see nobody; so I got in a rage, and cut with my saber right and left.' " . . .

This was enough for the dragoon-officers.   Hahn and Kern, meanwhile, had become so much accustomed to these marvels that they joked and amused themselves with them.   At last,—

"Hahn resolved that he would investigate them seriously.   He accordingly, one evening, sat down at his writing-table, with two lighted candles before him; being so placed that he could observe the whole room, and especially all the windows and doors.   He was left, for a time, entirely alone in the castle, the coachmen being in the stables, and Kern having gone out. Yet the very same occurrences took place as before; nay, the snuffers, under his very eyes, were raised and whirled about. He kept the strictest watch on the doors and windows; but nothing could be discovered.

"Several other persons witnessed these phenomena, at various times; a bookseller named Dörfel, and the Head Ranger Radezensky. This last remained with them all night. But no rest had he. He was kept awake with constant peltings. . . .

. "Inspector Knetch, from Koschentin, resolved to spend a night with Hahn and Kern. There was no end of the peltings they had during the evening; but finally they retired to rest, leaving the candles burning. Then all three saw two table-napkins rise to the ceiling in the middle of the room, there spread themselves out, and finally drop, fluttering, to the floor. A porcelain pipe-bowl, belonging to Kern, flew around and broke to pieces. Knives and forks flew about; a knife fell on Hahn's head, striking him, however, with the handle only. Thereupon it was resolved, as these disturbances had now continued throughout two months, to move out of the room. Kern and Hahn's servant carried a bed into the opposite chamber. No sooner had they gone, than a chalybeate water-bottle that was standing in the room moved close to the feet of the two who remained behind. A brass candlestick also, that appeared to come out of a corner of the room, fell to the ground, before them. In the room to which they removed, they spent a tolerably quiet night, though they could still hear noises in the room they had left. This was the last disturbance."

Hahn winds up his narration as follows:—

"The story remained a mystery. All reflection on these strange occurrences, all investigation, though most carefully made, to discover natural causes for them, left the observers in darkness. No one could suggest any possible means of effecting them, even had there been, which there was not, in the village or the neighborhood, any one capable of sleight of hand. And what motive could there be? The old castle was worth nothing, except to its owner. In short, one can perceive no imaginable purpose in the whole affair. It resulted but in the disturbing of some men, and in the frightening of others; but the occupants of the room became, during the two entire months that the occurrence lasted, as much accustomed to them as one can become to any daily recurring annoyance."*

The above narrative is subscribed and attested by Hahn as follows :—

"I saw and heard every thing, exactly as here set down; observing the whole carefully and quietly. I experienced no fear whatever; yet I am wholly unable to account for the occurrences narrated.

"Written this 19th of November, 1808.

"COUNCILOR HAHN."

Dr. Kerner, in the fourth edition of his " Seherin von Prevorst," informs us that the above narrative, when first printed by him, called forth various conjectured explanations of the mystery; the most plausible of which was, that Kern, being an adept in sleight of hand, had, for his amusement, thus made sport of his companion. When the doctor communicated this surmise to Hahn, the latter replied that, if there were no other cause for rejecting such a suspicion, the thing was rendered absolutely impossible by the fact that some of the manifestations occurred not only when he, Hahn, was entirely alone in the room, but even when Kern was temporarily absent on a journey. He adds, that Kern again and

---

* "*Die Seherin von Prevorst*," 4th ed., Stuttgart, 1846, pp. 495 to 504.

again urged him to leave the room; but that he, (Hahn,) still hoping to discover some natural explanation of these events, persisted in remaining. Their chief reason for leaving at last was Kern's regret for the destruction of his favorite pipe, an article of value, which he had bought in Berlin, and which he highly prized. He adds, that Kern died of a nervous fever, in the autumn of 1807.

Writing to Dr. Kerner on the subject, from Ingelfingen, under date 24th August, 1828, that is, more than twenty years after the events occurred, Hahn says, "I omitted no possible precautions to detect some natural cause. I am usually accused of too great skepticism rather than of superstition. Cowardice is not my fault, as those who know me intimately will testify. I could rely, therefore, on myself; and I can have been under no illusion as to the facts, for I often asked the spectators, 'What did you see?' and each time from their replies I learned that they had seen exactly the same as I did myself." . . . "I am at this moment entirely at a loss to assign any cause, or even any reasonable surmise, in explanation of these events. To me, as to all who witnessed them, they have remained a riddle to this day. One must expect hasty judgments to be passed on such occurrences; and even in relating what has not only been seen by oneself but also by others yet alive, one must be satisfied to incur the risk of being regarded as the dupe of an illusion."*

Dr. Kerner further adds, that, in the year 1830, a gentleman of the utmost respectability, residing in Stuttgart, visited Slawensik for the purpose of verifying the above narrative. He there found persons who ridiculed the whole as a deceit; but the only two men he met with, survivors of those who had actually witnessed the events, confirmed to him the accuracy of Hahn's narrative in every particular.

* "Seherin von Prevorst," pp. 506, 507.

This gentleman further ascertained that the Castle of Slawensik had been since destroyed, and that, in clearing away the ruins, there was found a male skeleton walled in and without coffin, with the skull split open. By the side of this skeleton lay a sword.

This being communicated to Hahn, he replies, very rationally, "One may imagine some connection between the discovered skeleton, the female image seen by Kern, and the disturbances we witnessed; but who can really know any thing about it?" And he adds, finally,—

"It matters nothing to me whether others believe my narrative or not. I recollect very well what I myself thought of such things before I had actually witnessed them, and I take it ill of nobody that he should pass upon them the same judgment which I would have passed previous to experience. A hundred witnesses will work no conviction in those who have made up their minds never to believe in any thing of the kind. I give myself no trouble about such persons; for it would be labor lost."

This last letter of Hahn's is dated May, 1831. During a quarter of a century, therefore, he retained, and reiterated, his conviction of the reality and unexplained character of the disturbances at Slawensik.

From the same source whence the above is derived, I select another example, of a later date, and which has the advantage of having been witnessed by Kerner himself.

THE SEERESS OF PREVORST.

Disturbances in the village of Oberstenfeld,

1825–26.

Amid the mountains of Northern Wurtemberg, in the village of Prevorst, there was born, in the year 1801, Madame Fredericke Hauffe, since well known to the

world through Dr. Kerner's history of her life and
sufferings, as the "Seeress of Prevorst."*

Even as a child Madame Hauffe was in the habit of
seeing what she believed to be disembodied spirits, not
usually perceptible, however, by those around her; and
this peculiarity, whether actual faculty or mere hallucination, accompanied her through life.

Kerner gives many examples. Throughout the year
1825, while residing in the village of Oberstenfeld, not
far from Löwenstein, in the northern portion of the
kingdom of Wurtemberg, Madame Hauffe was visited,
or believed herself to be so, by the appearance, usually
in the evening, about seven o'clock, of a male figure of
dark complexion, which, she alleged, constantly begged
for her prayers. With the question of the reality of
this appearance I have here nothing to do; but I invite
attention to the attendant circumstances. Kerner
says,—

"Each time before he appeared, his coming was announced to all present, without exception, by the sound
of knockings or rappings, sometimes on one wall, sometimes on another, sometimes by a sort of clapping in

---

* "*Die Seherin von Prevorst*, Eröffnungen über das innere Leben des
Menschen, und über das Hereinragen einer Geisterwelt in die unsere." By
Justinus Kerner, 4th ed., Stuttgart and Tubingen, 1846, 8vo, pp. 559.

This work, of which there is an English translation by Mrs. Crowe, attracted much attention and criticism at the time of its first appearance, and
since. It was reviewed in the "Revue des Deux Mondes" of July 15, 1842,
and there spoken of as "one of the most strange and most conscientiously
elaborated works that has ever appeared on such a subject." Of Dr. Kerner
himself the reviewer speaks as one of the ornaments of Germany.

Another Review, of February, 1846, notices in terms equally favorable
the work and its author. It accords to Kerner a high reputation in his
own country, not only as physician, but for his literary talents, and as a man
of learning and of piety,—a man whose sincerity and good faith cannot be
doubted even by the most skeptical. The reviewer further declares that the
book itself contains many truths which will have to be admitted into our
system of physiology and psychology.

the air, and other sounds, in the middle of the room. Of this there are still living more than twenty unimpeachable witnesses.

"By day and by night were heard the sounds of some one going up-stairs; but, seek as we would, it was impossible to discover any one. In the cellar the same knockings were heard, and they increased in loudness. If the knocking was heard behind a barrel, and if any one ran hastily to look behind it and detect the cause, the knockings immediately changed to the front of the barrel; and when one returned to the front they were again heard behind. The same thing occurred when it knocked on the walls of the room. If the knockings were heard outside, and one ran suddenly out to the spot, it immediately knocked inside; and *vice versa.*

"If the kitchen door was fastened at night ever so securely, even tied with twine, it stood open in the morning. It was constantly heard to open and shut; yet, though one might rush to it instantly, no one could be seen to enter or depart.

"Once, at about eleven o'clock at night, the disturbance was so violent that it shook the whole house; and the heavy beams and rafters moved back and forth. Madame Hauffe's father, on this occasion, had nearly decided to abandon the house the next day." . . .

"The poundings and cracking of the house were heard by passers-by in the street. At other times the knockings in the cellar had been such that all those who were passing stopped to listen.

"Glasses were often removed from the table, (and, on one occasion, the bottle,) as if by an invisible hand, and placed on the floor. So also the paper was taken from her father's writing-table, and thrown at him.

"Madame Hauffe visited Löwenstein; and there also the knockings and rappings were heard."

The last of the alleged visits of this spirit was on the

6tn of January, 1826. The above occurrences had been repeated, at intervals, throughout an entire year.

There are various other examples of similar character in Kerner's book; but it is useless to multiply them.

As we approach our own time, the records of such disturbances as we are here examining so increase in number that space fails me to reproduce them. I select the following as a sample, because the evidence adduced in proof that the phenomena were real, and that no mundane agency capable of producing them was ever discovered, is of a character such as daily decides questions touching men's property and lives.

THE LAW-SUIT.
Disturbances in a dwelling-house near Edinburgh,
1835.

This case is remarkable as having given rise to legal proceedings on the part of the owner of the house reputed to be haunted. It is related by Mrs. Crowe in her "Night Side of Nature;" and the particulars were communicated to her by the gentleman who conducted the suit for the plaintiff.* She does not give his name; but from an Edinburgh friend I have ascertained that it was Mr. Maurice Lothian, a Scottish solicitor, now Procurator Fiscal of the county of Edinburgh.

A certain Captain Molesworth rented the house in question, situated at Trinity, two miles from Edinburgh, from a Mr. Webster, in May, 1835. After two months' residence there, the captain began to complain of certain unaccountable noises, which, strangely enough, he took it into his head were made by his landlord, Mr. Webster, who occupied the adjoining dwelling. The latter naturally represented that it was not probable he should desire to damage the reputation of his own

---

* "Night Side of Nature," Routledge and Co.'s edition, pp. 445 to 447.

house, or drive a responsible tenant out of it; and re-torted the accusation. Meanwhile the disturbances continued daily and nightly. Sometimes there was the sound as of invisible feet; sometimes there were knock-ings, scratchings, or rustlings, first on one side, then on the other. Occasionally the unseen agent seemed to be rapping to a certain tune, and would answer, by so many knocks, any question to which the reply was in numbers; as, "How many persons are there in this room?" So forcible at times were the poundings that the wall trembled visibly. Beds, too, were occasionally heaved up, as by some person underneath. Yet, search as they would, no one could be found. Captain Moles-worth caused the boards to be lifted in the rooms where the noises were loudest and most frequent, and actually perforated the wall that divided his residence from that of Mr. Webster; but without the least result. Sheriff's officers, masons, justices of the peace, and the officers of the regiment quartered at Leith, who were friends of Captain Molesworth, came to his aid, in hopes of de-tecting or frightening away his tormentor; but in vain. Suspecting that it might be some one outside the house, they formed a cordon round it; but all to no purpose. No solution of the mystery was ever obtained.

Suit was brought before the Sheriff of Edinburgh, by Mr. Webster, against Captain Molesworth, for damages committed by lifting the boards, boring the walls, and firing at the wainscot, as well as for injury done in giving the house the reputation of being haunted, thus preventing other tenants from renting it. On the trial, the facts above stated were all elicited by Mr. Lothian, who spent several hours in examining numerous wit-nesses, some of them officers of the army and gentle-men of undoubted honor and capacity for observation.

It remains to be stated that Captain Molesworth had had two daughters; one of whom, named Matilda, had lately died, while the other, a girl between twelve and thirteen, named Jane, was sickly and usually kept her bed. It being observed that wherever the sick girl was, the noises more frequently prevailed, Mr. Webster declared that she made them; and it would seem that her father himself must, to some extent, have shared the suspicion; for the poor girl was actually tied up in a bag, so as to prevent all possible agency on her part. No cessation or diminution of the disturbance was, however, obtained by this harsh expedient.

The people in the neighborhood believed that the noises were produced by the ghost of Matilda warning her sister that she was soon to follow; and this belief received confirmation when that unfortunate young lady, whose illness may have been aggravated by the severe measures dictated by unjust suspicion, shortly after died.

Occasionally such narratives are published as mere specimens of a vulgar superstition, as by Mackay, in his work on "Popular Delusions." He notices, as one of the latest examples of the panic occasioned by a house supposed to be haunted, incidents that took place— like those just narrated—in Scotland, and that occurred some twenty years ago, regarding which he supplies the following particulars.

THE FARM-HOUSE OF BALDARROCH.

Disturbances in Aberdeenshire, Scotland,

1838.

" On the 5th of December, 1838, the inmates of the farm-house of Baldarroch, in the district of Banchory, Aberdeenshire, were alarmed by observing a great number of sticks, pebble-stones, and clods of earth flying about their yard and premises. They endeavored, but in vain, to discover who was the delinquent, and, the shower of stones continuing for five days in succession they came at last to the conclusion that the devil and his imps were alone the cause of it. The rumor soon spread all over that part of the country, and hundreds of persons came from far and near to witness the antics of the devils of Baldarroch. After the fifth day, the showers of clods and stones ceased on the outside of the premises, and the scene shifted to the interior. Spoons, knives, plates, mustard-pots, rolling-pins, and flat-irons appeared suddenly endued with the power of self-motion, and were whirled from room to room, and rattled down the chimneys, in a manner nobody could account for. The lid of a mustard-pot was put into a cupboard by a servant-girl, in the presence of scores of people, and in a few minutes afterward came bouncing down the chimney, to the consternation of everybody. There was also a tremendous knocking at the doors and on the roof, and pieces of stick and pebble-stones rattled against the windows and broke them. The whole neighborhood was a scene of alarm; and not only the vulgar, but persons of education, respectable farmers within a circle of twenty miles, expressed their belief in the supernatural character of these events."

The excitement, Mackay goes on to state, spread, within a week, over the parishes of Banchory-Ternan, Drumoak, Durris, Kincardine O'Neil, and all the adjacent district of Mearns and Aberdeenshire. It was affirmed and believed that all horses and dogs that approached the farm-house were immediately affected. The mistress of the house and the servant-girls said that whenever they went to bed they were pelted with pebbles and other missiles. The farmer himself traveled a distance of forty miles to an old conjurer, named Willie Foreman, to induce him, for a handsome fee, to remove the enchantment from his property. The heritor, the minister, and all the elders of the kirk instituted an investigation, which, however, does not appear to have had any result.

"After a fortnight's continuance of the noises," says Mackay, "the whole trick was discovered. The two servant-lasses were strictly examined, and then committed to prison. It appeared that they were alone at the bottom of the whole affair, and that the extraordinary alarm and credulity of their master and mistress in the first instance, and of the neighbors and country-people afterwards, made their task comparatively easy. A little common dexterity was all they had used; and, being themselves unsuspected, they swelled the alarm by the wonderful stories they invented. It was they who loosened the bricks in the chimneys and placed the dishes in such a manner on the shelves that they fell on the slightest motion."*

The proof that the girls were the authors of all the mischief appears to have rested on the fact that "no sooner were they secured in the county gaol than the noises ceased;" and thus, says Mackay, "most people were convinced that human agency alone had worked all the wonder." Others, however, he admits, still held out in their first belief, and were entirely dissatisfied with the explanation, as indeed they very well might be, if we are to trust to the details given by Mackay himself of these disturbances.

For five days a shower of sticks, stones, and clods of earth are seen flying about the yard and are thrown against the windows.† Hundreds of persons come to

---

* "*Popular Delusions*," vol. ii. pp. 133 to 136.

† This phenomenon, strange as it seems, is exactly paralleled in a recent case recorded in the "Gazette des Tribunaux" and noticed by De Mirville in his work "*Des Esprits*," pp. 381 to 384. It occurred in Paris, in the populous quarter of Montagne-Sainte-Geneviève. A house on the street des Grès was pelted, *for twenty-one nights in succession*, by a shower of heavy missiles, driven against it in such quantities, and with such violence, that

witness the phenomenon, and none of them can account for it. Is it credible, is it conceivable, that two girls, employed all day in menial duties under the eye of their mistress, should, by "a little common dexterity," have continued such a practical joke for five *hours*—to say nothing of five days—without being inevitably detected? Then various utensils in the house not only move, as if self-impelled, about the room, but are whirled from one room to another, or dropped down the chimney, in presence of crowds of witnesses. There is a tremendous knocking at the doors and on the roof, and the windows are broken by sticks and pebble-stones that rattle against them. This farce is kept up *for ten days more*, making the whole neighborhood a scene of alarm, baffling the ingenuity of heritor, minister, and elders; and we are asked to believe that it was all a mere prank of two servant-girls, effected by loosening a few bricks in the chimney and placing the crockery so that it fell on slight motion! A notable specimen, surely, of the credulousness of incredulity!

One can understand that a court of justice should ad-

---

the front of the house was actually pierced in some places, the doors and windows were shattered to atoms, and the whole exhibited the appearance of a building that had stood a siege against stones from catapults or discharges of grape-shot. The "Gazette" says, "Whence come these projectiles, which are pieces of pavement, fragments of old houses, entire blocks of building-stone, which, from their weight and from the distance whence they came, could not have been hurled by the hand of man? Up to this day it has been impossible to discover the cause." Yet the police, headed by the Chief of Police himself, was out every night, and placed a guard on the premises night and day. They employed, also, fierce dogs as guards; but all in vain.

De Mirville some time afterward called personally on the proprietor of the house, and on the Commissary of Police of that quarter. Both assured him in the most positive terms that, notwithstanding the constant precautions taken by a body of men unmatched for vigilance and sagacity, not the slightest clew to the mystery had ever been obtained. (pp. 384 to 386.)

mit, as presumptive proof against the girls, the fact that from the time they were lodged in jail the disturbances ceased. With the lights before them, the presumption was not unreasonable. But I have already adduced some proof, and shall hereafter add more,* that such disturbances appear to attach to individuals (or, in other words, to occur in certain localities in their presence) without any agency—at least, any conscious agency—on the part of those persons themselves.

Other narratives of this class, already in print, might here be introduced, did space permit. I instance one or two.

In "Douglas Jerrold's Journal" of March 26, 1847, is the narrative of disturbances in the family of a Mr. Williams, residing in Moscow Road. Utensils and furniture were moved about and destroyed, almost exactly as in the case of Mrs. Golding and her maid. There is no record, however, of any knockings on the walls or floor.

A similar case is detailed in the "*Revue Française*" for December, 1846, as having occurred in the house of a farmer at Clairefontaine, near Rambouillet.

A narrative more remarkable and detailed than either of these will be found in Spicer's ".Facts and Fantasies," as furnished in manuscript to the author by Mrs. E., a lady of fortune,—the disturbances running through *four years*, namely, from August, 1844, to September, 1848. Here there were knockings and trampings so loud as to shake the whole house, besides

---

* Of such examples, one of the most remarkable is that of the so-called "Electric Girl," examined by Arago. I had carefully prepared a narrative of this case from the original authorities, intending to introduce it here; but, finding this volume swelling beyond the dimensions to which I had resolved to restrict it, I threw the story out, and may publish it in a future work.

openings of doors and windows, ringing of bells, noises
as of moving of furniture, the rustling, in the very
room, of a silk dress, the shaking of the beds in which
they lay, the sound of carriages driving in the park
when none were there, &c. This narrative is supported by the certificates of servants and of a police
constable, who was summoned to remain at night on
the premises and to seek to discover the cause of these
annoyances. Some of the servants left the family,
unable to endure the terror and loss of sleep. Mr. E.
himself, after struggling for years against it, finally left
the estate of L——, where the disturbances took place,
with the intention never to return to it.*

These may be referred to by the curious. The following narrative, however, is so remarkable in itself,
and comes to me so directly from the original source,
that it would be doing injustice to the subject to omit
or abridge it.

THE CEMETERY OF AHRENSBURG.

Disturbances in a Chapel in the Island of Oesel,†
1844.

In the immediate vicinity of Ahrensburg, the only
town in the island of Oesel, is the public cemetery.
Tastefully laid out and carefully kept, planted with
trees and partly surrounded by a grove dotted with
evergreens, it is a favorite promenade of the inhabitants. Besides its tombs,—in every variety, from the
humblest to the most elaborate,—it contains several
private chapels, each the burying-place of some family
of distinction. Underneath each of these is a vault,

---

* *"Facts and Fantasies;"* a sequel to "Sights and Sounds, the Mystery
of the Day;" by Henry Spicer, Esq., London, 1853, pp. 76 to 101.

† The island of Oesel, in the Baltic, is possessed by Russia, having
been ceded to that Power, by the Treaty of Nystadt, in 1721. It constitutes
part of Livonia.

paved with wood, to which the descent is by a stairway from inside the chapel and closed by a door. The coffins of the members of the family more recently deceased usually remain for a time in the chapel. They are afterward transferred to the vaults, and there placed side by side, elevated on iron bars. These coffins it is the custom to make of massive oak, very heavy and strongly put together.

The public highway passes in front of the cemetery and at a short distance therefrom. Conspicuous, and to be seen by the traveler as he rides by, are three chapels, facing the highway. Of these the most spacious, adorned with pillars in front, is that belonging to the family of Buxhoewden, of patrician descent, and originally from the city of Bremen. It has been their place of interment for several generations.

It was the habit of the country-people, coming in on horseback or with carts on a visit to the cemetery, to fasten their horses, usually with very stout halters, immediately in front of this chapel, and close to the pillars that adorned it. This practice continued, notwithstanding that, for some eight or ten years previous to the incidents about to be narrated, there had been from time to time vague rumors of a mysterious kind connected with the chapel in question as being haunted,—rumors which, however, as they could not be traced to any reliable source, were little credited and were treated by its owners with derision.

The chief season of resort to the cemetery by persons from all parts of the island whose relatives lay buried there was on Pentecost Sunday and the succeeding days,—these being there observed much in the same manner as in most Catholic countries All-Souls Day usually is.*

---

* The religion of the island is the Protestant; though of late years attempts have been made to procure converts to the Greek Church.

On the second day of Pentecost, Monday, the 22d
of June, (New Style,) in the year 1844, the wife of a
certain tailor named Dalmann, living in Ahrensburg, had
come with a horse and small cart to visit, with her children, the tomb of her mother, situated behind the Buxhoewden family chapel, and had fastened her horse, as
usual, in front of it, without unharnessing him, proposing, as soon as she had completed her devotions, to
visit a friend in the country.

While kneeling in silent prayer by the grave, she had
an indistinct perception, as she afterward remembered,
that she heard some noises in the direction of the
chapel; but, absorbed in other thoughts, she paid at the
time no attention to it. Her prayers completed, and
returning to prosecute her journey, she found her
horse—usually a quiet animal—in an inexplicable state
of excitement. Covered with sweat and foam, its limbs
trembling, it appeared to be in mortal terror. When
she led it off, it seemed scarcely able to walk; and, instead of proceeding on her intended excursion, she found
herself obliged to return to town and to call a veterinary
surgeon. He declared that the horse must have been
excessively terrified from some cause or other, bled it,
administered a remedy, and the animal recovered.

A day or two afterward, this woman, coming to the
chateau of one of the oldest noble families of Livonia,
the Barons de Guldenstubbé, near Ahrensburg, as was
her wont, to do needle-work for the family, related to the
baron the strange incident which had occurred to her.
He treated it lightly, imagining that the woman exaggerated, and that her horse might have been accidentally
frightened.

The circumstance would have been soon forgotten
had it not been followed by others of a similar character. The following Sunday several persons, who
had attached their horses in front of the same

chapel, reported that they found them covered with sweat, trembling, and in the utmost terror; and some among them added that they had themselves heard, seeming to proceed from the vaults of the chapel, rumbling sounds, which occasionally (but this might have been the effect of imagination) assumed the character of groans.

And this was but the prelude to further disturbances, gradually increasing in frequency. One day in the course of the next month (July) it happened that eleven horses were fastened close to the columns of the chapel. Some persons, passing near by, and hearing, as they alleged, loud noises,* as if issuing from beneath the building, raised the alarm; and when the owners reached the spot they found the poor animals in a pitiable condition. Several of them, in their frantic efforts to escape, had thrown themselves on the ground, and lay struggling there; others were scarcely able to walk or stand; and all were violently affected, so that it became necessary immediately to resort to bleeding and other means of relief. In the case of three or four of them these means proved unavailing. They died within a day or two.

This was serious. And it was the cause of a formal complaint being made by some of the sufferers to the Consistory,—a court holding its sittings at Ahrensburg and having charge of ecclesiastical affairs.

About the same time, a member of the Buxhoewden family died. At his funeral, during the reading in the chapel of the service for the dead, what seemed groans and other strange noises were heard from beneath, to

---

* *Getöse* was the German word employed by the narrator in speaking to me of these sounds. It is the term often used to designate the rolling of distant thunder. Schiller says, in his " *Taucher*,"—

" Und wie mit des fernen Donner's Getöse—"

the great terror of some of the assistants, the servants especially. The horses attached to the hearse and to the mourning-coaches were sensibly affected, but not so violently as some of the others had been. After the interment, three or four of those who had been present, bolder than their neighbors, descended to the vault. While there they heard nothing; but they found, to their infinite surprise, that, of the numerous coffins which had been deposited there in due order side by side, almost all had been displaced and lay in a confused pile. They sought in vain for any cause that might account for this. The doors were always kept carefully fastened, and the locks showed no signs of having been tampered with. The coffins were replaced in due order.

This incident caused much talk, and, of course, attracted additional attention to the chapel and the alleged disturbances. Children were left to watch the horses when any were fastened in its vicinity; but they were usually too much frightened to remain; and some of them even alleged that they had seen some dark-looking specters hovering in the vicinity. The stories, however, related by them on this latter head were set down—reasonably enough, perhaps—to account of their excited fears. But parents began to scruple about taking their children to the cemetery at all.

The excitement increasing, renewed complaints on the subject reached the Consistory, and an inquiry into the matter was proposed. The owners of the chapel at first objected to this, treating the matter as a trick or a scandal set on foot by their enemies. But though they carefully examined the floor of the vault, to make sure that no one had entered from beneath, they could find nothing to confirm their suspicions. And, the Baron de Guldenstubbé, who was president of the Consistory, having visited the vaults privately in company with two members of the family, and having found the coffins again in the same disorder, they finally, after restoring the coffins to their places, assented to an official investigation of the affair.

The persons charged with this investigation were the Baron de Guldenstubbé, as president, and the bishop of the province, as vice-president, of the Consistory; two other members of the same body; a physician, named Luce; and, on the part of the magistracy of the town, the burgomeister, named Schmidt, one of the syndics, and a secretary.

They proceeded, in a body, to institute a careful examination of the vault. All the coffins there deposited, with the exception of three, were found this time, as before, displaced. Of the three coffins forming the exception, one contained the remains of a grandmother of the then representative of the family, who had died about five years previous; and the two others were of young children. The grandmother had been, in life, revered almost as a saint, for her great piety and constant deeds of charity and benevolence.

The first suggestion which presented itself, on discovering this state of things, was that robbers might have broken in for the sake of plunder. The vault of an adjoining chapel *had* been forcibly entered some time before, and the rich velvet and gold fringe which adorned the coffins had been cut off and stolen. But the most careful examination failed to furnish any grounds for such a supposition in the present case. The ornaments of the coffins were found untouched. The commission caused several to be opened, in order to ascertain whether the rings or other articles of jewelry which it was customary to bury with the corpses, and some of which were of considerable value,

23

had been taken. No indication of this kind, however, appeared. One or two of the bodies had moldered almost to dust; but the trinkets known to have formed part of the funeral apparel still lay there, at the bottom of the coffins.

It next occurred, as a possibility, to the commission, that some enemies of the Buxhoewden family, wealthy, perhaps, and determined to bring upon them annoyance and reproach, might have caused to be excavated a subterranean passage, its entrance at a distance and concealed so as to avoid observation, and the passage itself passing under the foundations of the building and opening into the vault. This might furnish sufficient explanation of the disarray of the coffins and of the noises heard from without.

To determine the point, they procured workmen, who took up the pavement of the vault and carefully examined the foundations of the chapel; but without any result. The most careful scrutiny detected no secret entrance.

Nothing remained but to replace every thing in due order, taking exact note of the position of the coffins, and to adopt especial precautions for the detection of any future intrusion. This, accordingly, was done. Both doors, the inner and the outer, after being carefully locked, were doubly sealed; first with the official seal of the Consistory, then with that bearing the arms of the city. Fine wood-ashes were strewed all over the wooden pavement of the vault, the stairs leading down to it from the chapel, and the floor of the chapel itself. Finally, guards, selected from the garrison of the town and relieved at short intervals, were set for three days and nights to watch the building and prevent any one from approaching it.

At the end of that time the commission of inquiry returned to ascertain the result. Both doors were found securely locked and the seals inviolate. They entered The coating of ashes still presented a smooth, unbroken surface. Neither in the chapel nor on the stairway leading to the vault was there the trace of a footstep, of man or animal. The vault was sufficiently lighted from the chapel to make every object distinctly visible. They descended. With beating hearts, they gazed on the spectacle before them. Not only was every coffin, with the same three exceptions as before, displaced, and the whole scattered in confusion over the place, but many of them, weighty as they were, had been set on end, so that the head of the corpse was downward. Nor was even this all. The lid of one coffin had been partially forced open, and there projected the shriveled right arm of the corpse it contained, showing beyond the elbow; the lower arm being turned up toward the ceiling of the vault!

The first shock over which this astounding sight produced, the commission proceeded carefully to take note, in detail, of the condition of things as they found them.

No trace of human footstep was discovered in the vault, any more than on the stairs or in the chapel. Nor was there detected the slightest indication of any felonious violation. A second search verified the fact that neither the external ornaments of the coffins nor the articles of jewelry with which some of the corpses had been decorated were abstracted. Every thing was disarranged; nothing was taken.

They approached, with some trepidation, the coffin from one side of which the arm projected; and, with a shudder, they recognized it as that in which had been placed the remains of a member of the Buxhoewden family who had committed suicide. The matter had been hushed up at the time, through the influence of the family, and the self-destroyer had been buried with the usual ceremonies; but the fact transpired, and was known all over the island, that he was found with his throat cut and the bloody razor still grasped in his right hand,—the same hand that was now thrust forth to human view from under the coffin-lid; a ghastly memorial, it seemed, of the rash deed which had ushered the unhappy man, uncalled, into another world!

An official report setting forth the state of the vault and of the chapel at the time when the commission set seals upon the doors, verifying the fact that the seals were afterward found unbroken and the coating of ashes intact, and, finally, detailing the condition of things as they appeared when the commission revisited the chapel at the end of the three days, was made out by the Baron de Guldenstubbé, as president, and signed by himself, by the bishop, the burgomeister, the physician, and the other members of the commission, as witnesses. This document, placed on record with the other proceedings of the Consistory, is to be found among its archives, and may be examined by any travelers, respectably recommended, on application to its secretary.

Never having visited the island of Oesel, I had not an opportunity of personally inspecting this paper. But the facts above narrated were detailed to me by Mademoiselle de Guldenstubbé,* daughter of the baron, who was residing in her father's house at the time and was cognizant of each minute particular. They were confirmed to me, also, on the same occasion, by her brother, the present baron.

This lady informed me that the circumstances produced so great an excitement throughout the whole island, that there could not have been found, among its fifty thousand inhabitants, a cottage inmate to whom they were not familiar. She added that the effect upon the physician, M. Luce, a witness of these marvels, was

---

* At Paris, on the 8th of May, 1859.

such as to produce a radical change in his creed. An able man, distinguished in his profession, familiar, too, with the sciences of botany, mineralogy, and geology, and the author of several works of repute on these subjects, he had imbibed the materialistic doctrines that were prevalent, especially among scientific men, throughout continental Europe, in his college days; and these he retained until the hour when, in the Buxhoewden vault, he became convinced that there are ultramundane as well as earthly powers, and that this is not our final state of existence.

It remains to be stated that, as the disturbances continued for several months after this investigation, the family, in order to get rid of the annoyance, resolved to try the effect of burying the coffins. This they did, covering them up, to a considerable depth, with earth. The expedient succeeded. From that time forth no noises were heard to proceed from the chapel; horses could be fastened with impunity before it; and the inhabitants, recovering from their alarm, frequented with their children, as usual, their favorite resort. Nothing remained but the memory of the past occurrences,—to fade away as the present generation dies out, and perhaps to be regarded by the next as an idle legend of the incredible.

To us, meanwhile, it is more than a legend. Fifteen years only have elapsed since the date of its occurrence. We have the testimony of living witnesses to its truth.

The salient points in the narrative are, first, the extreme terror of the animals, ending, in two or three cases, in death; and, secondly, the official character of the investigation, and the minute precautions taken by the commission of inquiry to prevent or detect deception.

23*

The evidence resulting from the first point is of the strongest kind. In such a case it is impossible that animals should simulate; equally impossible that they should be acted upon by imagination. Their terror was real, and had a real and adequate cause. But can the cause be considered adequate if we set down these noises as of an ordinary character? A common sound, much louder and more startling than we can suppose those from the chapel to have been,—thunder, for instance, when at no great distance,—often frightens horses, but never, so far as I know or have heard, to such a degree as to produce death.

To say nothing of the well-known case recorded in Scripture,* various examples more or less analogous to the above will be found throughout this volume.

As to the additional proof supplied by the result of the official inquiry, it is difficult, under any supposition, to explain it away. The only hypothesis, short of ultra-mundane interference, that seems left to us is that which occurred to the commission,—namely, the possibility of an underground passage. But, even if we consent to believe that these gentlemen, after the suggestion occurred to them and they had sent for workmen expressly to resolve their doubts, could yet suffer the work to be so carelessly done that the secret entrance escaped them at last, another difficulty remains. The vault had a wooden pavement. A portion of this, indeed, could be easily raised by a person desiring to effect an entrance. But, after a coat of ashes had been strewn over it, how could any one, working from beneath, replace it so as to leave on the surface of the ashes no trace of the operation?

Finally, if these disturbances are to be ascribed to trickery, why should the tricksters have discontinued

---

* Numbers xxii. 23.

their persecution as soon as the coffins were put under ground?

This last difficulty, however, exists equally in case we adopt the spiritual hypothesis. If to interference from another world these phenomena were due, why should that interference have ceased from the moment the coffins were buried?

And for what object, it may on the same supposition be further asked, such interference at all? It appears to have effected the conversion from materialism of the attendant physician,—possibly of others; but is that sufficient reply?

By many it will be deemed insufficient. But, even if it be, our ignorance of Divine motive cannot invalidate facts. We are not in the habit of denying such phenomena as an eruption of Vesuvius, or a devastating earthquake, on account of our inability to comprehend why Providence ordains them.

It remains at last, therefore, a simple question of fact. Having stated the circumstances exactly as I had them from a source as direct as can well be, and having added the suggestions to which in my mind they give rise, it rests with the reader to assign to each the weight which he may think it merits.

All these occurrences, it will be observed, date previous to the spring of March, 1848, when the first disturbances, the origin of Spiritualism in the United States, took place in the Fox family, and cannot, therefore, by possibility be imagined to have resulted from that movement. The same may be said of other European narratives of a somewhat later date; for it was not until the commencement of the year 1852 that the excitement which gradually followed the Rochester knockings attained such an extension as to cause the phenomena of rapping and table-turning to be known and talked of in Europe.

From the latter I select one, the circumstances connected with which gave rise, as in a previous example, to legal proceedings; and I restrict myself to the evidence given under oath in the course of trial. We can scarcely obtain stronger testimony for any past occurrence whatever.

THE CIDEVILLE PARSONAGE.

Disturbances in the Department of the Seine, France,

1850–51.

In the winter of 1850–51, certain disturbances of an extraordinary character occurred in the parsonage of Cideville, a village and commune near the town of Yerville, in the Department of Seine-Inférieure, about thirty-five miles east of Havre, and eighty miles northwest of Paris. This parsonage was occupied by M. Tinel, parish priest and curate of Cideville.

The rise and continuance of these disturbances appeared to depend on the presence of two children, then of the age of twelve and fourteen respectively, sons of respectable parents, themselves of amiable dispositions and good character, who had been intrusted to the care of the curate to be educated for the priesthood, and who resided in the parsonage.

The disturbances commenced, in the presence of these children, on the 26th of November, 1850, and continued daily, or almost daily,—usually in the room or rooms in which the children were,—for upward of *two months and a half*, namely, until the 15th of February, 1851, the day on which the children, by order of the Archbishop of Paris, were removed from the parsonage. From that day all noises and other disturbances ceased.*

---

* The children, when taken from M. Tinel, were intrusted to the care

It so happened, from certain circumstances preceding and attendant upon these strange phenomena,—chiefly, however, it would seem, in consequence of his own idle boasts of secret powers and knowledge of the black arts,—that a certain shepherd residing in the neighboring commune of Anzouville-l'Esvenal, named Felix Thorel, gradually came to be suspected, by the more credulous, of practicing sorcery against the children, and thus causing the disturbances at the parsonage which had alarmed and excited the neighborhood. It appears that the curate, Tinel, shared to some extent this popular fancy, and expressed the opinion that the shepherd was a sorcerer and the author of the annoyances in question.

Thereupon Thorel, having lost his place as shepherd in consequence of such suspicions, brought suit for defamation of character against the curate, laying the damages at twelve hundred francs. The trial was commenced before the justice of the peace of Yerville on the 7th of January, 1851, witnesses heard (to the number of eighteen for the prosecution and sixteen for the defense) on the 28th of January and succeeding days, and final judgment rendered on the 4th of February following.

In that document, after premising that, "whatever might be the cause of the extraordinary facts which occurred at the parsonage of Cideville, it is clear, from the sum total of the testimony adduced, that the cause of these facts still remains unknown;" after premising further "that although, on the one part, the defendant, (the curate,) according to several witnesses, did declare that the prosecutor (the shepherd) had boasted of producing the disturbances at the parsonage of Cideville,

of M. Fauvel, parish priest of St. Ouen du Breuil, who testifies to their good character and conduct. See his letter in De Mirville's pamphlet, "*Fragment d'un Ouvrage inédit.*" It does not appear that the disturbances followed them to their new home.

8

and did express his (the defendant's) own suspicions that he (the prosecutor) was the author of them, yet, on the other hand, it is proved by numerous witnesses that the said prosecutor had said and done whatever lay in his power to persuade the public that he actually had a hand in their perpetration, and particularly by his vaunts to the witnesses Cheval, Vareu, Lettellier, Foulongue, Le Hernault, and others;" and, further, after deciding that, in consequence, "the prosecutor cannot maintain a claim for damages for alleged defamation of which he was himself the first author," the magistrate gave judgment for the defendant, (the curate,) and condemned the prosecutor (the shepherd) to pay the expenses of the suit.

Within ten days after the rendition of this judgment, a gentleman who had visited the parsonage during these disturbances, had there witnessed many of the more extraordinary phenomena, and was himself one of the witnesses at the trial,—the Marquis de Mirville, well known to the literary world of Paris as the author of a recent work on Pneumatology,—collected from the legal record all the documents connected with the trial, including the *procès-verbal* of the testimony; this last being, according to the French forms of justice, taken down at the time of the deposition, then read over to each witness and its accuracy attested by him.

It is from these official documents, thus collected at the time as appendix to a pamphlet on the subject,* that I translate the following details of the disturbances in question, embodying those phenomena upon which the main body of the witnesses agreed, and omitting such portions of the testimony as are immaterial or uncor-

---

* "*Fragment d'un Ouvrage inédit*," published by Vrayet de Surcy, Paris, 1852. (The unpublished work here referred to is De Mirville's well-known volume on Pneumatology.)

roborated; also such as specially refer to the proofs for
and against the charge of defamation, and to the alleged
agency of the shepherd Thorel.

On Tuesday, the 26th of November, 1850, as the
two children were at work in one of the rooms in the
upper story of the parsonage, about five o'clock in the
afternoon, they heard knockings, resembling light blows
of a hammer, on the wainscoting of the apartment.
These knockings were continued daily throughout the
week, at the same hour of the afternoon.

On the next Sunday, the 1st of December, the blows
commenced at mid-day; and it was on that day that the
curate first thought of addressing them. He said,
"Strike louder!" Thereupon the blows were repeated
more loudly. They continued thus all that day.

On Monday, December 2, the elder of the two boys
said to the knockings, "Beat time to the tune of *Maître
Corbeau;*" and they immediately obeyed.

The next day, Tuesday, December 3, the boy having
related the above circumstances to M. Tinel, he, (Tinel,)
being much astonished, resolved to try, and said,
"Play us *Maître Corbeau;*" and the knockings obeyed.
The afternoon of that day, the knockings became so
loud and violent that a table in the apartment moved
somewhat, and the noise was so great that one could
hardly stay in the room. Later in the same afternoon,
the table moved from its place three times. The curate's
sister, after assuring herself that the children had not
moved it, replaced it; but twice it followed her back
again. The noises continued, with violence, all that
week.*

On Monday, December 9, there being present Auguste
Huet, a neighboring proprietor, the curate of Limesy,
and another gentleman, the younger child being also

---

* Testimony of Gustave Lemonier and of Clement Bunel.

present, but with his arms folded, Huet tapped with his finger on the edge of the table, and said, "Strike as many blows as there are letters in my name." Four blows were immediately struck, at the very spot, under his finger. He was convinced it could not be done by the child, nor by any one in the house. Then he asked it to beat time to the air of *"Au Clair de la Lune;"* and it did so.*

The Mayor of Cideville deposes to the fact that, being in the parsonage, he saw the tongs leap from the fire-place into the room. Then the shovel did the same thing. The Mayor said to one of the children, "How, Gustave! what is that?" The child replied, "I did not touch it." The tongs and shovel were then replaced, and a second time they leaped forward into the room. This time, as the Mayor testified, he had his eyes fixed upon them, so as to detect the trick in case any one pushed them; but nothing was to be seen.†

M. Leroux, curate of Saussay, deposes that, being at the parsonage, he witnessed things that were inexplicable to him. He saw a hammer fly, impelled by an invisible force, from the spot where it lay, and fall on the floor of the room without more noise than if a hand had lightly placed it there. He also saw a piece of bread that was lying on the table move of itself and fall below the table. He was so placed that it was impossible that any one could have thrown these things without his seeing him do it. He also heard the extraordinary noises, and took every possible precaution, even to placing himself under the table, to assure himself that the children did not produce them. So sure was he of this, that, to use his own expression, he would "sign it with his blood." (*"Je le signerais de mon sang."*) He

---

* Testimony of Auguste Huet.
† Testimony of Adolphe Cheval, Mayor of Cideville.

remarked that M. Tinel appeared exasperated by these noises and their continued repetition; and he added that, having slept several nights in the same room as M. Tinel, the latter awoke in a fright at the disturbances.*

The deposition of the Marquis de Mirville, proprietor at Gomerville, is one of the most circumstantial. He testifies to the following effect. Having heard much of the disturbances at Cideville, he suddenly resolved one day to go there. The distance from his residence is fourteen leagues. He arrived at the parsonage at nightfall, unexpected by its inmates, and passed the evening there, never losing sight of the curate nor leaving him a moment alone with the children. The curate knew the marquis's name, but only from a letter of introduction which the latter had brought.

M. de Mirville passed the night at the parsonage, the curate having given up to him his bed, in the same room in which the children slept. No disturbance during the night. The next morning one of the children awoke him, and said, "Do you hear, sir, how it scratches?"

"What, my child?"

"The spirit."

And the marquis heard, in effect, a strong scratching on the mattress of the children's bed. He notified the mysterious agent, however, that he should not think the noises worth listening to unless the theater of operations was removed from where the children were. Then the knockings were heard above the bed. "Too near yet!" said M. de Mirville. "Go and knock at that corner," (pointing to a distant corner of the room.) Instantly the knocking was heard there. "Ah!" said the marquis, "now we can converse: strike a single blow if you agree." A loud blow for answer.

---

* Testimony of Martin Tranquille Leroux, curate of Saussay.

So, after breakfast, the curate having gone to mass and the children being in the room at their studies, he carried out his intention, thus :—

"How many letters are there in my name? Answer by the number of strokes."

Eight strokes were given.

"How many in my given name?"

Five strokes. (*Jules.*)

"How many in my pre-name?" (*pré-nom*; a name, he remarked, by which he was never called, and which was only known from his baptismal record.)

Seven strokes. (*Charles.*)

"How many in my eldest daughter's name?"

Five strokes. (*Aline.*)

"How many in my younger daughter's name?"

Nine strokes. This time the first error, the name being *Blanche;* but the blows immediately began again and struck seven, thus correcting the original mistake.

"How many letters in the name of my commune? but take care and don't make a common mistake in spelling it."

A pause. Then ten strokes,—the correct number of *Gomerville;* often erroneously spelled *Gommerville.*

At the request of this witness, the knockings beat time to several airs. One, the waltz from " *Guillaume Tell,*" which it could not beat, was hummed by M. de Mirville. After a pause, the knockings followed the measure note by note; and it was several times repeated in the course of the day.

The witness, being asked if he thought the curate could be himself the author of these disturbances, replied, "I should be greatly astonished if any person in this neighborhood could entertain such an opinion."[*]

Madame de Saint-Victor, residing in a neighboring chateau, had frequently visited the parsonage,—at first,

---

[*] Testimony of Charles Jules de Mirville.

as she deposed, completely incredulous, and convinced that she could discover the cause of the disturbances. On the 8th of December, after vespers, being in the parsonage, and standing apart from any one, she felt her mantle seized by an invisible force, so as to give her a strong pull or shock, (*une forte sécousse.*) Among various other phenomena, just one week before she gave her evidence, (January 22,) while she was alone with the children, she saw two desks, at which they were then engaged in writing, upset on the floor, and the table upset on the top of them. On the 28th of January, she saw a candlestick take flight from the kitchen chimney-piece and strike her femme-de-chambre on the back. She also, in company with her son, heard the knockings beat the measure of various airs. When it beat "*Maître Corbeau,*" she said, "Is that all you know?" Whereupon it immediately beat the measure of "*Claire de Lune*" and "*J'ai du bon Tabac.*" During the beating of several of these airs, being alone with the children, she observed them narrowly,—their feet, their hands, and all their movements. It was impossible that they should have done it.*

Another important witness, M. Robert de Saint-Victor, son of the preceding witness, deposed as follows. On the invitation of the curate, several days after the disturbances began, he visited the parsonage, about half-past three in the afternoon. Going up-stairs, after a time he heard slight knockings on the wainscot. They resembled, yet were not exactly like, sounds produced by an iron point striking on hard wood. The witness arrived quite incredulous, and satisfied that he could discover the cause of these knockings. The first day they strongly excited his attention, but did not secure his conviction. The next day, at ten o'clock,

---

* Deposition of Marie-Françoise Adolphine Deschamps de Bois-Hebert, wife of M. de Saint-Victor.

he returned. Several popular songs were then, at his request, beaten in time. The same day, about three o'clock, he heard blows so heavy that he was sure a mallet striking on the floor would not have produced the like. Toward evening these blows were continued almost without interruption. At that time, M. Cheval, the Mayor of Cideville, and the witness, went over the house together. They saw, several times, the table at which the children were sitting move from its place. To assure themselves that this could not possibly be the children's doing, they placed both the children in the middle of the room; then M. Cheval and the witness sat down to the table, and felt it move away from the wall several times. They tried by main force to prevent it from moving; but their united efforts were unavailing. In spite of them, it moved from ten to twelve *centimetres*, (about four inches,) and that with a uniform motion, without any jerk. The witness's mother, who was present, had previously testified to the same fact.* While the curate was gone to the church, the witness remained alone with the children; and presently there arose such a clatter in the room that one could hardly endure it. Every piece of furniture there was set in vibration. And the witness confessed that he expected every moment that the floor of the apartment would sink beneath his feet. He felt convinced that if every person in the house had set to work, together, to pound with mallets on the floor, they could not have produced such a racket. The noise appeared especially to attach itself to the younger of the two children, the knockings being usually on that part of the wainscot nearest to where he happened to stand or sit. The child appeared in constant terror.

The witness finally became thoroughly convinced that

---

* See testimony of Madame de Saint-Victor.

the occult force, whatever its precise character, was intelligent. When he returned, several days later, to the parsonage, the phenomena continued with still increasing violence. One evening, desiring to enter the room where the children usually sat, the door resisted his efforts to open it,—a resistance which, the witness averred, he could not attribute to a natural cause; for when he succeeded in pushing it open and entering the room there was no one there. Another day, it occurred to him to ask for an air but little known,—the *Stabat Mater*, of Rossini; and it was given with extraordinary accuracy.

Returning, some days later, on the renewed invitation of the curate, this witness went up-stairs; and at the moment when he came opposite the door of the upper room, a desk that stood on the table at which the children usually studied (but they were not there at the time) started from its place, and came toward the witness with a swift motion, and following a line parallel with the floor, until it was about thirty centimetres (one foot) from his person, when it fell vertically to the floor. The place where it fell was distant about two metres (between six and seven feet) from the table.*

The witness Bouffay, vicar of St. Maclou, stated that he had been several times at the parsonage. The first time he heard continued noises in the apartments occupied by the children. These noises were intelligent and obedient. On one occasion, the witness sleeping in the children's room, the uproar was so violent that he thought the floor would open beneath him. He heard the noises equally in the presence and the absence of the curate; and he took especial notice that the children were motionless when the disturbances occurred, and evidently could not produce them. On one occa-

---

* Testimony of M. Raoul Robert de Saint-Victor.

sion, the witness, with the curate and the children, slept at a neighbor's house to escape the continued noises.*

The deposition of Dufour, land-agent at Yerville, was to the effect that, on the 7th of December, being at dinner in the parsonage, knockings were heard above. Mademoiselle Tinel said, "Do you hear? These are the noises that occur." The witness went up-stairs, and found the children sitting each at one end of the table, but distant from it fifty or sixty centimetres, (about two feet.) He heard strokes in the wall, which he is sure the children did not make. Then the table advanced into the room without any one touching it. The witness put it back in its place. It moved forward a second time about three metres (about ten feet) into the room, the children not touching it. As the witness was going down the stairs, he stopped on the first step to look round at the table, and saw it come forward to the edge of the stairway, impelled by an invisible force. The witness remarked that the table had no castors. This occurred while the curate was absent from the parsonage.†

The witness Gobert, vicar of St. Maclou, testified that when the curate of Cideville and the two children came to his (Gobert's) house, he heard, on the ceiling and walls of his apartment, noises similar to those which he (Gobert) had before heard at the Cideville parsonage.‡

Such are the main facts to which witnesses in this strange suit testified. I have omitted those which rested only on the testimony of the children. The industry of M. de Mirville has collected and embodied in the pamphlet referred to additional evidence, in the

---

* Testimony of Athanase Bouffay, vicar of St. Maclou, of Rouen.
† Testimony of Nicolas-Boniface Dufour, land-agent at Yerville.
‡ Testimony of Adalbert Honoré Gobert, vicar of St. Maclou, of Rouen.

shape of several letters written by respectable gentlemen who visited the parsonage during the disturbances.
One is from the assistant judge of a neighboring tribunal, M. Rousselin. He found the curate profoundly
afflicted by his painful position, and obtained from him
every opportunity of cross-questioning, separately, the
children, M. Tinel's sister, and his servant. Their entire
demeanor bore the impress of truthfulness. Their
testimony was clear, direct, and uniformly consistent.
He found the window-panes broken, and boards set up
against them. Another gentlemen states that, on his
arrival at the parsonage, he was struck with the sad and
unhappy look of the curate, who, he adds, impressed
him, from his appearance, as a most worthy man.

All these letters fully corroborate the preceding
testimony.

It would be difficult to find a case more explicit or
better authenticated than the foregoing. Yet it is certain that the phenomena it discloses, closely as these
resemble what has been occurring for ten years past
all over the United States, are not traceable, directly or
indirectly, through the influence of imitation, epidemic
excitement, or otherwise, to the Spiritual movement
among us. The history of the Rochester knockings,
then but commencing here, had never reached the humble parsonage of Cideville, and afforded no explanation
to its alarmed inmates of the annoyances which broke
their quiet and excited their fears.

I might go on, indefinitely, extending the number of
similar narratives, but a repetition would prove nothing
more than is established by the specimens already given.
I therefore here close my list of disturbances occurring
in Europe, and proceed to furnish, in conclusion, from
the most authentic sources, that example, already referred to, occurring in our own country, which has

become known, in Europe as well as America, under the name of the "ROCHESTER KNOCKINGS."

THE HYDESVILLE DWELLING-HOUSE.

Disturbances in Western New York,

1848.

There stands, not far from the town of Newark, in the county of Wayne and State of New York, a wooden dwelling,—one of a cluster of small houses like itself, scarcely meriting the title of a village, but known under the name of Hydesville; being so called after Dr. Hyde, an old settler, whose son is the proprietor of the house in question. It is a story and a half high, fronting south; the lower floor consisting, in 1848, of two moderate-sized rooms, opening into each other; east of these a bedroom, opening into the sitting-room, and a buttery, opening into the same room; together with a stairway, (between the bedroom and buttery,) leading from the sitting-room up to the half-story above, and from the buttery down to the cellar.

This humble dwelling had been selected as a temporary residence, during the erection of another house in the country, by Mr. John D. Fox.

The Fox family were reputable farmers, members of the Methodist Church in good standing, and much respected by their neighbors as honest, upright people. Mr. Fox's ancestors were Germans, the name being originally *Voss;* but both he and Mrs. Fox were native born. In Mrs. Fox's family, French by origin and Rutan by name, several individuals had evinced the power of second-sight,—her maternal grandmother, whose maiden name was Margaret Ackerman, and who resided at Long Island, among the number. She had, frequently, perceptions of funerals before they occurred, and was wont to follow these phantom processions to the grave as if they were material.

Mrs. Fox's sister also, Mrs. Elizabeth Higgins, had similar power. On one occasion, in the year 1823, the two sisters, then residing in New York, proposed to go to Sodus by canal. But Elizabeth said, one morning, "We shall not make this trip by water." "Why so?" her sister asked. "Because I dreamed last night that we traveled by land, and there was a strange lady with us. In my dream, too, I thought we came to Mott's tavern, in the Beech woods, and that they could not admit us, because Mrs. Mott lay dying in the house. I know it will all come true." "Very unlikely indeed," replied her sister; "for last year, when we passed there, Mr. Mott's wife lay dead in the house." "You will see. He must have married again; and he will lose his second wife." Every particular came to pass as Mrs. Higgins had predicted. Mrs. Johnson, a stranger, whom at the time of the dream they had not seen, *did* go with them, they made the journey by land, and were refused admittance into Mott's tavern, for the very cause assigned in Mrs. Higgins's dream.

Mr. and Mrs. Fox had six children, of whom the two youngest were staying with them when, on the 11th of December, 1847, they removed into the house I have described. The children were both girls: Margaret, then twelve years old; and Kate, nine.

Soon after they had taken up their residence in the dwelling referred to, they began to think it was a very noisy house; but this was attributed to rats and mice. During the next month, however, (January, 1848,) the noise began to assume the character of slight knockings heard at night in the bedroom; sometimes appearing to sound from the cellar beneath. At first Mrs. Fox sought to persuade herself this might be but the hammering of a shoemaker, in a house hard by, sitting up late at work. But further observation showed that the sounds, whencesoever proceeding, originated in the house. For not only did the knockings gradually become more distinct, and not only were they heard first in one part of the house, then in another, but the family finally remarked that these raps, even when not very loud, often caused a motion, tremulous rather than a sudden jar, of the bedsteads and chairs,—sometimes of the floor; a motion which was quite perceptible to the touch when a hand was laid on the chairs, which was sometimes sensibly felt at night in the slightly oscillating motion of the bed, and which was occasionally perceived as a sort of vibration even when standing on the floor.

After a time, also, the noises varied in their character, sounding occasionally like distinct footfalls in the different rooms.

Nor were the disturbances, after a month or two had passed, confined to sounds. Once something heavy, as if a dog, seemed to lie on the feet of the children; but it was gone before the mother could come to their aid. Another time (this was late in March) Kate felt as if a cold hand on her face. Occasionally, too, the bed-clothes were pulled during the night. Finally chairs were moved from their places. So, on one occasion, was the dining-table.

The disturbances, which had been limited to occasional knockings throughout February and the early part of March, gradually increased, toward the close of the latter month, in loudness and frequency, so seriously as to break the rest of the family. Mr. Fox and his wife got up night after night, lit a candle, and thoroughly searched every nook and corner of the house; but without any result. They discovered nothing. When the raps came on a door, Mr. Fox would stand, ready to open, the moment they were repeated. But this expedient, too, proved unavailing. Though he opened the door on the instant, there was no one to be seen. Nor did he or Mrs. Fox ever obtain the slightest clew to the cause of these disturbances.

The only circumstance which seemed to suggest the possibility of trickery or of mistake was, that these various unexplained occurrences never happened in daylight.

And thus, notwithstanding the strangeness of the thing, when morning came they began to think it must have been but the fancy of the night. Not being given to superstition, they clung, throughout several weeks of annoyance, to the idea that some natural explanation of these seeming accidents would at last appear. Nor did they abandon this hope till the night of Friday, the 31st of March, 1848.

The day had been cold and stormy, with snow on the ground. In the course of the afternoon, a son, David, came to visit them from his farm, about three miles distant. His mother then first recounted to him the particulars of the annoyances they had endured; for till now they had been little disposed to communicate these to any one. He heard her with a smile. "Well, mother," he said, "I advise you not to say a word to the neighbors about it. When you find it out, it will be one of the simplest things in the world." And in that belief he returned home.

Wearied out by a succession of sleepless nights and of fruitless attempts to penetrate the mystery, the Fox family retired on that Friday evening very early to rest, hoping for a respite from the disturbances that harassed them. But they were doomed to disappointment.

The parents had had the children's beds removed into their bedroom, and strictly enjoined them not to talk of noises even if they heard them. But scarcely had the mother seen them safely in bed, and was retiring to rest herself, when the children cried out, "Here they are again!" The mother chid them, and lay down

Thereupon the noises became louder and more startling
The children sat up in bed. Mrs. Fox called in her husband. The night being windy, it suggested itself to
him that it might be the rattling of the sashes. He
tried several, shaking them to see if they were loose.
Kate, the youngest girl, happened to remark that as
often as her father shook a window-sash the noises
seemed to reply. Being a lively child, and in a measure
accustomed to what was going on, she turned to where
the noise was, snapped her fingers, and called out, "Here,
old Splitfoot, do as I do!" *The knocking instantly responded.*

That was the very commencement. Who can tell
where the end will be?

I do not mean that it was Kate Fox who thus, half
in childish jest, first discovered that these mysterious
sounds seemed instinct with intelligence. Mr. Mompesson, two hundred years ago, had already observed a
similar phenomenon. Glanvil had verified it. So had
Wesley and his children. So, we have seen, had others.
But in all these cases the matter rested there, and the
observation was no further prosecuted. As, previous
to the invention of the steam-engine, sundry observers
had trodden the very threshold of the discovery and
there stopped, little thinking what lay close before
them, so, in this case, where the Royal Chaplain, disciple though he was of the inductive philosophy, and
where the founder of Methodism, admitting though he
did the probabilities of ultramundane interference,
were both at fault, a Yankee girl, but nine years old,
following up, more in sport than earnest, a chance observation, became the instigator of a movement which,
whatever its true character, has had its influence
throughout the civilized world. The spark had several
times been ignited,—once, at least, two centuries ago;
but it had died out each time without effect. It kindled
no flame till the middle of the nineteenth century.

And yet how trifling the step from the observation at Tedworth to the discovery at Hydesville! Mr. Mompesson, in bed with his little daughter, (about Kate's age,) whom the sound seemed chiefly to follow, "observed that it would exactly answer, in drumming, any thing that was beaten or called for." But his curiosity led him no further.

Not so Kate Fox. She tried, by silently bringing together her thumb and forefinger, whether she could still obtain a response. Yes! It could see, then, as well as hear! She called her mother. "Only look, mother!" she said, bringing together her finger and thumb as before. And as often as she repeated the noiseless motion, just so often responded the raps.

This at once arrested her mother's attention. "Count ten," she said, addressing the noise. Ten strokes, distinctly given! "How old is my daughter Margaret?" Twelve strokes! "And Kate?" Nine! "What can all this mean?" was Mrs. Fox's thought. Who was answering her? Was it only some mysterious echo of her own thought? But the next question which she put seemed to refute that idea. "How many children have I?" she asked, aloud. Seven strokes. "Ah!" she thought, "it can blunder sometimes." And then, aloud, 'Try again!' Still the number of raps was seven. Of a sudden a thought crossed Mrs. Fox's mind. "Are they all alive?" she asked. Silence, for answer. "How many are living?" Six strokes. "How many dead?" A single stroke. She *had* lost a child.

Then she asked, "Are you a man?" No answer. "Are you a spirit?" It rapped. "May my neighbors hear if I call them?" It rapped again.

Thereupon she asked her husband to call a neighbor, a Mrs. Redfield, who came in laughing. But her cheer was soon changed. The answers to her inquiries were

T   25

as prompt and pertinent as they had been to those of Mrs. Fox. She was struck with awe; and when, in reply to a question about the number of her children, by rapping four, instead of three as she expected, it reminded her of a little daughter, Mary, whom she had recently lost, the mother burst into tears.

But it avails not further to follow out in minute detail the issue of these disturbances, since the particulars have already been given, partly in the shape of formal depositions, in more than one publication,* and since they are not essential to the illustration of this branch of the subject.

It may, however, be satisfactory to the reader that I here subjoin to the above narrative—every particular of which I had from Mrs. Fox, her daughters Margaret and Kate, and her son David—a supplement, containing

---

* The earliest of these, published in Canandaigua only three weeks after the occurrences of the 31st of March, is a pamphlet of forty pages, entitled "*A Report of the Mysterious Noises heard in the house of Mr. John D. Fox, in Hydesville, Arcadia, Wayne County, authenticated by the certificates and confirmed by the statements of the citizens of that place and vicinity.*" Canandaigua, published by E. E. Lewis, 1848. It contains twenty-one certificates, chiefly given by the immediate neighbors, including those of Mr. and Mrs. Fox, of their son and daughter-in-law, of Mrs. Redfield, &c. &c., taken chiefly on the 11th and 12th of April. For a copy of the above pamphlet, now very scarce, I am indebted to the family of Mr. Fox, whom I visited in August, 1859, at the house of the son, Mr. David Fox, when I had an opportunity to visit the small dwelling in which the above-related circumstances took place; descending to its cellar, the alleged scene of dark deeds. The house is now occupied by a farm-laborer, who, Faraday-like, "does not believe in *spooks.*"

A more connected account, followed up by a history of the movement which had birth at Hydesville, is to be found in "*Modern Spiritualism: its Facts and Fanaticisms,*" by E. W. Capron, Boston, 1855, pp. 33 to 56.

Most of the witnesses signing the certificates above referred to offer to confirm their statements, if necessary, under oath; and they almost all expressly declare their conviction that the family had no agency in producing the sounds, that these were not referable to trick or deception or to any known natural cause, usually adding that they were no believers in the supernatural, and had never before heard or witnessed any thing not susceptible of a natural explanation.

a brief outline as well of the events which immediately succeeded, as those, connected with the dwelling in question, which preceded, the disturbances of the 31st of March.

On that night the neighbors, attracted by the rumor of the disturbances, gradually gathered in, to the number of seventy or eighty, so that Mrs. Fox left the house for that of Mrs. Redfield, while the children were taken home by another neighbor. Mr. Fox remained.

Many of the assembled crowd, one after another, put questions to the noises, requesting that assent might be testified by rapping. When there was no response by raps, and the question was reversed, there were always rappings; thus indicating that silence was to be taken for dissent.

In this way the sounds alleged that they were produced by a spirit; by an injured spirit; by a spirit who had been injured in that house; between four and five years ago; not by any of the neighbors, whose names were called over one by one, but by a man who formerly resided in the house,—a certain John C. Bell, a blacksmith. His name was obtained by naming in succession the former occupants of the house.

The noises alleged, further, that it was the spirit of a man thirty-one years of age; that he had been murdered in the bedroom, for money, on a Tuesday night, at twelve o'clock; that no one but the murdered man and Mr. Bell were in the house at the time; Mrs. Bell and a girl named Lucretia Pulver, who worked for them, being both absent; that the body was carried down to the cellar early next morning, not through the outside cellar-door, but by being dragged through the parlor into the buttery and thence down the cellar-stairs; that it was buried, ten feet deep, in the cellar, but not until the night after the murder.

Thereupon the party assembled adjourned to the

cellar, which had an earthen floor; and Mr. Redfield having placed himself on various parts of it, asking, each time, if that was the spot of burial, there was no response until he stood in the center: then the noises were heard, as from beneath the ground. This was repeated several times, always with a similar result, no sound occurring when he stood at any other place than the center. One of the witnesses describes the sounds in the cellar as resembling "a thumping a foot or two under ground."*

Then a neighbor named Duesler called over the letters of the alphabet, asking, at each, if that was the initial of the murdered man's first name; and so of the second name. The sounds responded at C and B. An attempt to obtain the entire name did not then succeed. At a later period the full name (as Charles B. Rosma) was given in the same way in reply to the questions of Mr. David Fox. Still it did not suggest itself to any one to attempt, by the raps, to have a communication spelled out. It is a remarkable fact, and one which in a measure explains the lack of further results at Tedworth and at Epworth, that it was not till about four months afterward, and at Rochester, that the very first brief

---

* "Report of the Mysterious Noises," p. 25. See also p. 17.

Mr. Marvin Losey and Mr. David Fox state, in their respective certificates, that on the night of Saturday, April 1, when the crowd were asking questions, it was arranged that those in the cellar should all stand in one place, except one, Mr. Carlos Hyde, while that one moved about to different spots; and that Mr. Duesler, being in the bedroom above, where of course he could not see Mr. Hyde nor any one else in the cellar, should be the questioner. Then, as Mr. Hyde stepped about in the cellar, the question was repeated by Mr. Duesler in the bedroom, "Is any one standing over the place where the body was buried?" In every instance, as soon as Mr. Hyde stepped to the center of the cellar the raps were heard, so that both those in the cellar and those in the rooms above heard them; but as often as he stood anywhere else there was silence. This was repeated, again and again —"Report of the Mysterious Noises," pp. 26 and 28.

communication by raps was obtained; the suggester being Isaac Post, a member of the Society of Friends, and an old acquaintance of the Fox family.

The report of the night's wonders at Hydesville spread all over the neighborhood; and next day, Saturday, the house was beset by a crowd of the curious. But while daylight lasted there were no noises.* These recommenced before seven o'clock in the evening. That night there were some three hundred people in and about the house.† Various persons asked questions; and the replies corresponded at every point to those formerly given.

Then it was proposed to dig in the cellar; but, as the house stands on a flat plain not far from a small sluggish stream, the diggers reached water at the depth of less than three feet, and had to abandon the attempt. It was renewed on Monday the 3d of April, and again the next day, by Mr. David Fox and others, baling and pumping out the water; but they could not reduce it much, and had to give up.‡

At a later period, when the water had much lowered, to wit, in the summer of 1848, Mr. David Fox, aided by Messrs. Henry Bush and Lyman Granger, of Rochester, and others, recommenced digging in the cellar. At the depth of five feet they came to a plank, through which they bored with an auger, when, the auger-bit being loose, it dropped through out of sight. Digging farther, they found several pieces of crockery and some charcoal and quicklime, indicating that the soil must at some time have been disturbed to a considerable depth; and finally they came upon some human hair and several bones, which, on examination by a medical man skilled

---

* The next day, however, Sunday, April 2, this was reversed. The noises responded throughout the day, but ceased in the evening and were not obtained throughout the night.—" Report of the Mysterious Noises," p. 9.

† " Report of the Mysterious Noises," p. 15.   ‡ Ibid. p. 29.

In anatomy, proved to be portions of a human skeleton, including two bones of the hand and certain parts of the skull; but no connected skull was found.*

It remains briefly to trace the antecedents of the disturbed dwelling.

William Duesler, one of those who gave certificates touching this matter, and who offers to confirm his testimony under oath, states that he inhabited the same house seven years before, and that during the term of his residence there he never heard any noise of the kind in or about the premises. He adds that a Mr. Johnson, and others, who, like himself, had lived there before Mr. Bell occupied the dwelling, make the same statement.†

Mrs. Pulver, a near neighbor, states that, having called one morning on Mrs. Bell while she occupied the house, she (Mrs. B.) told her she felt very ill, not having slept at all during the previous night; and, on being asked what the matter was, Mrs. Bell said she had thought she heard some one walking about from one room to another. Mrs. Pulver further deposes that she heard Mrs. Bell, on subsequent occasions, speak of noises which she could not account for.‡

The daughter of this deponent, Lucretia Pulver, states that she lived with Mr. and Mrs. Bell during part of the time they occupied the house, namely, for three months during the winter of 1843–44, sometimes working for them, sometimes boarding with them, and going to school, she being then fifteen years old. She says Mr. and Mrs. Bell "appeared to be very good folks, only rather quick-tempered."

She states that, during the latter part of her residence with them, one afternoon, about two o'clock, a peddler, on foot, apparently about thirty years of age, wearing a

---

* "*Modern Spiritualism,*" p. 53. Mr. David Fox, during my visit to him, confirmed to me the truth of this.

† "*Report of the Mysterious Noises,*" p. 16.   ‡ Ibid pp. 37, 38.

black frock-coat and light-colored pantaloons, and having with him a trunk and a basket, called at Mr. Bell's. Mrs. Bell informed her she had known him formerly. Shortly after he came in, Mr. and Mrs. Bell consulted together for nearly half an hour in the buttery. Then Mrs. Bell told her—very unexpectedly to her—that they did not require her any more; that she (Mrs. B.) was going that afternoon to Lock Berlin, and that she (Lucretia) had better return home, as they thought they could not afford to keep her longer. Accordingly, Mrs. Bell and Lucretia left the house, the peddler and Mr. Bell remaining. Before she went, however, Lucretia looked at a piece of delaine, and told the peddler she would take a dress off it if he would call the next day at her father's house, hard by, which he promised to do; but he never came. Three days afterward, Mrs. Bell returned, and, to Lucretia's surprise, sent for her again to stay with them.

A few days after this, Lucretia began to hear knocking in the bedroom—afterward occupied by Mr. and Mrs. Fox—where she slept. The sounds seemed to be under the foot of the bed, and were repeated during a number of nights. One night, when Mr. and Mrs. Bell had gone to Lock Berlin, and she had remained in the house with her little brother and a daughter of Mr. Losey, named Aurelia, they heard, about twelve o'clock, what seemed the footsteps of a man walking in the buttery. They had not gone to bed till eleven, and had not yet fallen asleep. It sounded as if some one crossed the buttery, then went down the cellar-stair, then walked part of the way across the cellar, and stopped. The girls were greatly frightened, got up and fastened doors and windows.

About a week after this, Lucretia, having occasion to go down into the cellar, screamed out. Mrs. Bell asked what was the matter. Lucretia exclaimed, "What *has*

Mr. Bell been doing in the cellar?" She had sunk in the soft soil and fallen. Mrs. Bell replied that it was only rat-holes. A few days afterward, at nightfall, Mr. Bell carried some earth into the cellar, and was at work there some time. Mrs. Bell said he was filling up the rat-holes.*

Mr. and Mrs. Weekman depose that they occupied the house in question, after Mr. Bell left it, during eighteen months, namely, from the spring of 1846 till the autumn of 1847.

About March, 1847, one night as they were going to bed they heard knockings on the outside door; but when they opened there was no one there. This was repeated, till Mr. Weekman lost patience; and, after searching all round the house, he resolved, if possible, to detect these disturbers of his peace. Accordingly, he stood with his hand on the door, ready to open it at the instant the knocking was repeated. It *was* repeated, so that he felt the door jar under his hand; but, though he sprang out instantly and searched all round the house, he found not a trace of any intruder.

They were frequently afterward disturbed by strange and unaccountable noises. One night Mrs. Weekman heard what seemed the footsteps of some one walking in the cellar. Another night one of her little girls, eight years old, screamed out, so as to wake every one in the house. She said something cold had been moving over her head and face; and it was long ere the terrified child was pacified, nor would she consent to sleep in the same room for several nights afterward.

Mr. Weekman offers to repeat his certificate, if required, under oath.†

---

* *"Report of the Mysterious Noises,"* pp. 35, 36, 37. I have added a few minor particulars, related by Lucretia to Mrs. Fox.

† Ibid. pp. 33, 34.

But it needs not further to multiply extracts from these depositions. Nothing positive can be gathered from them. It is certain, however, that the peddler never reappeared in Hydesville nor kept his promises to call. On the other hand, Mr. Bell, who had removed early in 1846 to the town of Lyons, in the same county, on hearing the reports of the above disclosures, came forthwith to the scene of his former residence, and obtained from the neighbors, and made public, a certificate setting forth that "they never knew any thing against his character," and that when he lived among them "they thought him, and still think him, a man of honest and upright character, incapable of committing crime." This certificate is dated April 5, (six days after the first communications,) and is signed by forty-four persons. The author of the "Report of the Mysterious Noises," in giving it entire, adds that others besides the signers are willing to join in the recommendation.*

It is proper also to state, in this connection, that, a few months afterward,—to wit, in July or August, 1848,—a circumstance occurred at Rochester, New York, somewhat analogous in character, and indicating the danger of indulging, without corroborating evidence, in suspicions aroused by alleged spiritual information. A young peddler, with a wagon and two horses, and known to be possessed of several hundred dollars, having put up at a tavern in that city, suddenly disappeared. Public opinion settled down to the belief that he was murdered. An enthusiastic Spiritualist had the surmise confirmed by the raps. Through the same medium the credulous inquirer was informed that the body lay in the canal, several spots being successively indicated where it could be found. These were anxiously dragged, but to no purpose. Finally the dupe's wife was required to go into

---

* "Report of the Mysterious Noises," pp. 38, 39.

the canal at a designated point, where she would certainly discover the corpse; in obeying which injunction she nearly lost her life. Some months afterward, the alleged victim reappeared : he had departed secretly for Canada, to avoid the importunities of his creditors.*

In the Hydesville case, too, there was some rebutting evidence. The raps had alleged that, though the peddler's wife was dead, his five children lived in Orange County, New York; but all efforts to discover them there were fruitless. Nor does it appear that any man named Rosma was ascertained to have resided there.

It remains to be added that no legal proceedings were ever instituted, either against Mr. Bell, in virtue of the suspicions aroused, or by him against those who expressed such suspicions. He finally left the country.

It is evident that no sufficient case is made out against him. The statements of the earthly witnesses amount to circumstantial evidence only; and upon unsupported ultramundane testimony no dependence can be placed. It may supply hints; it may suggest inquiries; but assurance it cannot give.

The Hydesville narrative, however, as one of unexplained disturbances, like those at Cideville, at Ahrensburg, at Slawensik, at Epworth, and at Tedworth, rests for verification on the reality of the phenomena themselves, not on the accuracy of the extrinsic information alleged to be thereby supplied.

---

* For details, see " *Modern Spiritualism,*" pp. 60 to 62. If we concede the reality of the spirit-rap, and if we assume to judge of ultramundane intentions, we may imagine that the purpose was, by so early and so marked a lesson, to warn men, even from the commencement, against putting implicit faith in spiritual communications.

It is worthy of remark, however, that there is this great difference in these two cases, that the Hydesville communications came by spontaneous agency, uncalled for, unlooked for, while those obtained at Rochester were evoked and expected.

With this case I close the list of these narrations; for to follow up similar examples, since occurring throughout our country,* would lead me, away from my object, into the history of the rise and progress of the Spiritual movement itself.

---

* As that occurring at Stratford, Connecticut, in the house of the Rev Dr. Eliakim Phelps, more whimsical, and also more surprising, in many of its modifications, than any of those here related; commencing on the 10th of March, 1850, and continuing, with intervals, a year and nine months; namely, till the 15th of December, 1851. A detailed account of this case will be found in "*Modern Spiritualism*," pp. 132 to 171.

CHAPTER III.

SUMMING UP.

I HAVE few words to add, in summing up the foregoing evidence that the disturbances which give rise to rumors of haunted houses are, in certain cases, actual and unexplained phenomena.

Little comment is needed, or is likely to be useful. There are men so hard-set in their preconceptions on certain points that no evidence can move them. Time and the resistless current of public sentiment alone avail to urge them on. They must wait. And as to those whose ears are still open, whose convictions can still be reached, few, I venture to predict, will put aside, unmoved and incredulous, the mass of proof here brought together. Yet a few considerations, briefly stated, may not be out of place.

The testimony, in most of the examples, is direct and at first hand, given by eye and ear witnesses and placed on record at the time.

It is derived from reputable sources. Can we take exception to the character and standing of such witnesses as Joseph Glanvil, John Wesley, Justinus Kerner? Can we object to the authority of Mackay, a skeptic and a derider? Does not the narrative of Hahn evince in the observer both coolness and candor? As to the Ahrensburg story, it is the daughter of the chief magistrate concerned in its investigation who testifies. And where shall we find, among a multitude of witnesses, better proof of honesty than in the agreement in the depositions at Cideville and at Hydesville?

The phenomena were such as could be readily observed. Many of them were of a character so palpable and notorious that for the observers to imagine them was a sheer impossibility. The thundering blows at Mr. Mompesson's shook the house and awoke the neighbors in an adjoining village. The poundings at Madame Hauffe's displaced the rafters and arrested the attention of passers-by in the street. At Epworth, let them make what noises they might, the "dead, hollow note would be clearly heard above them all." At Hydesville, the house was abandoned by its occupants, and hundreds of the curious assembled, night after night, to test the reality of the knockings which sounded from every part of it.

There was ample opportunity to observe. The occurrences were not single appearances, suddenly presenting themselves, quickly passing away: they were repeated day after day, month after month, sometimes year after year. They could be tested and re-tested. Nor did they produce in the witnesses an evanescent belief, fading away after sober reflection. Mr. Mompesson, Councilor Hahn, Emily Wesley, when half a lifetime had passed by, retained, and expressed, the same unwavering conviction as at first.

The narratives fail neither in minute detail of circumstance, nor in specifications of person, of time, and of place.

The observers were not influenced by expectancy, nor biased by recital of previous examples. The phenomena, indeed, have been of frequent occurrence; exhibiting an unmistakable family likeness, constituting a class. Yet not in a single instance does this fact appear to have been known to the observers. That which each witnessed he believed to be unexampled. Neither at Tedworth, nor Epworth, nor Slawensik, nor Baldarroch, nor Ahrensburg, nor Cideville, nor Hydesville, do the sufferers seem to have known that others had suffered by similar annoyance before. The more reliable, on that account, is their testimony.

There was not only no motive for simulation, but much temptation to conceal what actually occurred. Mr. Mompesson suffered in his name and estate. Mrs. Wesley strictly enjoined her son to impart the narrative to no one. Judge Rousselin found the curate of Cideville profoundly afflicted by his painful position. Mrs. Fox's health (as I learned) suffered seriously from grief. "What have we done," she used to say, "to deserve this?" We can readily conceive that such must have been the feeling. What more mortifying or painful than to be exposed to the suspicion of being either a willful impostor, or else the subject of punishment, from Heaven, for past misdeeds?

Finally, the phenomena were sometimes attested by the official records of public justice. So, during the trial of the drummer, the suit of Captain Molesworth, and the legal proceedings instituted, at Cideville, against the shepherd Thorel. Where shall we seek a higher grade of human evidence?

If such an array of testimony as this, lacking no element of trustworthiness, converging from numerous independent sources, yet concurrent through two centuries, be not entitled to credit, then what dependence can we place on the entire records of history? What becomes of the historical evidence for any past event whatever? If we are to reject, as fable, the narratives here submitted, are we not tacitly indorsing the logic of those who argue that Jesus Christ never lived? Nay, must we not accept as something graver than pleasantry that pamphlet in which a learned and ingenious Churchman sets forth plausible reasons for the belief that rumor, in her most notorious iterations, may be but a lying witness, and that it is doubtful whether Napoleon Buonaparte ever actually existed?*

---

* *"Historic Doubts relative to Napoleon Buonaparte,"* by Archbishop Whately, 12th ed., London, 1855.

BOOK IV.

OF APPEARANCES COMMONLY CALLED APPARITIONS

CHAPTER I.

TOUCHING HALLUCINATION.

The evidence for a future life derived from an occasional appearance of the dead, provided that appearance prove to be an objective phenomenon, and provided we do not misconceive its character, is of the highest grade. If it be important, then, to obtain a valuable contribution to the proofs of the soul's immortality, what more worthy of our attention than the subject of apparitions?

But in proportion to its importance and to its extraordinary character is the urgent propriety that it be scrupulously, even distrustfully, examined, and that its reality be tested with dispassionate care.

For its discussion involves the theory of hallucination; a branch of inquiry which has much engaged, as indeed it ought, the attention of modern physiologists.

That pure hallucinations occur, we cannot rationally doubt; but what are, and what are not, hallucinations, it may be more difficult to determine than superficial observers are wont to imagine.

Hallucination, according to the usual definition, consists of ideas and sensations conveying unreal impressions. It is an example of false testimony (not always credited) apparently given by the senses in a diseased or abnormal state of the human organization.

"It is evident," says Calmeil, "that if the same material combination which takes place in the brain of a man at the sight of a tree, of a dog, of a horse, is capable of being reproduced at a moment when these objects are no longer within sight, then that man will persist in believing that he still sees a horse, a dog, or a tree."*

It is a curious question, not yet fully settled by medical writers on the subject, whether hallucinations of the sight cause an actual image on the retina. Burdach, Müller,† Baillarger,‡ and others, who maintain the affirmative, remind us that patients who have recovered from an attack of hallucination always say, 'I saw; I heard;' thus speaking as of actual sensations. Dechambre§ and De Boismont, who assume the negative, adduce in support of their opinion the facts that a patient who has lost his leg will still complain of cold or pain in the toes of the amputated foot, and that men blind from amaurosis, where there is paralysis of the optic nerve, are still subject to visual hallucinations. The latter seems the better opinion. How can a mere mental conception (as Dechambre has argued) produce an image in the eye? And to what purpose? For, if the conception is already existing in the brain, what need of the eye to convey it thither? If it could be proved, in any given case, that a real image had been produced on the surface of the retina, it would, I think, go far to prove,

---

* "De la Folie," vol. i. p. 113.

† I have not access to the German originals; but both Burdach and Müller have been translated into French by Jourdain; see Burdach's "Traité de Physiologie," Paris, 1839, vol. v. p. 206, and Müller's "Manuel de Physiologie," Paris, 1845, vol. ii. p. 686.

‡ Baillarger; "Des Hallucinations, &c.," published in the "Mémoires de l'Academie Royale de Médecine," vol. xii. p. 369.

§ Dechambre's "Analyse de l'Ouvrage du Docteur Szafkowski sur les Hallucinations," published in the "Gazette Médicale" for 1850, p. 274.

I am indebted to De Boismont for most of these references. See his work, "Des Hallucinations," Paris, 1852, chap. 16.

also, that an objective reality must have been present to produce it. And so also of sonorous undulations actually received by the tympanum.

This will more clearly appear if we take instances of hallucination of other senses,—as of smell and touch Professor Bennett, of Scotland, in a pamphlet against Mesmerism,* vouches for two examples adduced by him to prove the power of imagination. He relates the first as follows:—"A clergyman told me that, some time ago, suspicions were entertained in his parish of a woman who was supposed to have poisoned her newly-born infant. The coffin was exhumed, and the procurator-fiscal, who attended with the medical men to examine the body, declared that he already perceived the odor of decomposition, which made him feel faint; and, in consequence, he withdrew. But on opening the coffin it was found to be empty; and it was afterward ascertained that no child had been born, and, consequently, no murder committed." Are we to suppose that the olfactory nerve was acted upon by an odor when the odor was not there? But here is the other case, from the same pamphlet. "A butcher was brought into the shop of Mr. McFarlane, the druggist, from the market-place opposite, laboring under a terrible accident. The man, in trying to hook up a heavy piece of meat above his head, slipped, and the sharp hook penetrated his arm, so that he himself was suspended. On being examined, he was pale, almost pulseless, and expressed himself as suffering acute agony. The arm could not be moved without causing excessive pain, and in cutting off the sleeve he frequently cried out; yet when the arm was exposed it was found to be perfectly uninjured, the hook having only traversed the sleeve of his coat!" What acted, in this case, on the nerves of sensation? There

---

* "*The Mesmeric Mania of* 1851," Edinburgh, 1851.

U   26*

was not the slightest lesion to do this; yet the effect on the brain was exactly the same as if these nerves had been actually irritated, and that, too, in the most serious manner.

The senses which most frequently seem to delude us are sight and hearing. Dr. Carpenter mentions the case of a lady, a near relative of his, who, "having been frightened in childhood by a black cat which sprang up from beneath her pillow just as she was laying her head upon it, was accustomed for many years afterward, whenever she was at all indisposed, to see a black cat on the ground before her; and, although perfectly aware of the spectral character of the appearance, yet she could never avoid lifting her foot as if to step over the cat when it appeared to be lying in her path."* Another lady, mentioned by Calmeil, continued, for upward of ten years, to imagine that a multitude of birds were constantly on the wing, flying close to her head; and she never sat down to dinner without setting aside crumbs of bread for her visionary attendants.†

So of auditory hallucinations, where the sense of hearing appears to play us false. Writers on the subject record the cases of patients who have been pursued for years, or through life, by unknown voices, sounds of bells, strains of music, hissing, barking, and the like. In many cases the sounds seemed, to the hallucinated, to proceed from tombs, from caverns, from beneath the ground; sometimes the voice was imagined to be internal, as from the breast or other portions of the body.‡

---

* "*Principles of Human Physiology,*" 5th ed., London, 1855, p. 564.

† *Calmeil,* vol. i. p. 11. I do not cite more apocryphal cases, as when Pic, in his life of the noted Benedictine Savonarola, tells us that the Holy Ghost, on several occasions, lit on the shoulders of the pious monk, who was lost in admiration of its golden plumage; and that when the divine bird introduced its beak into his ear he heard a murmur of a most peculiar description.—*J. F. Pic, in Vitâ Savonarolæ,* p. 124.

‡ *Calmeil,* work cited, vol. i. p. 8.

Calmeil relates the example of an aged courtier who, imagining that he heard rivals continually defaming him in presence of his sovereign, used constantly to exclaim, "They lie! you are deceived! I am calumniated, my prince."* And he mentions the case of another monomaniac who could not, without a fit of rage, hear pronounced the name of a town which recalled to him painful recollections. Children at the breast, the birds of the air, bells from every clock-tower, repeated, to his diseased hearing, the detested name.

These all appear to be cases of simple hallucination; against which, it may be remarked, perfect soundness of mind is no guarantee. Hallucination is not insanity: It is found, sometimes, disconnected not only from insanity, but from monomania in its mildest type. I knew well a lady who, more than once, distinctly saw feet ascending the stairs before her. Yet neither her physician nor she herself ever regarded this apparent marvel in other light than as an optical vagary dependent on her state of health.

In each of the cases above cited, it will be remarked that one person only was misled by deception of sense. And this brings me to speak of an important distinction made by the best writers on this subject: the difference, namely, between hallucination and illusion: the former being held to mean a false perception of that which has no existence whatever; the latter, an incorrect perception of something which actually exists. The lady who raised her foot to step over a black cat, when, in point of fact, there was nothing there to step over, is deemed to be the victim of a hallucination. Nicolai, the Berlin bookseller, is usually cited as one of the most noted cases; and his memoir on the subject, addressed to the Royal Society of Berlin, of which he

---

* *Calmeil,* work cited, vol i. p. 7.

was a member, is given as a rare example of philosophical and careful analysis of what he himself regarded
as a series of false sensations.* He imagined (so he relates) that his room was full of human figures, moving
about; all the exact counterpart of living persons, except that they were somewhat paler; some known to
him, some strangers; who occasionally spoke to each
other and to him; so that at times he was in doubt
whether or not some of his friends had come to visit him.

An illusion, unlike a hallucination, has a foundation
in reality. We actually see or hear something, which
we mistake for something else.† The mirage of the
Desert, the Fata Morgana of the Mediterranean, are
well-known examples. Many superstitions hence take
their rise. Witness the Giant of the Brocken, aerial
armies contending in the clouds, and the like.‡

---

* Nicolai read his memoir on the subject of the specters or phantoms
which disturbed him, with psychological remarks thereon, to the Royal
Society of Berlin, on the 28th of February, 1799. The translation of this
paper is given in *Nicholson's Journal*, vol. vi. p. 161.

† In actual mania, hallucinations are commonly set down as much more
frequent than illusions. De Boismont mentions that, out of one hundred
and eighty-one cases of mania observed by Messrs. Aubanel and Thore,
illusions showed themselves in sixteen instances, while hallucination
supervened in fifty-four. The exact list was as follows: *Illusions* of sight,
nine; of hearing, seven; *hallucinations* of hearing, twenty-three; of sight,
twenty-one; of taste, five; of touch, two; of smell, one; internal, two.—
"Des Hallucinations," p. 168.

‡ In the "Philosophical Magazine" (vol. i. p. 232) will be found a
record of the observations which finally explained to the scientific world
the nature of the gigantic appearance which, from the summit of the
Brocken, (one of the Hartz Mountains,) for long years excited the wondering credulity of the inhabitants and the astonishment of the passing
traveler. A Mr. Haue devoted some time to this subject. One day, while
he was contemplating the giant, a violent puff of wind was on the point
of carrying off his bat. Suddenly clapping his hand upon it, the giant did
the same. Mr. Haue bowed to him, and the salute was returned. He then
called the proprietor of the neighboring inn and imparted to him his discovery. The experiments were renewed with the same effect. It became
evident that the appearance was but an optical effect produced by a strongly

There are collective illusions; for it is evident that the same false appearance which deceives the senses of one man is not unlikely to deceive those of others also. Thus, an Italian historian relates that the inhabitants of the city of Florence were for several hours the dupes of a remarkable deception. There was seen, in the air, floating above the city, the colossal figure of an angel; and groups of spectators, gathered together in the principal streets, gazed in adoration, convinced that some miracle was about to take place. After a time it was discovered that this portentous appearance was but a simple optical illusion, caused by the reflection, on a cloud, of the figure of the gilded angel which surmounts the celebrated Duomo, brightly illuminated by the rays of the sun.

But I know of no well-authenticated instance of collective hallucinations. No two patients that I ever heard of imagined the presence of the same cat or dog at the same moment. None of Nicolai's friends perceived the figures which showed themselves to him. When Brutus's evil genius appeared to the Roman leader, no one but himself saw the colossal presence or heard the warning words, "We shall meet again at Philippi." It was Nero's eyes alone that were haunted with the specter of his murdered mother.*

---

illuminated body placed amid light clouds, reflected from a considerable distance, and magnified till it appeared five or six hundred feet in height.

In Westmoreland and other mountainous countries the peasants often imagine that they see in the clouds troops of cavalry and armies on the march,—when, in point of fact, it is but the reflection of horses pasturing on a hill-side, and peaceful travelers or laborers passing over the landscape.

* There is no proof that the appearances which presented themselves to Nicolai, to Brutus, and to Nero were other than mere hallucinations; yet, if it should appear that apparitions, whether of the living or the dead, are sometimes of objective character, we are assuming too much when we receive it as certain that nothing appeared to either of these men.

This is a distinction of much practical importance. If two persons perceive at the same time the same phenomenon, we may conclude that that phenomenon is an objective reality,—has, in some phase or other, actual existence.

The results of what have been usually called electro-biological experiments cannot with any propriety be adduced in confutation of this position. The biologized patient knowingly and voluntarily subjects himself to an artificial influence, of which the temporary effect is to produce false sensations; just as the eater of hasheesh, or the chewer of opium, conjures up the phantasmagoria of a partial insanity, or the confirmed drunkard exposes himself to the terrible delusions of delirium-tremens. But all these sufferers know, when the fit has passed, that there was nothing of reality in the imaginations that overcame them.

If we could be biologized without ostensible agency, in a seemingly normal and quiet state of mind and body, unconsciously to ourselves at the time, and without any subsequent conviction of our trance-like condition, then would Reason herself cease to be trustworthy, our very senses become blind guides, and men would but grope about in the mists of Pyrrhonism. Nothing in the economy of the universe, so far as we have explored it, allows us for a moment to entertain the idea that its Creator has permitted, or will ever permit, such a source of delusion.

We are justified in asserting, then, as a general rule, that what the senses of two or more persons perceive at the same time is not a hallucination; in other words, that there is *some* foundation for it.

But it does not follow that the converse of the proposition is true. It is not logical to conclude that, in every instance in which some strange appearance can be perceived by one observer only among many, it is a hallucination. In some cases where certain persons perceive phenomena which escape the senses of others, it is certain that the phenomena are, or may be, real. An every-day example of this is the fact that persons endowed with strong power of distant vision clearly distinguish objects which are invisible to the short-sighted. Again, Reichenbach reports that his sensitives saw, at the poles of the magnet, odic light, and felt, from the near contact of large free cystals, odic sensations, which by Reichenbach himself, and others as insensible to odic impressions as he, were utterly unperceived.* It is true that before such experiments can rationally produce conviction they must be repeated again and again, by various observers and with numerous subjects, each subject unknowing the testimony of the preceding, and the result of these various experiments must be carefully collated and compared. But, these precautions scrupulously taken, there is nothing in the nature of the experiments themselves to cause them to be set aside as untrustworthy.

There is nothing, then, absurd or illogical in the supposition that some persons may have true perceptions of which we are unconscious. We may not be able to comprehend *how* they receive these; but our ignorance of the mode of action does not disprove the reality of the effect. I knew an English gentleman who, if a cat had been secreted in a room where he was, invariably and infallibly detected her presence. *How* he perceived this, except by a general feeling of uneasiness, he could never explain; yet the fact was certain.

---

* Reichenbach, in his *"Sensitive Mensch,"* (vol. i. p. 1,) estimates the number of sensitives, including all who have any perception whatever of odic sights and feelings, at nearly one-half the human race. Cases of high sensitiveness are, he says, most commonly found in the diseased; sometimes, however, in the healthy. In both he considers them comparatively rare.

If we were all born deaf and dumb, we could not imagine how a human being should be able to perceive that a person he did not see was in an adjoining room, or how he could possibly become conscious that a town-clock, a mile off and wholly out of sight, was half an hour faster than the watch in his pocket. If to a deaf-mute, congenitally such, we say, in explanation, that we know these things because we *hear* the sound of the person's voice and of the clock striking, the words are to him without significance. They explain to him nothing. He believes that there *is* a perception which those around him call hearing, because they all agree in informing him of this. He believes that, under particular circumstances, they *do* become conscious of the distant and the unseen. But, if his infirmity continue till death, he will pass to another world with no conviction of the reality of hearing save that belief alone, unsustained except by the evidence of testimony.

What presumption is there against the supposition that, as there are exceptional cases in which some of our fellow-creatures are inferior to us in the range of their perceptions, there may be exceptional cases also in which some of them are superior? And why may not we, like the life-long deaf-mute, have to await the enlightenment of death before we can receive as true, except by faith in others' words, the allegations touching these superior perceptions?

There is, it is true, between the case of the deaf-mute and ours this difference: he is in the minority, we in the majority: his witnesses, therefore, are much more numerous than ours. But the question remains, are our witnesses, occasional only though they be, sufficient in number and in credibility?

That question, so far as it regards what are commonly called apparitions, it is my object in the next chapter to discuss.

Before doing so, however, one or two remarks touching current objections may here be in place.

It has usually been taken for granted that, if medicine shall have removed a perception, it was unreal. This does not follow. An actual perception may, for aught we know, depend on a peculiar state of the nervous system, and may be possible during that state only; and that state may be changed or modified by drugs. Our senses frequently are, for a time, so influenced; the sense of sight, for example, by belladonna. I found in England several ladies, all in the most respectable class of society, who have had, to a greater or less extent, the perception of apparitions; though they do not speak of this faculty or delusion (let the reader select either term) beyond the circle of their immediate friends. One of these ladies, in whose case the perception has existed from early infancy, informed me that it was suspended by indisposition, even by a severe cold. In this case, any medicine which removed the disease restored the perception.

Some writers have attempted to show that hallucination is epidemical, like the plague or the small-pox. If this be true at all, it is to an extent so trifling and under circumstances so peculiar that it can only be regarded as a rare exception to a general rule.* De Gasparin

* I find in De Boismont's elaborate work on Hallucinations but a single example detailed of what may be regarded as a collective hallucination, and that given (p. 72) on the authority of Bovet, and taken from his "*Pandemonium, or The Devil's Cloyster*," published in 1684, (p. 202;) not the most conclusive evidence, certainly. It is, besides, but the case of two men alleged to have seen, at the same time, the same apparition of certain richly-dressed ladies. But one of these men was at the time in a stupor, apparently suffering from nightmare, and did not speak of the vision at all until it was suggested to him by the other. We know, however, that suggestions made to a sleeping man sometimes influence his dreams. (See Abercrombie's "*Intellectual Powers*," 15th ed., London, 1857, pp. 202, 203.) A case cited and vouched for by Dr. Wigan ("*Duality of the Mind*," Lon-

314 IS THERE EVIDENCE

seeks to prove the contrary of this* by reminding us
that in Egypt, in the time of Justinian, all the world is
said to have seen black men without heads sailing in
brazen barks; that during an epidemic that once de-
populated Constantinople the inhabitants saw demons
passing along the streets from house to house, dealing
death as they passed; that Thucydides speaks of a
general invasion of specters which accompanied the
great plague at Athens; that Pliny relates how, during
the war of the Romans against the Cimbrians, the clash
of arms and the sound of trumpets were heard, as if
coming from the sky; that Pausanias writes that, long
after the action at Marathon, there were heard each
night on the field of battle the neighing of horses and
the shock of armies; that at the battle of Platæa the
heavens resounded with fearful cries, ascribed by the
Athenians to the god Pan; and so on.

Of these appearances some were clearly illusions, not
hallucinations; and as to the rest, M. de Gasparin is too
sensible a writer not to admit that "many of these
anecdotes are false and many are exaggerated."† For
myself, it would be almost as easy to convince me, on
the faith of a remote legend, that these marvelous
sights and sounds had actually existed, as that large
numbers of men concurred in the conviction that they

don, 1844, pp. 166 *et seq.*) does not prove that hallucination may be of a
collective character, though sometimes adduced t prove it.

Writers who believe in second-sight (as Martin, in his "*Description of
the Western Islands of Scotland*") allege that if two men, gifted with that
faculty, be standing together, and one of them, perceiving a vision, design-
edly touch the other, he also will perceive it. But we have no better evidence for this than for the reality of the faculty in question. And if second-
sight be a real phenomenon, then such seers are not deceived by a hallucination.

* "*Des Tables Tournantes, du Surnaturel en Général, et des Esprits,*" par
le Comte Agénor de Gasparin, Paris, 1855, vol. i. pp. 537 *et seq.*

† De Gasparin's work already cited, vol. i. p. 538.

saw and heard them. The very details whicn accompany many of them suffice to discredit the idea they are adduced to prove. In the relation of Pausanias, for example, touching the nightly noises on the battle-field of Marathon, we read that those who were attracted to the spot by curiosity heard them not: it was to the chance traveler only, crossing the haunted spot without premeditation, that the phantom horses neighed and the din of arms resounded. Imagination or expectation, it would seem, had nothing to do with it. It was a local phenomenon. Can we believe it to have been a perversion of the sense of hearing? If we do, we admit that hallucination may be endemic as well as epidemic.

I would not be understood as denying that there have been times and seasons during which instances of hallucination have increased in frequency beyond the usual rate. That which violently excites the mind often reacts morbidly on the senses. But this does not prove the position I am combating. The reaction consequent upon the failure of the first French Revolution, together with the horrors of the reign of terror, so agitated and depressed the minds of many, that in France suicides became frequent beyond all previous example. Yet it would be a novel doctrine to assert that suicide is of a contagious or epidemical character.

De Boismont reminds us that considerable assemblages of men ("des réunions considérables") have been the dupes of the same illusions. "A cry," he says, "suffices to affright a multitude. An individual who thinks he sees something supernatural soon causes others, as little enlightened as he, to share his conviction."* As to *illusions*, both optical and oral, this is undoubtedly true; more especially when these present themselves in times

---

* *"Des Hallucinations,"* p. 128.

of excitement,—as during a battle or a plague,—or when they are generated in twilight gloom or midnight darkness. But that the contagion of example, or the belief of one individual under the actual influence of hallucination, suffices to produce, in others around, disease of the retina or of the optic or auditory nerve, or, in short, any abnormal condition of the senses, is a supposition which, so far as my reading extends, is unsupported by any reliable proof whatever.

The hypothesis of hallucination, then, is, in a general way, untenable in cases where two or more independent observers perceive the same or a similar appearance. But, since we know that hallucination does occur, that hypothesis may, in cases where there is but a single observer, be regarded as the more natural one, to be rebutted only by such attendant circumstances as are not explicable except by supposing the appearance real.

Bearing with us these considerations, let us now endeavor to separate, in this matter, the fanciful from the real. In so doing, we may find it difficult to preserve the just mean between too ready admission and too strenuous unbelief. If the reader be tempted to suspect in me easy credulity, let him beware on his part of arrogant prejudgment. " Contempt before inquiry," says Paley, " is fatal." Discarding alike prejudice and superstition, adopting the inductive method, let us seek to determine whether, even if a large portion of the thousand legends of ghosts and apparitions that have won credence in every age be due to hallucination, there be not another portion—the records of genuine phenomena—observed by credible witnesses and attested by sufficient proof.

CHAPTER II.

APPARITIONS OF THE LIVING.

When, in studying the subject of apparitions, I first met an alleged example of the appearance of a living person at a distance from where that person actually was, I gave to it little weight. And this the rather because the example itself was not sufficiently attested. It is related and believed by Jung Stilling as having occurred about the years 1750 to 1760, and is to this effect.

There lived at that time, near Philadelphia, in a lonely house and in a retired manner, a man of benevolent and pious character, but suspected to have some occult power of disclosing hidden events. It happened that a certain sea-captain having been long absent and no letter received from him, his wife, who lived near this man, and who had become alarmed and anxious, was advised to consult him. Having heard her story, he bade her wait a little and he would bring her an answer. Thereupon he went into another room, shutting the door; and there he stayed so long that, moved by curiosity, she looked through an aperture in the door to ascertain what he was about. Seeing him lying motionless on a sofa, she quickly returned to her place. Soon after, he came out, and told the woman that her husband was at that time in London, in a certain coffeehouse which he named, and that he would soon return. He also stated the reasons why his return had been delayed and why he had not written to her; and she went home somewhat reassured. When her husband did return, they found, on comparing notes, that every thing she had been told was exactly true. But the strangest part of the story remains. When she took her husband to see the alleged seer, he started back in surprise, and afterward confessed to his wife that, on a certain day, (the same on which she had consulted the person in question,) he was in a coffee-house in London, (the same that had been named to her,) and that this very man had there accosted him, and had told him that his wife was in great anxiety about him; that then the sea-captain had replied informing the stranger why his return was delayed and why he had not written, whereupon the man turned away, and he lost sight of him in the crowd.*

This story, however, came to Stilling through several hands, and is very loosely authenticated. It was brought from America by a German who had emigrated to the United States, and had been many years manager of some mills on the Delaware. He related it, on his return to Germany, to a friend of Stilling's, from whom Stilling had it. But no names nor exact dates are given; and it is not even stated whether the German emigrant obtained the incident directly either from the sea-captain or his wife.

It is evident that such a narrative, coming to us with no better vouchers than these, (though we may admit Stilling's entire good faith,) cannot rationally be accepted as authority.

Yet it is to be remarked that, in its incidents, the above story is but little more remarkable than the Joseph Wilkins dream or the case of Mary Goffe, both already given in the chapter on Dreams. If true, it evidently belongs to the same class, with this variation: that the phenomena in the two cases referred to occurred spontaneously, whereas, according to the Stilling narra-

---

* "*Theorie der Geisterkunde,*" vol. iv. of Stilling's "*Sämmtliche Werke,*" pp. 501 to 503. I have somewhat abridged in translating it.

tive, they were called up by the will of the subject and could be reproduced at pleasure.

The next narrative I am enabled to give as perfectly authentic.

APPARITION IN IRELAND.

There was living, in the summer of the year 1802, in the south of Ireland, a clergyman of the Established Church, the Rev. Mr. ——, afterward Archdeacon of ——, now deceased. His first wife, a woman of great beauty, sister of the Governor of ——, was then alive. She had been recently confined, and her recovery was very slow. Their residence—an old-fashioned mansion, situated in a spacious garden—adjoined on one side the park of the Bishop of ——. It was separated from it by a wall, in which there was a private door.

Mr. —— had been invited by the bishop to dinner; and as his wife, though confined to bed, did not seem worse than usual, he had accepted the invitation. Returning from the bishop's palace about ten o'clock, he entered, by the private door already mentioned, his own premises. It was bright moonlight. On issuing from a small belt of shrubbery into a garden walk, he perceived, as he thought, in another walk, parallel to that in which he was, and not more than ten or twelve feet from him, the figure of his wife, in her usual dress. Exceedingly astonished, he crossed over and confronted her. It *was* his wife. At least, he distinguished her features, in the clear moonlight, as plainly as he had ever done in his life. "What *are* you doing here?" he asked. She did not reply, but receded from him, turning to the right, toward a kitchen-garden that lay on one side of the house. In it there were several rows of peas, staked and well grown, so as to shelter any person passing behind them. The figure passed round one end of these. Mr. —— followed quickly, in increased astonishment, mingled with alarm; but when he reached the open space beyond the peas the figure was nowhere to be seen. As there was no spot where, in so short a time, it could have sought concealment, the husband concluded that it was an apparition, and not his wife, that he had seen. He returned to the front door, and, instead of availing himself of his pass-key as usual, he rung the bell. While on the steps, before the bell was answered, looking round, he saw the same figure at the corner of the house. When the servant opened the door, he asked him how his mistress was. "I am sorry to say, sir," answered the man, "she is not so well. Dr. Osborne has been sent for." Mr. —— hurried up-stairs, found his wife in bed and much worse, attended by the nurse, who had not left her all the evening. From that time she gradually sank, and within twelve hours thereafter expired.

The above was communicated to me by Mr. ——, now of Canada, son of the archdeacon.* He had so often heard his father narrate the incident that every particular was minutely imprinted on his memory. I inquired of him if his father had ever stated to him whether, during his absence at the bishop's, his wife had slept, or had been observed to be in a state of swoon or trance; but he could afford me no information on that subject. It is to be regretted that this had not been observed and recorded. The wife knew where her husband was and by what route he would return. We may imagine, but cannot prove, that this was a case similar to that of Mary Goffe,—the appearance of the wife, as of the mother, showing itself where her thoughts and affections were.

The following narrative I owe to the kindness of a

---

* On the 1st of June, 1859.

friend, Mrs. D——, now of Washington, the daughter of a Western clergyman of well-known reputation, recently deceased.

TWO APPARITIONS OF LIVING PERSONS, IN THE SAME HOUSE, ON THE SAME DAY.

"I resided for several years in a spacious old stone house, two stories high, agreeably situated, amid fruit-trees and shrubbery, on the banks of the Ohio River, in Switzerland County, Indiana. Two verandas, above and below, with outside stairs leading up to them, ran the entire length of the house on the side next the river. These, especially the upper one with its charming prospect, were a common resort of the family.

"On the 15th of September, 1845, my younger sister, J——, was married, and came with her husband, Mr. H—— M——, to pass a portion of the honeymoon in our pleasant retreat.

"On the 18th of the same month, we all went, by invitation, to spend the day at a friend's house about a mile distant. As twilight came on, finding my two little ones growing restless, we decided to return home. After waiting some time for my sister's husband, who had gone off to pay a visit in a neighboring village, saying he would soon return, we set out without him. Arrived at home, my sister, who occupied an upper room, telling me she would go and change her walking-dress, proceeded up-stairs, while I remained below to see my drowsy babes safe in bed. The moon, I remember, was shining brightly at the time.

"Suddenly, after a minute or two, my sister burst into the room, wringing her hands in despair, and weeping bitterly. 'Oh, sister, sister!' she exclaimed; 'I shall lose him! I know I shall! Hugh is going to die.' In the greatest astonishment, I inquired what was the

V

matter; and then, between sobs, she related to me the cause of her alarm, as follows :—

"As she ran up-stairs to their room she saw her husband seated at the extremity of the upper veranda, his hat on, a cigar in his mouth, and his feet on the railing, apparently enjoying the cool river-breeze. Supposing, of course, that he had returned before we did, she approached him, saying, 'Why, Hugh, when did you get here? Why did you not return and come home with us?' As he made no reply, she went up to him, and, bride-like, was about to put her arms round his neck, when, to her horror, the figure was gone and the chair empty. She had barely strength left (so great was the shock) to come down-stairs and relate to me what her excited fears construed into a certain presage of death.

"It was not till more than two hours afterward, when my brother-in-law actually returned, that she resumed her tranquillity. We rallied and laughed at her then, and, after a time, the incident passed from our minds.

"Previously to this, however,—namely, about an hour before Hugh's return,—while we were sitting in the parlor, on the lower floor, I saw a boy, some sixteen years of age, look in at the door of the room. It was a lad whom my husband employed to work in the garden and about the house, and who, in his leisure hours, used to take great delight in amusing my little son Frank, of whom he was very fond. He was dressed, as was his wont, in a suit of blue summer-cloth, with an old palm-leaf hat without a band, and he advanced, in his usual bashful way, a step or two into the room, then stopped, and looked round, apparently in search of something. Supposing that he was looking for the children, I said to him, 'Frank is in bed, Silas, and asleep long ago.' He did not reply, but, turning with a quiet smile that was common to him, left the room, and I noticed, from the window, that he lingered near the outside door, walking backward and forward before it once or twice. If I had afterward been required to depose, on oath, before a court of justice, that I had seen the boy enter and leave the room, and also that I had noticed him pass and repass before the parlor-window, I should have sworn to these circumstances without a moment's hesitation. Yet it would seem that such a deposition would have conveyed a false impression.

"For, shortly after, my husband, coming in, said, 'I wonder where Silas is?' (that was the boy's name.)

" 'He must be somewhere about,' I replied: 'he was here a few minutes since, and I spoke to him.' Thereupon Mr. D—— went out and called him, but no one answered. He sought him all over the premises, then in his room, but in vain. No Silas was to be found; nor did he show himself that night; nor was he in the house the next morning when we arose.

"At breakfast he first made his appearance. 'Where have you been, Silas?' said Mr. D——.

"The boy replied that he had been 'up to the island, fishing.'

" 'But,' I said, 'you were here last night.'

" 'Oh, no,' he replied, with the simple accent of truth. 'Mr. D—— gave me leave to go fishing yesterday; and I understood I need not return till this morning: so I stayed away all night. I have not been near here since yesterday morning.'

"I could not doubt the lad's word. He had no motive for deceiving us. The island of which he spoke was two miles distant from our house; and, under all the circumstances, I settled down to the conclusion that as, in my sister's case, her husband had appeared where he was not, so in the case of the boy also it was the appearance only, not the real person, that I had seen that evening. It was remarkable enough that both the incidents should have occurred in the same house and on the same day.

"It is proper I should add that my sister's impression that the apparition of her husband foreboded death did not prove true. He outlived her; and no misfortune which they could in any way connect with the appearance happened in the family.

"Nor did Silas die; nor, so far as I know, did any thing unusual happen to him."*

This case is, in some respects, a strong one. There was evidently no connection between the appearance to the one sister and that to the other. There was no excitement preceding the apparitions. In each case, the evidence, so far as one sense went, was as strong as if the real person had been present. The narrator expressly says she would unhesitatingly have sworn, in a court of justice, to the presence of the boy Silas. The sister addressed the appearance of her husband, unexpected as it was, without doubt or hesitation. The theory of hallucination *may* account for both cases; but, whether it does or not, the phenomenon is one which ought to challenge the attention of the jurist as well as of the psychologist. If appearances so exactly counterfeiting reality as these can, occasionally, cheat human sense, their possible occurrence ought not to be ignored in laying down rules of evidence. The presumption, of course, is, in every case, very strongly against them. Yet cases *have* occurred in which an *alibi*, satisfactorily proved yet conflicting with seemingly unimpeachable evidence, has completely puzzled the courts. An example, related and vouched for by Mrs. Crowe, but witn-

---

* Communicated to me, in Washington, June 24, 1859

out adducing her authority, and which I have not myself verified, is, in substance, as follows:—

In the latter part of the last century, in the city of Glasgow, Scotland, a servant-girl, known to have had illicit connection with a certain surgeon's apprentice, suddenly disappeared. There being no circumstances leading to suspicion of foul play, no special inquiry was made about her.

In those days, in Scottish towns, no one was allowed to show himself in street or public ground during the hours of church-service; and this interdiction was enforced by the appointment of inspectors, authorized to take down the names of delinquents.

Two of these, making their rounds, came to a wall, the lower boundary of "The Green," as the chief public park of the city is called. There, lying on the grass, they saw a young man, whom they recognized as the surgeon's assistant. They asked him why he was not at church, and proceeded to register his name; but, instead of attempting an excuse, he merely rose, saying, "I am a miserable man; look in the water!" then crossed a style and struck into a path leading to the Rutherglen road. The inspectors, astonished, *did* proceed to the river, where they found the body of a young woman, which they caused to be conveyed to town. While they were accompanying it through the streets, they passed one of the principal churches, whence, at the moment, the congregation were issuing; and among them they perceived the apprentice. But this did not much surprise them, thinking he might have had time to go round and enter the church toward the close of the service.

The body proved to be that of the missing servant-girl. She was found pregnant, and had evidently been murdered by means of a surgeon's instrument, which had remained entangled in her clothes. The apprentice, who proved to have been the last person seen in her company before she disappeared, was arrested, and would, on the evidence of the inspectors, have been found guilty, had he not, on his trial, established an incontrovertible *alibi;* showing, beyond possible doubt, that he had been in church during the entire service. The young man was acquitted. The greatest excitement prevailed in the public mind at the time; but all efforts to obtain a natural explanation failed.*

If this story can be trusted, it is conclusive of the question. Both inspectors saw, or believed they saw, the same person; a person of whom they were not in search and whom they did not expect to find there. Both heard the same words; and these words directed them to the river, and were the cause of their finding the dead body; the body, too, of a girl with whom the apprentice had been on the most intimate and suspicious terms, whether he was her murderer or not. When did hallucination lead to such a discovery as that?

In the next case, if it be one of hallucination, two senses were deceived.

SIGHT AND SOUND.

During the winter of 1839–40, Dr. J—— E—— was residing, with his aunt Mrs. L——, in a house on Fourteenth Street, near New York Avenue, in the city of Washington.

Ascending one day from the basement of the house to the parlor, he saw his aunt descending the stairs. He stepped back to let her pass, which she did, close to him, but without speaking. He instantly ascended the stairs and entered the parlor, where he found his aunt sitting quietly by the side of the fire.

---

* *"Night Side of Nature,"* by Catherine Crowe, 16th ed., London, 1854, pp. 183 to 186.

The distance from where he first saw the figure to the spot where his aunt was actually sitting was between thirty and forty feet. The figure seemed dressed exactly as his aunt was; and he distinctly heard the rustle of her dress as she passed.

As the figure, when descending the stairs and passing Dr. E——, bore the very same appearance as a real person, and as the circumstance occurred in broad daylight, Dr. E—— long thought that, if not a mere hallucination, it might augur death; but nothing happened to justify his anticipations.*

The next example is of a much more conclusive character than any of the foregoing, if we except the narrative of Mrs. Crowe.

APPARITION OF THE LIVING,

Seen by Mother and Daughter.

In the month of May and in the year 1840, Dr. D——, a noted physician of Washington, was residing with his wife and his daughter Sarah (now Mrs. B——) at their country-seat, near Piney Point, in Virginia, a fashionable pleasure-resort during the summer months.

One afternoon, about five o'clock, the two ladies were walking out in a copse-wood not far from their residence; when, at a distance on the road, coming toward them, they saw a gentleman. "Sally," said Mrs. D——, "there comes your father to meet us." "I think not," the daughter replied: "that cannot be papa: it is not so tall as he."

As he neared them, the daughter's opinion was confirmed. They perceived that it was not Dr. D——, but a Mr. Thompson, a gentleman with whom they were well

---

* The above was related to me by Dr. E—— himself, in Washington, on the 5th of July, 1859; and the MS. was submitted to him for revision.

acquainted, and who was at that time, though they then knew it not, a patient of Dr. D——'s. They observed also, as he came nearer, that he was dressed in a blue frock-coat, black satin waistcoat, and black pantaloons and hat. Also, on comparing notes afterward, both ladies, it appeared, had noticed that his linen was particularly fine and that his whole apparel seemed to have been very carefully adjusted.

He came up so close that they were on the very point of addressing him; but at that moment he stepped aside, as if to let them pass; and then, *even while the eyes of both the ladies were upon him,* he suddenly and entirely disappeared.

The astonishment of Mrs. D—— and her daughter may be imagined. They could scarcely believe the evidence of their own eyes. They lingered, for a time, on the spot, as if expecting to see him reappear; then, with that strange feeling which comes over us when we have just witnessed something unexampled and incredible, they hastened home.

They afterward ascertained, through Dr. D——, that his patient Mr. Thompson, being seriously indisposed, was confined to his bed; and that *he had not quitted his room, nor indeed his bed, throughout the entire day.*

It may properly be added that, though Mr. Thompson was familiarly known to the ladies and much respected by them as an estimable man, there were no reasons existing why they should take any more interest in him, or he in them, than in the case of any other friend or acquaintance. He died just six weeks from the day of this appearance.

The above narrative is of unquestionable authenticity. It was communicated in Washington, in June, 1859, by Mrs. D—— herself; and the manuscript, being submitted to her for revision, was assented to as accurate. It had been frequently related, both by mother and daughter, to the lady—a friend of theirs—who first brought it to my notice.

What shall we say to it? What element of authenticity does it lack? The facts are of comparatively recent occurrence. They are reported directly by the observers of the phenomenon. The circumstances preclude even the hypothesis of suggestion. The mother's remark to the daughter was, "There comes your father." The daughter dissents, remarking that it was a shorter man. When the appearance approaches, both ladies distinguish the same person, and that so unmistakably that they advance to meet him and speak to him, without the least mistrust. It was evidently an appearance seen independently by both the observers.

It was seen, too, in broad daylight, and under no excitement whatever. The ladies were enjoying a quiet afternoon's walk. There was no terror to blind, no anxiety of affection to conjure up (as skepticism might imagine it can) the phantom of the absent. The incident is (as they suppose) of the most commonplace character. The gentleman whom they see advancing to meet them is an ordinary acquaintance,—ill at the time, it is true; but even that fact is unknown to them. They both continue to see him until he is within speaking-distance. Both observe his dress, even the minute particulars of it; so that on the senses of both precisely the same series of impressions is produced. They ascertain this by a subsequent comparison of their sensations.

Nor do they lose sight of him in any doubtful way, or while their attention is distracted. He disappears before their eyes at the very moment they are about to address him.

How strong in this case is the presumptive evidence against hallucination! Even setting aside the received doctrine of the books, that there is no collective hallucination, how can we imagine that there should be produced, at the very same moment, without suggestion, or expectation, or unusual excitement of any kind, on the brain of two different persons, a perception of the self-same image, minutely detailed, without any external object to produce it? Was that image imprinted on the retina in the case both of mother and daughter? How could this be if there was nothing existing in the outside world to imprint it? Or was there no image on the retina? Was it a purely subjective impression? that is, a false perception, due to disease? But among the millions of impressions which *may* be produced, if imagination only is the creative agent, how infinite the probabilities *against* the contingency that, out of these millions, this one especial object should present itself in two independent cases!—not only a particular person, dressed in a particular manner, but that person advancing along a road, approaching within a few steps of the observers, and then disappearing! Yet even this is not the limit of the adverse chances. There is not only identity of object, but exact coincidence of time. The two perceive the very same thing at the very same moment; and this coincidence continues throughout several minutes.

What is the natural and necessary conclusion? That there *was* an image produced on the retina, and that there *was* an objective reality there to produce it.

It may seem marvelous, it may appear hard to believe, that the appearance of a human being, in his usual dress, should present itself where that human being is not. It would be a thing a thousand times more marvelous, ten thousand times harder to believe, that the fortuitous action of disease, freely ranging throughout the infinite variety of contingent possibilities, should produce, by mere chance, a mass of coincidences such as make up, in this case, the concurrent and cotemporaneous sensations of mother and daughter

I might here adduce an example which several writers have noticed; that, namely, of the apparition to Dr Donne, in Paris, of his wife, with her hair hanging loose and a dead child in her arms, on the very day and at the very hour that she was delivered of a still-born child at Drewry House, the residence of Dr. Donne's patron, Sir Robert Drewry, then ambassador at the French Court. It is related and vouched for by "honest Izaak," as his friends used to call the author of "The Compleat Angler;"* but it is two hundred and fifty years old. Therefore I prefer to pass on to the following, of modern date and direct authentication.

APPARITION AT SEA.

During the autumn of 1857, Mr. Daniel M——, a young American gentleman, after having traveled throughout Germany, was returning to the United States in a Bremen packet.

One tempestuous evening his mother, Mrs. A—— M——, residing near New York, knowing that her son was probably then at sea, became much alarmed for his safety, and put up in secret an earnest prayer that he might be preserved to her.

There was residing in the same house with her, at that time, one of her nieces, named Louisa, who was in the habit of receiving impressions of what might be called a clairvoyant character. This niece had heard the expression of her aunt's fears, but, like the rest of the family, she was ignorant that these fears had found expression in prayer for her cousin's safety. The day after the tempest, she had an impression so vivid and distinct that she was induced to record it in writing. It was to the effect that her aunt had no cause to fear, seeing that the object of her anxiety was in safety, and that at the

* "The Lives of Dr. John Donne, Sir Henry Wotton, &c." By Isaac Walton, Oxford edition, 1824, pp. 16 to 19.

very hour of the previous evening when the mother had so earnestly put up a secret prayer for him, *her son, being at the time in his state-room, had been conscious of his mother's presence.*

This she read to her aunt the same day, thinking it might tend to comfort her.

And then she waited with great anxiety for her cousin's return, when she might have her doubts resolved as to the truth or falsehood of the mysterious impression regarding him.

He arrived three weeks afterward, safe and well; but during the afternoon and evening that succeeded his arrival, no allusion whatever was made by any one to the above circumstances. When the rest of the family retired, Louisa remained, proposing to question him on the subject. He had stepped out; but after a few minutes he returned to the parlor, came up to the opposite side of the table at which she was sitting, looking agitated, and, before she herself could proffer a word, he said, with much emotion, "Cousin, I must tell you a most remarkable thing that happened to me." And with that, to her astonishment, he burst into tears.

She felt that the solution of her doubts was at hand; and so it proved. He told her that one night during the voyage, soon after he had lain down, he saw, on the side of the state-room opposite his berth, the appearance of his mother. It was so startlingly like a real person that he rose and approached it. He did not, however, attempt to touch it, being ultimately satisfied that it was an apparition only. But on his return to his berth he still saw it, for some minutes, as before.

On comparing notes, it was ascertained that the evening on which the young man thus saw the appearance of his mother at sea was the same on which she had so earnestly prayed for his safety,—the very same, too, which his cousin Louisa had designated in writing, three weeks before, as the time when he had seen the apparition in question. And, as nearly as they could make it out, the hour also corresponded.

The above narrative was communicated to me* by the two ladies concerned, the mother and her niece, both being together when I obtained it. They are highly intellectual and cultivated. I am well acquainted with them, and I know that entire reliance may be placed on their statement.

In this case, as in that in which the apparition of Mr. Thompson showed itself to mother and daughter, there are two persons having coincident sensations; Louisa impressed that her cousin was conscious of his mother's presence, and the cousin impressed with that very consciousness. Unlike the Thompson case, the cousins were many hundred miles distant from each other at the time. Suggestion was impossible; equally so was any mistake by after-thought. Louisa committed her impression to writing at the time, and read it to her aunt. The writing remained, real and definite, in proof of that impression. And she made no inquiry of her cousin, put no leading question, to draw out a confirmation or refutation of her perceptions regarding him. The young man volunteered his story; and his tears of emotion attested the impression which the apparition had made.

Chance coincidence, as every one must see, was out of the question. Some other explanation must be sought.

The following narrative, drawn from nautical life, exhibits coincidences as unmistakably produced by some agency other than chance.

THE RESCUE.

Mr. Robert Bruce, originally descended from some branch of the Scottish family of that name, was born,

---

* On the 8th of August, 1859.

in humble circumstances, about the close of the last century, at Torbay, in the south of England, and there bred
up to a seafaring life.

When about thirty years of age, to wit, in the year
1828, he was first mate on a bark trading between
Liverpool and St. John's, New Brunswick.

On one of her voyages bound westward, being then
some five or six weeks out and having neared the eastern portion of the Banks of Newfoundland, the captain
and mate had been on deck at noon, taking an observation of the sun; after which they both descended to
calculate their day's work.

The cabin, a small one, was immediately at the stern
of the vessel, and the short stairway descending to it
ran athwart-ships. Immediately opposite to this stairway, just beyond a small square landing, was the mate's
state-room; and from that landing there were two
doors, close to each other, the one opening aft into the
cabin, the other, fronting the stairway, into the state-
room. The desk in the state-room was in the forward
part of it, close to the door; so that any one sitting at
it and looking over his shoulder could see into the cabin.

The mate, absorbed in his calculation, which did not
result as he expected, varying considerably from the
dead-reckoning, had not noticed the captain's motions.
When he had completed his calculations, he called out,
without looking round, "I make our latitude and longitude so and so. Can that be right? How is yours?"

Receiving no reply, he repeated his question, glancing
over his shoulder and perceiving, as he thought, the
captain busy writing on his slate. Still no answer.
Thereupon he rose; and, as he fronted the cabin-door,
the figure he had mistaken for the captain raised its
head and disclosed to the astonished mate the features
of an entire stranger.

Bruce was no coward; but, as he met that fixed gaze

looking directly at him in grave silence, and became assured that it was no one whom he had ever seen before, it was too much for him; and, instead of stopping to question the seeming intruder, he rushed upon deck in such evident alarm that it instantly attracted the captain's attention. "Why, Mr. Bruce," said the latter, "what in the world is the matter with you?"

"The matter, sir? Who is that at your desk?"

"No one that I know of."

"But there *is*, sir: there's a stranger there."

"A stranger! Why, man, you must be dreaming. You must have seen the steward there, or the second mate. Who else would venture down without orders?"

"But, sir, he was sitting in your arm-chair, fronting the door, writing on your slate. Then he looked up full in my face; and, if ever I saw a man plainly and distinctly in this world, I saw him."

"Him! Whom?"

"God knows, sir: I don't. I saw a man, and a man I had never seen in my life before."

"You must be going crazy, Mr. Bruce. A stranger, and we nearly six weeks out!"

"I know, sir; but then I saw him."

"Go down and see who it is."

Bruce hesitated. "I never was a believer in ghosts," he said; "but, if the truth must be told, sir, I'd rather not face it alone."

"Come, come, man. Go down at once, and don't make a fool of yourself before the crew."

"I hope you've always found me willing to do what's reasonable," Bruce replied, changing color; "but if it's all the same to you, sir, I'd rather we should both go down together."

The captain descended the stairs, and the mate followed him. Nobody in the cabin! They examined the state-rooms. Not a soul to be found!

"Well, Mr. Bruce," said the captain, "did not I tell you you had been dreaming?"

"It's all very well to say so, sir; but if I didn't see that man writing on your slate, may I never see my home and family again!"

"Ah! writing on the slate! Then it should be there still." And the captain took it up.

"By God," he exclaimed, "here's something, sure enough! Is that your writing, Mr. Bruce?"

The mate took the slate; and there, in plain, legible characters, stood the words, "STEER TO THE NOR'WEST."

"Have you been trifling with me, sir?" added the captain, in a stern manner.

"On my word as a man and as a sailor, sir," replied Bruce, "I know no more of this matter than you do. I have told you the exact truth."

The captain sat down at his desk, the slate before him, in deep thought. At last, turning the slate over and pushing it toward Bruce, he said, "Write down, 'Steer to the nor'west.'"

The mate complied; and the captain, after narrowly comparing the two handwritings, said, "Mr. Bruce, go and tell the second mate to come down here."

He came; and, at the captain's request, he also wrote the same words. So did the steward. So, in succession, did every man of the crew who could write at all. But not one of the various hands resembled, in any degree, the mysterious writing.

When the crew retired, the captain sat deep in thought. "Could any one have been stowed away?" at last he said. "The ship must be searched; and if I don't find the fellow he must be a good hand at hide-and-seek. Order up all hands."

Every nook and corner of the vessel, from stem to stern, was thoroughly searched, and that with all the eagerness of excited curiosity,—for the report had gone out that a stranger had shown himself on board; but not a living soul beyond the crew and the officers was found.

Returning to the cabin after their fruitless search, "Mr. Bruce," said the captain, "what the devil do you make of all this?"

"Can't tell, sir. *I* saw the man write; *you* see the writing. There must be something in it."

"Well, it would seem so. We have the wind free, and I have a great mind to keep her away and see what will come of it."

"I surely would, sir, if I were in your place. It's only a few hours lost, at the worst."

"Well, we'll see. Go on deck and give the course nor'west. And, Mr. Bruce," he added, as the mate rose to go, "have a look-out aloft, and let it be a hand you can depend on."

His orders were obeyed. About three o'clock the look-out reported an iceberg nearly ahead, and, shortly after, what he thought was a vessel of some kind close to it.

As they approached, the captain's glass disclosed the fact that it was a dismantled ship, apparently frozen to the ice, and with a good many human beings on it. Shortly after, they hove to, and sent out the boats to the relief of the sufferers.

It proved to be a vessel from Quebec, bound to Liverpool, with passengers on board. She had got entangled in the ice, and finally frozen fast, and had passed several weeks in a most critical situation. She was stove, her decks swept,—in fact, a mere wreck; all her provisions and almost all her water gone. Her crew and passengers had lost all hopes of being saved, and their gratitude for the unexpected rescue was proportionately great.

As one of the men who had been brought away in

the third boat that had reached the wreck was ascending the ship's side, the mate, catching a glimpse of his face, started back in consternation. It was the very face he had seen, three or four hours before, looking up at him from the captain's desk.

At first he tried to persuade himself it might be fancy; but the more he examined the man the more sure he became that he was right. Not only the face, but the person and the dress, exactly corresponded.

As soon as the exhausted crew and famished passengers were cared for, and the bark on her course again, the mate called the captain aside. "It seems that was not a ghost I saw to-day, sir: the man's alive."

"What do you mean? Who's alive?"

"Why, sir, one of the passengers we have just saved is the same man I saw writing on your slate at noon. I would swear to it in a court of justice."

"Upon my word, Mr. Bruce," replied the captain, "this gets more and more singular. Let us go and see this man."

They found him in conversation with the captain of the rescued ship. They both came forward, and expressed, in the warmest terms, their gratitude for deliverance from a horrible fate,—slow-coming death by exposure and starvation.

The captain replied that he had but done what he was certain they would have done for him under the same circumstances, and asked them both to step down into the cabin. Then, turning to the passenger, he said, "I hope, sir, you will not think I am trifling with you; but I would be much obliged to you if you would write a few words on this slate." And he handed him the slate, with that side up on which the mysterious writing was not. "I will do any thing you ask," replied the passenger; "but what shall I write?"

"A few words are all I want. Suppose you write, 'Steer to the nor'west.'"

The passenger, evidently puzzled to make out the motive for such a request, complied, however, with a smile. The captain took up the slate and examined it closely; then, stepping aside so as to conceal the slate from the passenger, he turned it over, and gave it to him again with the other side up.

"You say that is your handwriting?" said he.

"I need not say so," rejoined the other, looking at it, "for you saw me write it."

"And this?" said the captain, turning the slate over.

The man looked first at one writing, then at the other, quite confounded. At last, "What is the meaning of this?" said he. "I only wrote one of these. Who wrote the other?"

"That's more than I can tell you, sir. My mate here says you wrote it, sitting at this desk, at noon to-day."

The captain of the wreck and the passenger looked at each other, exchanging glances of intelligence and surprise; and the former asked the latter, "Did you dream that you wrote on this slate?"

"No, sir, not that I remember."

"You speak of dreaming," said the captain of the bark. "What was this gentleman about at noon to-day?"

"Captain," rejoined the other, "the whole thing is most mysterious and extraordinary; and I had intended to speak to you about it as soon as we got a little quiet. This gentleman," (pointing to the passenger,) "being much exhausted, fell into a heavy sleep, or what seemed such, some time before noon. After an hour or more, he awoke, and said to me, 'Captain, we shall be relieved this very day.' When I asked him what reason he had for saying so, he replied that he had dreamed that he was on board a bark, and that she was coming to our rescue. He described her appearance and rig; and, to our utter astonishment, when your vessel hove in sight she corresponded exactly to his description of her. We had not put much faith in what he said; yet still we hoped there might be something in it, for drowning men, you know, will catch at straws. As it has turned out, I cannot doubt that it was all arranged, in some incomprehensible way, by an overruling Providence, so that we might be saved. To Him be all thanks for His goodness to us."

"There is not a doubt," rejoined the other captain, "that the writing on the slate, let it have come there as it may, saved all your lives. I was steering at the time considerably south of west, and I altered my course to nor'west, and had a look-out aloft, to see what would come of it. But you say," he added, turning to the passenger, "that you did not dream of writing on a slate?"

"No, sir. I have no recollection whatever of doing so. I got the impression that the bark I saw in my dream was coming to rescue us; but *how* that impression came I cannot tell. There is another very strange thing about it," he added. "Every thing here on board seems to me quite familiar; yet I am very sure I never was in your vessel before. It is all a puzzle to me. What did your mate see?"

Thereupon Mr. Bruce related to them all the circumstances above detailed. The conclusion they finally arrived at was, that it was a special interposition of Providence to save them from what seemed a hopeless fate.

The above narrative was communicated to me by Capt. J. S. Clarke, of the schooner Julia Hallock,* who

---

* In July, 1859. The Julia Hallock was then lying at the foot of Rutgers Slip, New York. She trades between New York and St. Jago, in the

had it directly from Mr. Bruce himself. They sailed together for seventeen months, in the years 1836 and '37; so that Captain Clarke had the story from the mate about eight years after the occurrence. He has since lost sight of him, and does not know whether he is yet alive. All he has heard of him since they were shipmates is, that he continued to trade to New Brunswick, that he became the master of the brig Comet, and that she was lost.

I asked Captain Clarke if he knew Bruce well, and what sort of man he was.

"As truthful and straightforward a man," he replied, "as ever I met in all my life   We were as intimate as brothers; and two men can't be together, shut up for seventeen months in the same ship, without getting to know whether they can trust one another's word or not. He always spoke of the circumstance in terms of reverence, as of an incident that seemed to bring him nearer to God and to another world. I'd stake my life upon it that he told me no lie."

This story, it will be observed, I had at second hand only, and related after an interval of more than twenty years from the time it was told to Captain Clarke. I had no opportunity of cross-examining the main witness. Inaccuracies, therefore, may, with the best intentions on the part of all concerned, have crept into it. Yet the evidence, with the drawback above stated, is direct enough. And Captain Clark furnishes the best proof of his sincerity when he permits me to use his name as reference in support of what I have here related.

---

island of Cuba. The captain allowed me to use his name, and to refer to him as evidence for the truth of what is here set down.

Evidence at second hand, how reliable soever it appear, might properly be deemed inconclusive if the story stood alone. But if we find others, as we have, directly authenticated, of the same class, furnishing proof of phenomena strictly analogous to those which lie at the bottom of this narrative, there seems no sufficient reason why we should regard it as apocryphal, or, setting it down as some idle forecastle yarn, should refuse to admit it as a valid item of evidence.

It is not, for example, characterized by phenomena more marvelous than those presented in the following story, of much later date, and directly authenticated by the chief witness :—

THE DYING MOTHER AND HER BABE.

In November of the year 1843, Miss H——, a young lady then between thirteen and fourteen years of age, was on a visit to a family of her acquaintance (Mr. and Mrs. E——) residing at their country-seat in Cambridgeshire, England. Mrs. E—— was taken ill; and, her disease assuming a serious form, she was recommended to go to London for medical advice. She did so; her husband accompanied her; and they left their guest and their two children, the youngest only ten weeks old, at home.

The journey, however, proved unavailing: the disease increased, and that so rapidly that, after a brief sojourn in the metropolis, the patient could not bear removal.

In the mean time the youngest child, little Fannie, sickened, and, after a brief illness, died. They wrote immediately to the father, then attending on what he felt to be the death-bed of his wife; and he posted down at once. It was on a Monday that the infant died; on Tuesday Mr. E—— arrived, made arrangements for the funeral, and left on Wednesday to return to his wife, from whom, however, he concealed the death of her infant.

On Thursday, Miss H—— received from him a letter, in which he begged her to go into his study and take from his desk there certain papers which were pressingly wanted. It was in this study that the body of the infant lay in its coffin; and, as the young lady proceeded thither to execute the commission, one of the servants said to her, "Oh, miss, are you not afraid?" She replied that there was nothing to be afraid of, and entered the study, where she found the papers required. As she turned, before leaving the room, to look at the babe, she saw, reclining on a sofa near to it, the figure of a lady whom she recognized as the mother. Having from infancy been accustomed to the occasional sight of apparitions, she was not alarmed, but approached the sofa to satisfy herself that it *was* the appearance of her friend. Standing within three or four feet of the figure for several minutes, she assured herself of its identity. It did not speak, but, raising one arm, it first pointed to the body of the infant, and then signed upward. Soon afterward, and before it disappeared, the young lady left the room.

This was a few minutes after four o'clock in the afternoon. Miss H—— particularly noticed the time, as she heard the clock strike the hour a little before she entered the study.

The next day she received from Mr. E—— a letter, informing her that his wife had died the preceding day (Thursday) at half-past four. And when, a few days later, that gentleman himself arrived, he stated that Mrs. E——'s mind had evidently wandered before her death; for, but a little time previous to that event, seeming to revive as from a swoon, she had asked her husband "why he had not told her that her baby was in heaven." When he replied evasively, still wishing to conceal from her the fact of her child's death, lest the shock might hasten her own, she said to him, "It is useless to deny it, Samuel; *for I have just been home, and have seen her in her little coffin.* Except for your sake, I am glad she is gone to a better world; for I shall soon be there to meet her myself." Very shortly after this she expired.

This narrative was related to me in January, 1859, by the lady who saw the apparition. She is now the wife of a learned professor, and the active and respected mother of a family, with as little, apparently, of the idle enthusiast or dreamy visionary about her as possible. She resides near London.*

It will be observed that, as the young lady entered the study a few minutes after four, and as the mother spoke of her alleged visit very shortly before her death, which occurred at half-past four, the coincidence as to time is, as nearly as may be, exact.

In the preceding narrative, as in most of those which reach us touching apparitions of the living, the subject of the phenomenon was insensible during its occurrence. But this does not seem to be a necessary condition. Examples may be found in which not only the person of whom the double appears is not asleep nor in a trance, but is present at the moment of that appearance, and himself witnesses it. Such an example I have been

---

* This story was submitted by me, in manuscript, to the lady in question, and its accuracy assented to by her.

In exemplification of the manner in which such phenomena are often kept hushed up, I may state that Miss H——, though with an instinctive feeling of how it would be received, ventured, soon after she left the study, to say to a lady then residing in the house, that *she thought* she had just seen Mrs. E——, and hoped there would be no bad news from London the next day. For this she was so sharply chidden, and so peremptorily bid not to nurse such ridiculous fancies, that, even when the confirmatory news arrived and Mr. E—— returned home, she was deterred from stating the circumstance to him. To this day he does not know it.

fortunate enough to obtain, directly authenticated by two of the witnesses present. Here it is:—*

THE TWO SISTERS.

In the month of October, 1833, Mr. C——, a gentleman, several members of whose family have since become well and favorably known in the literary world, was residing in a country-house, in Hamilton County, Ohio. He had just completed a new residence, about seventy or eighty yards from that in which he was then living, intending to move into it in a few days. The new house was in plain sight of the old, no tree or shrub intervening; but they were separated, about half-way, by a small, somewhat abrupt ravine. A garden stretched from the old house to the hither edge of this ravine, and the farther extremity of this garden was about forty yards from the newly-erected building. Both buildings fronted west, toward a public road, the south side of the old dwelling being directly opposite to the north side of the new. Attached to the rear of the new dwelling was a spacious kitchen, of which a door opened to the north.

---

* In the first editions of this work, another narrative, bearing upon the habitual appearance of a living person, was here given. It is now replaced by that of the "Two Sisters," for the following reasons. A friend of one of the parties concerned, having made inquiries regarding the story, kindly furnished me with the result; and the evidence thus adduced tended to invalidate essential portions of it. A recent visit to Europe enabled me to make further inquiries into the matter; and though, in some respects, these were confirmatory, yet I learned that a considerable portion of the narrative in question, which had been represented to me as directly attested, was in reality sustained only by second-hand evidence. This circumstance, taken in connection with the conflicting statements above referred to, places the story outside the rule of authentication to which, in these pages, I have endeavored scrupulously to conform; and I therefore omit it altogether.

It is very gratifying to find that, after the test of six months' publicity, the authenticity of but a single narrative, out of the seventy or eighty that are embraced in this volume, has been called in question.—*Note to tenth thousand, September,* 1860.

The family, at that time, consisted of father, mother, uncle, and nine children. One of the elder daughters, then between fifteen and sixteen years old, was named Rhoda; and another, the youngest but one, Lucy, was between three and four years of age.

One afternoon in that month of October, after a heavy rain, the weather had cleared up; and between four and five o'clock the sun shone out. About five o'clock, Mrs. C—— stepped out into a yard on the south side of the dwelling they were occupying, whence, in the evening sun, the new house, including the kitchen already referred to, was distinctly visible. Suddenly she called a daughter, A——, saying to her, "What can Rhoda possibly be doing there, with the child in her arms? She ought to know better, this damp weather." A——, looking in the direction in which her mother pointed, saw, plainly and unmistakably, seated in a rocking-chair just within the kitchen-door of the new residence, Rhoda, with Lucy in her arms. "What a strange thing!" she exclaimed: "it is but a few minutes since I left them up-stairs." And, with that, going in search of them, she found both in one of the upper rooms, and brought them down. Mr. C—— and other members of the family soon joined them. Their amazement—that of Rhoda especially—may be imagined. The figures seated at the hall-door, and the two children now actually in their midst, were absolutely identical in appearance, even to each minute particular of dress.

Five minutes more elapsed, in breathless expectation, and there still sat the figures; that of Rhoda appearing to rock with the motion of the chair on which it seemed seated. All the family congregated, and every member of it—therefore twelve persons in all—saw the figures, noticed the rocking motion, and became convinced, past all possible doubt, that it *was* the appearance of Rhoda and Lucy.

Then the father, Mr. C——, resolved to cross over and endeavor to obtain some solution of the mystery; but, having lost sight of the figures in descending the ravine, when he ascended the opposite bank they were gone.

Meanwhile the daughter A—— had walked down to the lower end of the garden, so as to get a closer view; and the rest remained gazing from the spot whence they had first witnessed this unaccountable phenomenon.

Soon after Mr. C—— had left the house, they all saw the appearance of Rhoda rise from the chair with the child in its arms, then lie down across the threshold of the kitchen-door; and, after it had remained in that recumbent position for a minute or two, still embracing the child, the figures were seen gradually to sink down, out of sight.

When Mr. C—— reached the entrance there was not a trace nor appearance of a human being. The rocking-chair, which had been conveyed across to the kitchen some time before, still stood there, just inside the door, but it was empty. He searched the house carefully, from garret to cellar; but nothing whatever was to be seen. He inspected the clay, soft from the rain, at the rear exit of the kitchen, and all around the house, but not a footstep could he discover. There was not a tree or bush anywhere near behind which any one could secrete himself, the dwelling being erected on a bare hill-side.

The father returned from his fruitless search, to learn, with a shudder, what the family, meanwhile, had witnessed. The circumstance, as may be supposed, made upon them a profound impression; stamping itself, in indelible characters, on the minds of all. But any mention of it was usually avoided, as something too serious to form the topic of ordinary conversation.

I received it directly from two of the witnesses,[*] Miss A——, and her sister, Miss P——. They both stated to me that their recollections of it were as vivid as if it had occurred but a few weeks since.

No clew or explanation of any kind was ever obtained; unless we are to accept as such the fact that Rhoda, a very beautiful and cultivated girl, at the time in blooming health, died very unexpectedly on the 11th of November of the year following, and that Lucy, then also perfectly well, followed her sister on the 10th of December, the same year: both deaths occurring, it will be observed, within a little more than a year of that day on which the family saw the apparition of the sisters.

There is a sequel to this story, less conclusive, but which may be worth relating.

The new house was, after a time, tenanted by a son of Mr. C——; and, even from the time it was first occupied, it began to acquire the reputation of being occasionally, and to a slight extent, what is called haunted. The most remarkable incident occurred in this wise :—

A son of Mr. C——'s brother, seven years old, Alexander by name, was playing one day, in the year 1858, in an upper room, when, all at once, he noticed a little girl, seemingly about four years old, with a bright red dress. Though he had never seen her before, he approached her, hoping to find a playmate, when she suddenly vanished before his eyes, or, as the child afterward expressed it, she "went right out." Though a bold, fearless boy, he was very much frightened by this sudden disappearance, and came running down-stairs to relate it in accents of terror to his mother.

It was afterward recollected that, during little Lucy's

---

[*] In New York, on February 22, 1860. On February 27, I submitted to these ladies the manuscript of the narrative, and they assented to its accuracy.

last illness, they had been preparing for her a red dress, which greatly pleased the child's fancy. She was very anxious that it should be completed.

One day she had said to a sister, "You will finish my dress, even if I am ill: will you not?" To which her sister had replied, "Certainly, my dear, we shall finish it, of course." "Oh, not of coarse," said the child: "finish it of fine." This expression, at which they laughed at the time, served to perpetuate in the family the remembrance of the anxiety constantly evinced by the little sufferer about her new red dress; which, however, she never lived to wear.

It need hardly be added, that the little Alexander had never heard of his aunt Lucy, dying as she did in infancy twenty-five years before. The impression produced by this incident on the boy's mind, bold as was his natural character, was so deep and lasting that, for months afterward, nothing could induce him to enter the room again.

Perhaps we ought not to pass by unheedingly a hint even so slightly indicated as that suggested by this last incident. The "ruling passion strong in death" has become a proverbial expression; and, to a four-years infant, the longing after a bright new dress might take the place of maturer yearnings,—of love, in the youth; of ambition, in the man of riper years. Why a childish fancy cherished up to the last moment of earth-life should so operate in another phase of being as to modify a spirit-appearance, is not clear; perhaps it is unlikely that it should do so; it may not have been Lucy who appeared; the coincidence may have been purely fortuitous. Yet I do not feel sure that it was so, or that no connection exists between the death-bed longing and the form selected (if it was selected) by the child-aunt when she appeared (if she did really appear) to her startled nephew.

In the above example, as in that already given of Mr. Thompson appearing to mother and daughter, it is evident that the apparition of the two sisters, whatever its exact character, must have been, in some sense, objective; in other words, it must have produced an image on the retina; for upon the senses of twelve witnesses precisely the same impression was made. Each one recognised, in the figures seated at the open door, at seventy or eighty yards' distance, the sisters Rhoda and Lucy. All witnessed the motion of the rocking-chair. All, with the exception of Mr. C——, saw the appearance of Rhoda rise from that chair, lie down across the threshold of the door, and then disappear, as if sinking into the earth. Of the persons thus present, Miss A——, one of the two ladies whose personal deposition to me attests this narrative, witnessed the apparent rising from the chair and sinking into the ground from the lower end of the garden, a distance of forty yards only. Finally, the actual presence of Rhoda and Lucy, in bodily form, among the spectators, precluded the possibility of trick or optical deception.

This presence of the two sisters, in their normal condition, suggests also a wholesome lesson. We must not generalize too hastily from a few facts. In most of the preceding examples, the person appearing was asleep or in a trance; and the theory which the most readily suggests itself is that, while the " brother of death" held sway, the spiritual body, partially detached, might assume, at distance from the natural body, the form of its earthly associate. But in the present case that theory seems inapplicable. The counterpart of the two sisters, seen by themselves as well as others, appears to be a phenomenon of a different character,—more in the nature of a picture, or representation, perhaps; by what agency or for what object presented we shall, it may be, inquire in vain.

Indeed, it is altogether illogical, in each particular instance of apparition, or other rare and unexplained phenomenon, to deny its reality until we can explain the purpose of its appearance; to reject, in fact, every extraordinary occurrence until it shall have been clearly explained to us for what great object God ordains or permits it. In the present example we discover no sufficient reason why two deaths not to occur for more than a year should be thus obscurely foreshadowed, if, indeed, foreshadowed they were. The only effect we may imagine to have been produced would be a vague apprehension of evil, without certain cause or definite indication. But what then? The phenomenon is one of a class, governed, doubtless, by general laws. There is good reason, we may justly infer, for the existence of that class; but we ought not to be called upon to show the particular end to be effected by each example. As a general proposition, we believe in the utility of thunderstorms, as tending to purify the atmosphere; but who has a right to require that we disclose the designs of Providence, if, during the elemental war, Amelia be stricken down a corpse from the arms of Celadon?

Space fails me, and it might little avail, to multiply examples attesting apparitions of the living. I close the series, therefore, by placing before the reader a narrative wherein, perhaps, he may find some traces, vague if they be, indicating the character of so many of the preceding examples as relate to appearances which show themselves during sleep or trance, and hinting to us, if even slightly, how these may occur. I am enabled to furnish it at first hand.

THE VISIONARY EXCURSION.

In June of the year 1857, a lady whom I shall designate as Mrs. A—— (now Lady ——) was residing with

her husband, a colonel in the British army, and their
infant child, on Woolwich Common, near London.

One night in the early part of that month, suddenly
awaking to consciousness, she felt herself as if standing
by the bedside and looking upon her own body, which
lay there by the side of her sleeping husband. Her
first impression was that she had died suddenly; and
the idea was confirmed by the pale and lifeless look of
the body, the face void of expression, and the whole
appearance showing no sign of vitality. She gazed at it
with curiosity for some time, comparing its dead look
with that of the fresh countenances of her husband and
of her slumbering infant in a cradle hard by. For a
moment she experienced a feeling of relief that she had
escaped the pangs of death; but the next she reflected
what a grief her death would be to the survivors, and
then came a wish that she could have broken the news
to them gradually. While engaged in these thoughts,
she felt herself carried to the wall of the room, with a
feeling that it must arrest her farther progress. But
no: she seemed to pass through it into the open air.
Outside the house was a tree; and this also she appeared
to traverse, as if it interposed no obstacle. All this
occurred without any desire on her part. Equally without having wished or expected it, she found herself,
after a time, on the opposite side of the Common, at
Woolwich, close to the entrance of what is called the
Repository.* She saw there, as is usual, a sentry, and
narrowly observed his uniform and appearance. From
his careless manner, she felt sure that, though she seemed
to herself to be standing near him, he did not perceive
her. Then, first passing to the arsenal, where she saw
another sentinel, she returned to the barracks, and there
heard the clock strike three. Immediately after this she
found herself in the bedchamber of an intimate friend,

---

* A storehouse of arms and ammunition.

Miss L—— M——, then residing at Greenwich. With her she seemed to commence a conversation, but its purport she did not afterward distinctly recollect; for soon after it began she was conscious of seeing and hearing nothing more.

Her first words on awaking next morning were, "So I am not dead, after all?" When her husband questioned her as to the meaning of so strange an exclamation, she related to him the vision (if vision it was) of the night.

The above occurred during a Wednesday night; and they expected Miss L—— M—— on a visit on the next Friday. The husband exacted from his wife a promise that she would not write to, or in any way communicate with, this young lady in the mean time; and she gave him her word of honor to that effect.

So far there appeared to be nothing beyond an ordinary phenomenon, such as constantly occurs during sleep. It is not, indeed, customary to dream of seeing oneself; but who shall set limits to the vagaries of the sleeping fancy?

The sequel, however, contains the puzzle, and, some may think, one of those explanatory hints that are worth noting and reflecting on.

Colonel A—— was in company with his wife when, on the next Friday, she met her friend, Miss L—— M——. It ought to be stated that this lady has from her childhood habitually seen apparitions. No allusion whatever was made to the subject uppermost in their thoughts; and after a while they all three walked out into the garden. There the two ladies began conversing about a new bonnet; and Mrs. A—— said, "My last was trimmed with violet; and I like the color so much I think I shall select it again." "Yes," her friend replied, "I know that is your color." "How so?" Mrs. A—— asked. "Because when you came to me the other

X   30*

night—let me see: when was it?—ah, I remember, the night before last—it was robed in violet that you appeared to me." "I appeared to you the other night?" "Yes, about three o'clock; and we had quite a conversation together. Have you no recollection of it?"

This was deemed conclusive, both by husband and wife, in proof that something beyond the usual hypothesis of dreaming fancy was necessary to explain the visionary excursion to Woolwich.

This is the only time that any similar occurrence has happened to Mrs. Colonel A———. Her husband is now in India, a brigadier-general; and she has often earnestly longed that her spirit might be permitted, during the watches of the night, to visit him there. For a time, encouraged by what had already happened, she expected this. But longing and expectation have proved alike unavailing. Unthought of, unwished for, the phenomenon came; earnestly desired, fondly expected, it failed to appear. Expectant attention, then, is evidently not the explanation in this case.

It was related to me in February, 1859, by the one lady, the nightly visitant, and confirmed to me, a few days afterward, by the other, the receiver of the visit.

Resembling in its general character the Wilkins dream, the above differs from it chiefly in this, that the narrator appears to have observed more minutely the succession of her sensations; thus suggesting to us the idea that the apparently lifeless body which seemed to her to remain behind might, for the time, have parted with what we may call a spiritual portion of itself;* which

---

* Dr. Kerner relates that on the 28th of May, 1827, about three o'clock in the afternoon, being with Madame Hauffe, who was ill in bed at the time, that lady suddenly perceived the appearance of herself, seated in a chair, wearing a white dress; not that which she then wore, but another belonging to her. She endeavored to cry out, but could neither speak nor move. Her

portion, moving off without the usual means of locomotion, might make itself perceptible, at a certain distance, to another person.

Let him who may pronounce this a fantastical hypothesis, absurd on its face, suggest some other sufficient
to explain the phenomenon we are here examining.

This phenomenon, whatever its exact character, is
evidently the same as that which, under the name of
wraith, has for centuries formed one of the chief items
in what are usually considered the superstitions of Scotland. In that country it is popularly regarded as a
forewarning of death.* This, doubtless, *is* a superstition;
and by the aid of the preceding examples one may
rationally conjecture how it originated.

The indications are:—

That during a dream or a trance, partial or complete,
the counterpart of a living person may show itself, at
a greater or less distance from where that person actually is.

And that, as a general rule, with probable exceptions,
this counterpart appears where the thoughts or the
affections, strongly excited, may be supposed to be.†

---

eyes remained wide open and fixed; but she saw nothing except the appearance and the chair on which it sat. After a time she saw the figure rise
and approach her. Then, as it came quite close to her, she experienced
what seemed an electric shock, the effect of which was perceptible to Dr.
Kerner; and, with a sudden cry, she regained the power of speech, and
related what she had seen and felt. Dr. Kerner saw nothing.—*Seherin von
Prevorst*, pp. 138, 139.

* "Barbara MacPherson, Relict of the deceast Mr. Alexander MacLeod,
late Minister of St. Kilda, informed me the Natives of that Island have a
particular kind of Second Sight, which is always a Forerunner of their
approaching End. Some Months before they sicken, they are haunted
with an Apparition resembling themselves in all Respects, as to their
Person, Features, or Cloathing."—*Treatise on Second Sight, Dreams, and
Apparitions*, Edinburgh, 1763, by THEOPHILUS INSULANUS, Relation X.

† "Examples have come to my knowledge in which sick persons, over-

In the case of Mary Goffe* the type is very distinct. Hers was that uncontrollable yearning which a mother only knows. "If I cannot sit, I will lie all along upon the horse; for I *must* go to see my poor babes." So when the thoughts of Mrs. E——, dying in London, reverted to her infant, then lying in its coffin in Cambridgeshire. So, again, when the Irish clergyman went to dine with his bishop, leaving his wife sick at home, and she seemed to come forth to meet the returning absentee. To the apprentice, the probable murderer, we cannot ascribe what merits the name of affection. But we can imagine with what terrible vividness his feelings and apprehensions may have dwelt, throughout the protracted Scottish church-service, on the spot where lay the body of his victim and of his unborn child.

Less distinctly marked are some of the other cases, as that of Joseph Wilkins, not specially anxious about his mother; the Indiana bridegroom, Hugh, separated but an hour or two from his bride; the servant-boy, Silas, gone a-fishing; finally, Mrs. A——, with no prompting motive more than the ordinary wish to visit a friend. In some of these cases, it will be observed, death speedily followed; in others it did not. Joseph Wilkins lived forty-five years after his dream. Hugh survived his wife. Silas is alive, a prosperous tradesman. Mrs. A—— still lives, in excellent health. It is evident that a speedy death does not *necessarily* follow such an apparition.

The reasons why it is in many cases the precursor of death probably are, that during a fatal illness the patient frequently falls into a state of trance, favorable, in all probability, to such a phenemenon; then, again, that, in

---

come with an unspeakable longing to see some absent friend, have fallen into a swoon, and during that swoon have appeared to the distant object of their affection."—JUNG STILLING: *Theorie der Geisterkunde,* § 100.

* Chapter on Dreams.

anticipation of death, the thoughts recur with peculiar liveliness to absent objects of affection; and, finally, perhaps, that the spiritual principle, soon to be wholly freed from its fleshly incumbrance, may, as it approaches the moment of entire release, the more readily be able to stray off for a time, determined in its course by the guiding influence of sympathy.

But it is evident that the vicinity of death is not needed to confer this power, and that anxiety, arising from other cause than the anticipation of approaching dissolution, may induce it. A tempest aroused the fears of the mother for her son on the Bremen packet. She appeared to him in his cabin. Yet both mother and son are alive at this day.

In this, as in a hundred other cases, the dispassionate examination of an actual phenomenon, and of its probable cause, is the most effectual cure for superstitious excitement and vulgar fears.

CHAPTER III.

APPARITIONS OF THE DEAD.

———" Dare I say
No spirit ever brake the band
That stays him from the native land
   Where first he walked when clasped in clay?

" No visual shade of some one lost,
But he, the spirit himself, may come,
Where all the nerve of sense is dumb,
   Spirit to spirit, ghost to ghost."—TENNYSON.

IF, as St. Paul teaches and Swedenborgians believe, there go to make up the personality of man a natural body and a spiritual body;* if these co-exist, while earthly life endures, in each one of us; if, as the apostle further intimates† and the preceding chapter seems to prove, the spiritual body—a counterpart, it would seem, to human sight, of the natural body—may, during life, occasionally detach itself, to some extent or other and for a time, from the material flesh and blood which for a few years it pervades in intimate association; and if death be but the issuing forth of the spiritual body from its temporary associate; then, at the moment of its exit, it is that spiritual body which through life may have been occasionally and partially detached from the natural body, and which at last is thus entirely and forever

---

* 1 Corinthians xv. 44. The phrase is not, " a natural body and *a spirit;*" it is expressly said, " There is a natural body, and there is a spiritual *body.*"

† 2 Corinthians xii. 2.

358

divorced from it, that passes into another state of existence.

But if that spiritual body, while still connected with its earthly associate, could, under certain circumstances, appear, distinct and distant from the natural body, and perceptible to human vision, if not to human touch, what strong presumption is there against the supposition that after its final emancipation the same spiritual body may still at times show itself to man?*

If there be no such adverse presumption, then we ought to approach the subject, not as embodying some wild vagary barely worth noticing, just within the verge of possibility, but as a respectable and eminently serious question, worthy of our gravest attention, and as to which, let us decide as we will, there is much to be said on both sides before reaching a decision.

Nor is an apparition of the dead a phenomenon (or alleged phenomenon) of which the reality can be settled, affirmatively or negatively, by speculation in the closet. A hundred theorists, thus speculating, may decide, to their own satisfaction, that it ought not to be, or that it cannot be. But if sufficient observation show that it *is*, it only follows that these closet theorists had no correct conception of the proper or the possible.

---

* The Rev. George Strahan, D.D., in his preface to his collection of the *"Prayers and Meditations"* of his friend Dr. Samuel Johnson, (London, 1785,) has the following passage :—

"The improbability arising from rarity of occurrence or singularity of nature amounts to no disproof: it is a presumptive reason of doubt too feeble to withstand the conviction induced by positive credible testimony, such as that which has been borne to shadowy reappearances of the dead." . . . "One true report that a spirit has been seen may give occasion and birth to many false reports of similar incidents; but universal and unconcerted testimony to a supernatural casualty cannot always be untrue. An appearing spirit is a prodigy too singular in its nature to become a subject of general invention." . . . "To a mind not influenced by popular prejudice, it will be scarcely possible to believe that apparitions would have been vouched for in all countries had they never been seen in any."

It was in the field, not in the closet, that the question was decided whether aerolites occasionally fall upon our earth. Chladni and Howard might have theorized over their desks for a lifetime: they would have left the question open still. But they went out into the world. They themselves saw no aerolite fall. But they inspected meteoric masses *said* to have fallen. They made out lists of these. They examined witnesses; they collected evidence. And finally they convinced the world of scientific skeptics that the legends in regard to falling stones which have been current in all ages, ever since the days of Socrates, were something more than fabulous tales.

I propose, in prosecuting a more important inquiry, to follow the example of Chladni and Howard, with what success time and the event must determine.

Innumerable examples may be met with of persons who allege that they have seen apparitions,—among these, men eminent for intelligence and uprightness. A noted example is that of Oberlin, the well-known Alsatian philanthropist, the benevolent pastor of Ban-de-la-Roche.

He was visited, two years before his death,—namely, in 1824,—by a Mr. Smithson, who published an account of his visit.* Thence are gleaned the following particulars.

OBERLIN.

The valley of Ban-de-la-Roche, or Steinthal, in Alsace, the scene for more than fifty years of Oberlin's labors of love, surrounded by lofty mountains, is for more than half the year cut off from the rest of the world by snows obstructing the passes.

---

* " *Intellectual Repository*" for April, 1840, pp. 151 to 162.

There Oberlin found the peasantry with very peculiar opinions. He said to Mr. Smithson that when he first came to reside among the inhabitants of Steinthal they had what he then considered "many superstitious notions respecting the proximity of the spiritual world, and of the appearance of various objects and phenomena in that world, which from time to time were seen by some of the people belonging to his flock. For instance, it was not unusual for a person who had died to appear to some individual in the valley." . . . "The report of every new occurrence of this kind was brought to Oberlin, who at length became so much annoyed that he was resolved to put down this species of superstition, as he called it, from the pulpit, and exerted himself for a considerable time to this end, but with little or no desirable effect. Cases became more numerous, and the circumstances so striking as even to stagger the skepticism of Oberlin himself." (p. 157.)

Ultimately the pastor came over to the opinions of his parishioners in this matter. And when Mr. Smithson asked him what had worked such conviction, he replied "that he himself had had ocular and demonstrative experience respecting these important subjects." He added that "he had a large pile of papers which he had written on this kind of spiritual phenomena, containing the facts, with his own reflections upon them." (p. 158.) He stated further to Mr. Smithson that such apparitions were particularly frequent after that well-known and terrible accident which buried several villages, (the fall of the Rossberg, in 1806.) Soon after, as Oberlin expressed it, a considerable number of the inhabitants of the valley "had their spiritual eyesight opened" (p. 159) and perceived the apparitions of many of the sufferers.

Stöber, the pupil and biographer of Oberlin, and throughout his life the intimate friend of the family, states that the good pastor was fully persuaded of the

31

actual presence of his wife for several years after her decease. His unswerving conviction was that, like an attendant angel, she watched over him, held communion with him, and was visible to his sight; that she instructed him respecting the other world and guarded him from danger in this; that, when he contemplated any new plan of utility, in regard to the results of which he was uncertain, she either encouraged his efforts or checked him in his project. He considered his interviews with her not as a thing to be doubted, but as obvious and certain,—as certain as any event that is witnessed with the bodily eyes. When asked how he distinguished her appearance and her communications from dreams, he replied, " How do you distinguish one color from another ?"*

I myself met, when in Paris, during the month of May, 1859, Monsieur Matter, a French gentleman holding an important official position in the Department of Public Instruction, who had visited Oberlin some time before his death, and to whom the worthy pastor submitted the "large pile of papers" referred to by Mr. Smithson.† He found it to contain, among other things, a narrative of a series of apparitions of his deceased wife, and of his *interviews* with her.‡

Monsieur Matter, who kindly furnished me with notes, in writing, on this matter, adds, " Oberlin was convinced that the inhabitants of the invisible world can appear to us, and we to them, when God wills; and that we are apparitions to them, as they to us."§

Neither the intelligence nor the good faith of Oberlin

---

* *"Vie de J. F. Oberlin,"* par Stöber, p. 223.

† The manuscript was entitled *"Journal des Apparitions et Instructions par Rêves."*

‡ *Entretiens* was the word employed.

§ This appears to have been the opinion of Jung Stilling, with whom Oberlin was well acquainted. See *" Theorie der Geisterkunde,'* § 3.

can be called in question. But it will be said that intelligence and honesty are no security against hallucination, and that the pastor, in his secluded valley, after the loss of a wife whom he tenderly loved, might gradually have become infected with the superstitions of his parishioners. Although the opinions of such a man as Oberlin must ever count for something, yet it is to be admitted that we have not the means of disproving such surmises as these.

We need some circumstantial link, connecting the alleged apparition with the material world. Can we obtain such?

The following is from a respectable source:—

LORENZO THE MAGNIFICENT AND THE IMPROVISATORE.

"Condivi relates an extraordinary story respecting Piero de' Medici, (son of Lorenzo 'the Magnificent,') communicated to him by Michael Angelo, who had, it seems, formed an intimacy with one Cardiere, an improvisatore that frequented the house of Lorenzo and amused his evenings with singing to the lute. Soon after the death of Lorenzo, Cardiere informed Michael Angelo that Lorenzo had appeared to him, habited only in a black and ragged mantle thrown over his naked limbs, and had ordered him to acquaint Piero de' Medici that he would in a short time be banished from Florence. Cardiere, who seems judiciously to have feared the resentment of the living more than of the dead, declined the office; but soon afterward Lorenzo, entering his chamber at midnight, awoke him, and, reproaching him with his inattention, gave him a violent blow on the cheek. Having communicated this second visit to his friend, who advised him no longer to delay his errand, he set out for Careggi, where Piero then resided; but, meeting him with his attendants about midway between that place and Florence, he there delivered his message, to the great amusement of Piero and his followers, one of whom—Bernardo Divizio, afterward Cardinal da Bibbiena—sarcastically asked him 'whether, if Lorenzo had been desirous of giving information to his son, it was likely he would have preferred such a messenger to a personal communication.' The biographer adds, 'La vision del Cardiere, o delusion diabolica, o predizion divina, o forte immaginazione, ch'ella si fosse, si verificò.' "*

Here is an alleged prediction and its fulfillment. But the course of policy pursued by Piero was such that it needed not prophetic instinct to discern the probability that he might one day lose his position in Florence. On the other hand, those who know Italian society will feel assured that a dependant like Cardiere was not likely to venture on such a liberty, unless driven to it by what *he* thought an actual injunction.

As to the cardinal's objection, it is a common one, often flippantly expressed. " It is somewhat remarkable," says Mr. Grose, " that ghosts do not go about their business like persons of this world. In cases of murder, a ghost, instead of going to the next justice of the peace and laying its information, or to the nearest relation of the person murdered, appears to some poor laborer who knows none of the parties, draws the curtains of some decrepit nurse or almswoman, or hovers about the place where his body is deposited."†

---

* " The vision of Cardiere, be it diabolical delusion, or divine forewarning, or vivid imagination, was verified." The anecdote is extracted from " *The Life of Lorenzo de' Medici,*" by William Roscoe, chap. 10.

† " *Provincial Glossary and Popular Superstitions,*" by Francis Grose, Esq., F.A.S., 2d ed., London, 1790, p. 10.

If the cardinal or the antiquary merit a serious answer, it is this: If the appearance of apparitions be an actual phenomenon, it is without doubt, regulated by some general law. And, to judge from the examples on record, it would seem that, under that law, it is only rarely, under certain conditions and to certain persons, that such appearance is possible.

Somewhat more remarkable is the coincidence in the following case:—

ANNA MARIA PORTER'S VISITOR.

When the celebrated Miss Anna Maria Porter was residing at Esher, in Surrey, an aged gentleman of her acquaintance, who lived in the same village, was in the habit of frequenting her house, usually making his appearance every evening, reading the newspaper, and taking his cup of tea.

One evening Miss Porter saw him enter as usual and seat himself at the table, but without speaking. She addressed some remark to him, to which he made no reply; and, after a few seconds, she saw him rise and leave the room without uttering a word.

Astonished, and fearing that he might have been suddenly taken ill, she instantly sent her servant to his house to make inquiries. The reply was, that the old gentleman had died suddenly about an hour before.

This was related by Miss Porter herself to Colonel H——, of the Second Life Guards, and by Colonel H——'s widow repeated to me, in London, during the month of February, 1859.

Unless we imagine, in this case, an escape from the nurse's care resembling that of the member of the Plymouth Club in the example already cited from Sir Walter Scott,* it is difficult to avoid the conclusion

---

* See chapter on Dreams.

31*

that this was an apparition of the dead. Miss Porter herself believed it such; and it appears that she had sent *immediately*, and that the old gentleman had died *an hour before.*

It will be admitted that the following is quite as difficult to explain away.

THE DEAD BODY AND THE BOAT-CLOAK.

We shall not find, in any other class of society, so sensitive an aversion to be taxed with any thing that may be construed into superstition as in the fashionable man of the world. For that reason the following, from the private diary of such a one, who passed his life in the most aristocratic circles of London and Paris, the intimate of nobles and princes of the blood, is the rather entitled to credit. The reserve with which such narratives are communicated, when the subjects belong to what is called *good society*, is evinced by the substitution of initials for the full names. The narrative is communicated in the most direct manner by one who had the best opportunities of knowing the exact facts of the case.

" *Wednesday, December* 26, 1832.—Captain —— recounted a curious anecdote that had happened in his own family. He told it in the following words:—

"It is now about fifteen months ago that Miss M——, a connection of my family, went with a party of friends to a concert at the Argyle rooms. She appeared there to be suddenly seized with indisposition, and, though she persisted for some time to struggle against what seemed a violent nervous affection, it became at last so oppressive that they were obliged to send for their carriage and conduct her home. She was for a long time unwilling to say what was the cause of her indisposition; but, on being more earnestly questioned, she at length confessed that she had, immediately on arriving in the concert-room, been terrified by a horrible vision, which unceasingly presented itself to her sight. It seemed to her as though a naked corpse was lying on the floor at her feet; the features of the face were partly covered by a cloth mantle, but enough was apparent to convince her that the body was that of Sir J—— Y——. Every effort was made by her friends at the time to tranquilize her mind by representing the folly of allowing such delusions to prey upon her spirits, and she thus retired to bed; but on the following day the family received the tidings of Sir J—— Y—— having been drowned in Southampton River that very night by the oversetting of his boat; and the body was afterwards found entangled in a *boat-cloak*. Here is an authenticated case of second-sight, and of very recent date."*

For the following I am indebted to the kindness of my friend Dr. Ashburner, of London.

APPARITION IN INDIA.

"In the year 1814 I became acquainted with Colonel Nathan Wilson, a man of strong intellectual powers, who had served many years in India under Sir Arthur Wellesley, afterward Duke of Wellington. I was introduced to him by Sir Charles Forbes, at a shooting-lodge at Strathdon, and there we had an opportunity of becoming intimate. I had, from his own lips, the narrative I am about to relate to you, and which I may preface by a few words touching the opinions of the narrator.

"Colonel Wilson made no secret of his atheism. In India especially, as I have myself observed, the ten-

---

* *"A Portion of the Journal kept by Thomas Raikes, Esq., from* 1831 *to* 1847," 2d ed., London, 1856, vol. i. p. 131.

dency of many minds, influenced by considering the great diversities of religious belief around them, is toward skepticism. Colonel Wilson, fortified by the perusal of Volney, D'Holbach, Helvetius, Voltaire, and others of similar stamp, rejected, as untenable, the doctrine of a future state of existence, and even received with some impatience any arguments on a subject as to which, he seemed to think, no one could any further enlighten him.

"In the year 1811, being then in command of the 19th regiment of dragoons,* stationed at Tellicherry, and delighting in French literature, he formed an intimacy with Monsieur Dubois, a Roman Catholic missionary priest, an ardent and zealous propagandist and an accomplished man. Notwithstanding the great difference in their creeds, so earnest and yet liberal-minded was the Frenchman, so varied his store of information, and so agreeable and winning his manner, that the missionary and the soldier associated much together, and finally formed a strong attachment to each other. The former did not fail to avail himself of this intimacy by endeavoring to bring about the conversion of his friend. They conversed often and freely on religious subjects; but Colonel Wilson's skepticism remained unshaken.

"In July, 1811, the priest fell ill, much to the regret of the little circle at Tellicherry, where he was greatly beloved. At the same time, a mutiny having broken out at Vellore, Colonel Wilson was summoned thither, and, proceeding by forced marches, encamped on an extensive plain before the town.

"The night was sultry; and Colonel Wilson, arrayed as is common in that climate, in shirt and long light calico drawers with feet, sought repose on a couch within his tent; but in vain. Unable to sleep, his

---

* Or possibly the 17th dragoons; for he had commanded both.

attention was suddenly attracted to the entrance of his tent: he saw the purdah raised and the priest Dubois present himself. The pale face and earnest demeanor of his friend, who stood silent and motionless, riveted his attention. He called him by name, but without reply: the purdah fell, and the figure had disappeared.

"The colonel sprang up, and, hastily donning his slippers, rushed from the tent. The appearance was still in sight, gliding through the camp, and making for the plain beyond. Colonel Wilson hastened after it, and at so rapid a pace that when his brother officers, roused by the sentries, went in pursuit of him, it was with difficulty he was overtaken. The apparition having been seen by Captain Wilson only, his comrades concluded that it was the effect of slight delirium produced by fatigue. But when the surgeon of the regiment felt the colonel's pulse, he declared that it beat steadily, without acceleration.

"Colonel Wilson felt assured that he had received an intimation of the death of his friend the missionary, who had repeatedly promised, in case he died first, to appear to him as a spirit. He requested his brother officers to note the time. They did so; and when subsequent letters from Tellicherry announced the decease of Dubois, it was found that he had died at the very hour when his likeness appeared to his friend.

"Desirous to ascertain what effect this apparition had produced on Colonel Wilson's opinions touching a future state, I put the question directly to him. 'I think it a very curious phenomenon,' he replied, 'not to be accounted for in the present state of our knowledge, and requiring investigation. But it is not sufficient to alter my convictions. Some energetic projection from Dubois's brain, at the moment of approaching annihilation,

Y

might perhaps suffice to account for the appearance which I undoubtedly witnessed.' "*

We can scarcely find a stronger proof of the vivid reality, to the observer, of this appearance than the shift to which he is reduced to explain it. He "undoubtedly witnessed it," he tells us; but, he argues, "it might, perhaps, be a projection from Dubois's brain at the moment of dissolution." What a *perhaps* is this! A projection from the brain of a dying man is to appear miles away from his dying bed, and, having assumed human form, is to imitate human locomotion! What sort of projection? Not a soul or a spiritual body, for an atheist admits no such entities,—nothing that inhabits, or is to inhabit, a future world of which an atheist denies the existence. What then? A portion of the physical substance of the brain, detached from it, and shot off, like some military projectile, from Tellicherry to Vellore? Concede the monstrous assumption. What directs it precisely to the friend to whom the owner of the brain had promised, in the event of death, to appear as a spirit? But suppose it to have arrived at Colonel Wilson's tent: what gave a detached portion of a brain the power to clothe itself in the complete form of a man, with a head and recognizable countenance, with arms, legs, a body?—the power, too, to glide away from a person pursuing it?

But it is sheer waste of time to track to its source a hypothesis so preposterous as this. In what a maze of absurdity may a man, reputed intelligent, involve himself when governed by a settled predetermination to ignore the possibility of a future world, where our

* Extracted from a letter in my possession, addressed to me by Dr. Ashburner, dated No. 7, Hyde Park Place, London, March 12, 1859.

spirits may hereafter exist, and whence they may occasionally return!

Narratives of apparitions at or about the moment of death are perhaps the most frequent of any. For a striking and directly authenticated example of this class I am indebted to my friend William Howitt, whose name is almost as familiar on this side of the Atlantic as in his own country. I give it in his own words.

THE BROTHER'S APPEARANCE TO THE SISTER.

"The circumstance you desire to obtain from me is one which I have many times heard related by my mother. It was an event familiar to our family and the neighborhood, and is connected with my earliest memories; having occurred, about the time of my birth, at my father's house at Heanor, in Derbyshire, where I myself was born.

"My mother's family name, Tantum, is an uncommon one, which I do not recollect to have met with except in a story of Miss Leslie's. My mother had two brothers, Francis and Richard. The younger, Richard, I knew well, for he lived to an old age. The elder, Francis, was, at the time of the occurrence I am about to report, a gay young man, about twenty, unmarried; handsome, frank, affectionate, and extremely beloved by all classes throughout that part of the country. He is described, in that age of powder and pigtails, as wearing his auburn hair flowing in ringlets on his shoulders, like another Absalom, and was much admired, as well for his personal grace as for the life and gayety of his manners.

"One fine calm afternoon, my mother, shortly after a confinement, but perfectly convalescent, was lying in bed, enjoying, from her window, the sense of summer beauty and repose; a bright sky above, and the quiet

village before her. In this state she was gladdened by
hearing footsteps which she took to be those of her
brother Frank, as he was familiarly called, approaching
the chamber-door. The visitor knocked and entered.
The foot of the bed was toward the door, and the curtains at the foot, notwithstanding the season, were
drawn, to prevent any draught. Her brother parted
them, and looked in upon her. His gaze was earnest,
and destitute of its usual cheerfulness, and he spoke not
a word. 'My dear Frank,' said my mother, 'how glad
I am to see you! Come round to the bedside: I wish to
have some talk with you.'

"He closed the curtains, as complying; but, instead of
doing so, my mother, to her astonishment, heard him
leave the room, close the door behind him, and begin to
descend the stairs. Greatly amazed, she hastily rang,
and when her maid appeared she bade her call her
brother back. The girl replied that she had not seen
him enter the house. But my mother insisted, saying,
'He was here but this instant. Run! quick! Call him
back! I must see him.'

"The girl hurried away, but, after a time, returned,
saying that she could learn nothing of him anywhere;
nor had any one in or about the house seen him either
enter or depart.

"Now, my father's house stood at the bottom of the
village, and close to the highroad, which was quite
straight; so that any one passing along it must have
been seen for a much longer period than had elapsed.
The girl said she had looked up and down the road, then
searched the garden,—a large, old-fashioned one, with
shady walks. But neither in the garden nor on the
road was he to be seen. She had inquired at the nearest
cottages in the village; but no one had noticed him pass.

"My mother, though a very pious woman, was far
from superstitious; yet the strangeness of this circum-

stance struck her forcibly. While she lay pondering upon it, there was heard a sudden running and excited talking in the village street. My mother listened: it increased, though up to that time the village had been profoundly still; and she became convinced that something very unusual had occurred. Again she rang the bell, to inquire the cause of the disturbance. This time it was the monthly nurse who answered it. She sought to tranquilize my mother, as a nurse usually does a patient. 'Oh, it is nothing particular, ma'am,' she said, 'some trifling affair,'—which she pretended to relate, passing lightly over the particulars. But her ill-suppressed agitation did not escape my mother's eye. 'Tell me the truth,' she said, 'at once. I am certain something very sad has happened.' The woman still equivocated, greatly fearing the effect upon my mother in her then situation. And at first the family joined in the attempt at concealment. Finally, however, my mother's alarm and earnest entreaties drew from them the terrible truth that her brother had just been stabbed at the top of the village, and killed on the spot.

"The melancholy event had thus occurred. My uncle, Francis Tantum, had been dining at Shipley Hall, with Mr. Edward Miller Mundy, member of Parliament for the county. Shipley Hall lay off to the left of the village as you looked up the main street from my father's house, and about a mile distant from it; while Heanor Fall, my uncle's residence, was situated to the right; the road from the one country-seat to the other crossing, nearly at right angles, the upper portion of the village street, at a point where stood one of the two village inns, the Admiral Rodney, respectably kept by the widow H——ks. I remember her well,—a tall, fine-looking woman, who must have been handsome in her youth, and who retained, even past middle age, an air superior to her condition. She had one only child, a son, then scarcely twenty. He was a good-looking, brisk young fellow, and bore a very fair character. He must, however, as the event showed, have been of a very hasty temper.

"Francis Tantum, riding home from Shipley Hall after the early country dinner of that day, somewhat elate, it may be, with wine, stopped at the widow's inn and bade the son bring him a glass of ale. As the latter turned to obey, my uncle, giving the youth a smart switch across the back with his riding-whip, cried out, in his lively, joking way, 'Now be quick, Dick; be quick!'

"The young man, instead of receiving the playful stroke as a jest, took it as an insult. He rushed into the house, snatched up a carving-knife, and, darting back into the street, stabbed my uncle to the heart, as he sat on his horse, so that he fell dead, on the instant, in the road.

"The sensation throughout the quiet village may be imagined. The inhabitants, who idolized the murdered man, were prevented from taking summary vengeance on the homicide only by the constables carrying him off to the office of the nearest magistrate.

"Young H——ks was tried at the next Derby assizes; but (justly, no doubt, taking into view the sudden irritation caused by the blow) he was convicted of manslaughter only, and, after a few months' imprisonment, returned to the village; where, notwithstanding the strong popular feeling against him, he continued to keep the inn, even after his mother's death. He is still present to my recollection, a quiet, retiring man, never guilty of any other irregularity of conduct, and seeming to bear about with him the constant memory of his rash deed,—a silent blight upon his life.

"So great was the respect entertained for my uncle, and such the deep impression of his tragic end, that so long as that generation lived the church-bells of the village were regularly tolled on the anniversary of his death.

"On comparing the circumstances and the exact time at which each occurred, the fact was substantiated that the apparition presented itself to my mother almost instantly after her brother had received the fatal stroke."*

Almost the only desirable condition left unfulfilled in the preceding narrative is that more than one person, and each influenced independently, should have witnessed the apparition. This additional voucher is supplied in the following.

THE NOBLEMAN AND HIS SERVANT.

The late Lord M——, having gone to the Highlands about the end of the last century, left his wife perfectly well in London. The night of his arrival at his Highland home, he was awakened by seeing a bright light in his room. The curtains of his bed opened, and he saw the appearance of Lady M—— standing there. He rang for his servant, and inquired of him what he saw; upon which the man exclaimed, in terror, "It's my lady!" Lady M—— had died suddenly in London that night. The story made a great noise at the time; and George the Third, sending for Lord M—— and ascertaining from him the truth of it, desired him to write out the circumstances as they happened; and the servant countersigned the statement.

About a year afterward, a child five years old, the youngest daughter of Lord M——, rushed breathlessly into the nursery, exclaiming, "I have seen mamma standing at the top of the stair and beckoning to me." That night the child, little Annabella M——, was taken ill, and died.

---

* Extracted from a letter addressed to me by Mr. Howitt, dated Highgate, March 28, 1859.

I can vouch, in an unqualified manner, for the authen‐ticity of both the above circumstances; having received the account, in writing, from a member of Lord M——'s family.

In the following example the testimony of two wit‐nesses to the same apparition is obtained under circum‐stances quite as conclusive. It was related to me in Naples, January 2, 1857, by one of these witnesses, (an intelligent English lady, of highly respectable family, who had spent many years in Russia,) as follows.

LOUISE.

In the early part of the year 1856, Mrs. F—— resided for some months in the family of Prince ——, a noble‐man who had occupied a high official position under the Emperor Nicholas.

One evening, between eleven and twelve, Mrs. F—— was in a small cabinet adjoining the bedroom of the Princess —— and separated from it by hangings only, when she heard the door of the bedchamber open, and the princess (as she supposed) enter the room, set down her candle, and walk about. Expecting her to come into the cabinet, as was her wont, she waited; but in vain. Then she heard her again open the door and descend the stairs. Some twenty minutes afterward, steps re‐ascended the stairs, and the princess herself entered and spoke to her. Mrs. F—— ascertained, to her surprise, that the princess had not been in her room before; yet the latter testified no astonishment when Mrs. F—— mentioned what she had heard.

Learning, next morning, that the lady's maid had not entered the room, and that no one else had access to it, Mrs. F—— again adverted to the extraordinary occur‐rence; and the princess told her frankly, what Mrs F—— then learned for the first time, that they were accustomed to such mysterious visits; that they commonly portended some unusual occurrence in the family; and that her husband had disposed of a palace they formerly owned in another street, for no other reason than to endeavor to escape the repeated noises and other disturbances by which they had been there tormented. One of these was the frequent sounding of heavy steps, during the dead of night, along a certain corridor. The prince had repeatedly, during the occurrence of these sounds, caused every egress from the corridor in question to be closed and guarded; but in vain. No solution of the mystery was ever obtained.

The princess added that to their new palace, in which they then were, and the windows of which looked out on the beautiful Neva, the noises had followed them, occurring at intervals. One of her daughters, previous to her marriage, had constantly experienced the sensation as of some one approaching her side, preceded by the tread of steps and what seemed the rustling of a silk dress, and sometimes accompanied by the sound as of water poured on the table.

At this time there was in the house a femme-de-chambre named Louise, a young German girl of respectable family, cultivated much beyond the station she then occupied, and which she had been induced to accept in consequence of a disappointment in love produced by the obstinate opposition of the young man's relatives to the proposed match. In consequence of her obliging, cheerful disposition, and her intelligence, she was a great favorite in the household, particularly with Mrs. F——, whom she had nursed during an illness.

When, subsequently, she herself fell ill, much interest was felt for her by all the family, and Mrs. F—— was frequently at her bedside.

One evening the family physician, after visiting Louise, reported that she was doing very well, and would doubtless recover; so that Mrs. F—— retired to rest without any anxiety on her account.

About two o'clock that night she was disturbed by the feeling as of something touching her; and, thinking it to be a rat, she became thoroughly awake with the fright. Then she felt, most distinctly, the touch as it were of a human hand pressing gently on different parts of her body and limbs. The sensation was so positive and unmistakable that she became convinced there was some one in the room. But she could see or hear nothing; and after a time it ceased. The next morning the servant awoke her with the intelligence that Louise had died suddenly about two o'clock the preceding night.

The girl's effects, including her clothes and letters, (some of them from her lover, who still cherished affection for her,) together with her lover's portrait, were collected together and placed, until they should be claimed by her family, *not* in the room in which she died, but in another, which became the bedroom of the femme-de-chambre who succeeded her.

As the family had frequently lost their servants through terror of the mysterious disturbances, they took measures to prevent the report of these from reaching this woman's ears. She heard, however, at various times, disturbing noises at night, and declared that on several occasions she had distinctly seen move silently across the floor a form, her description of which tallied exactly with the usual appearance of poor Louise, whom in life she had never seen. This apparition caused her to ask if it was not the room in which her predecessor had died. But being reassured on that point, and having boasted, when the noises first occurred, that no ghost could inspire her with any fear, she was ashamed of yielding to her wish to sleep with one of the servant-girls, and continued to occupy her own bedroom.

Some five weeks after the death of Louise, and a few

minutes after midnight, Mrs F—— had ascended the stairs with a candle; and, as she reached the landing, a dim form flitted suddenly past from left to right,—not so rapidly, however, but that she could distinguish that it was transparent; for she distinctly perceived through it the opposite window. As she passed her hands over her eyes,—the thought flashing across her mind that this might be a hallucination only,—she was startled by a violent scream as of agony from the bedroom of the femme-de-chambre, situated on the left of the stair-landing. The scream was so loud that it aroused the household, and Princess —— and others hastened with Mrs. F—— to ascertain its cause. They found the maid in violent convulsions; and when, after some time, they recovered her, she declared, in accents of extreme terror, that the figure she had already several times seen had appeared to her in the most distinct form, approached the bed and bent over her, so that she seemed to feel its very breath and touch, upon which she lost consciousness and knew not what happened further. She could not be persuaded again to sleep in that room; and the disturbances continued there after she left it.

But, after a time, the young man who had been engaged to Louise wrote for her effects, requesting that they might be sent home, overland, at his expense. The new femme-de-chambre assisted in packing them. In taking up one of Louise's dresses, she dropped it in sudden terror, declaring that in exactly such a dress had the figure been clothed that bent over her when she swooned away.

From the day these effects were taken from the room where they had been placed, and sent off, all noises and disturbances therein entirely ceased.*

---

* I read over the above narrative to Mrs. F——, made a few corrections at her suggestion, and then she assented to its accuracy in every particular

We are gradually reaching a point in this series of narratives at which it becomes very difficult to explain away the phenomena they embrace, or to account for these on any other than the spiritual hypothesis. In the preceding example, for instance, what can possibly explain the coincident visions of Louise's successor and Mrs. F——, except the supposition of an objective reality?

We find narratives as conclusive as the above current throughout society,—usually discredited by superficial commentators,—sometimes justly, for many of them are apocryphal enough; sometimes, as I believe, unjustly.

I select, as a specimen of this latter class, from among what are called modern ghost-stories, one which, on account of the rank and character of the two seers, (Sir John Sherbroke and General Wynyard,) has been as much talked of throughout England as perhaps any other. It was published in the newspapers of the day; and the narrative, in a somewhat diffuse form, has been preserved in at least one modern publication.* It is alluded to, but the initials only given, in Archdeacon Wrangham's edition of Plutarch, in a note, thus:—" A very singular story, however, could be told on this head by Generals S—— and W——, both men of indisputable honor and spirit, and honorably distinguished by their exertions in their country's service." It is related, in a succinct manner, by Dr. Mayo in his work on Popular Superstitions; and he accompanies it with the following voucher:—"I have had opportunities of inquiring of two near relations of General Wynyard upon what evidence the above story rests. They told me they had each heard it from his own mouth. More recently a gentleman whose accuracy of information exceeds that of most people told me that he had heard the late Sir

* *Signs before Death,*" collected by Horace Welby, London, 1825, pp 77 to 82.

John Sherbroke, the other party in the ghost-story, tell it, much in the same way, at a dinner-table."* Here it is :—

THE WYNYARD APPARITION.

In the year 1785, Sir John Sherbroke and General Wynyard, then young men, were officers in the same regiment, stationed at that time in the island of Cape Breton, off Nova Scotia.

On the 15th of October of that year, between eight and nine o'clock P.M., these two young officers were seated before the fire, at coffee, in Wynyard's parlor. It was a room in the new barracks, with two doors,— the one opening on an outer passage, the other into that officer's bedroom, from which bedroom there was no exit except by returning through the parlor.

Sherbroke, happening to look up from his book, saw beside the door which opened on the passage the figure of a tall youth, apparently about twenty years of age, but pale and much emaciated. Astonished at the presence of a stranger, Sherbroke called the attention of his brother officer, sitting near him, to the visitor. "I have heard," he said, in afterward relating the incident, "of a man's being as pale as death; but I never saw a living face assume the appearance of a corpse except Wynyard's at that moment." Both remained silently gazing on the figure as it passed slowly through the room and entered the bed-chamber, casting on young Wynyard, as it passed, a look, as his friend thought, of melancholy affection. The oppression of its presence was no sooner removed than Wynyard, grasping his friend's arm, exclaimed,

* "On the Truths contained in Popular Superstitions," by Herbert Mayo, M.D., Professor of Anatomy and Physiology in King's College, &c. &c., 3d ed., Edinburgh and London, 1851, pp. 63, 64.

in scarcely articulate tones, "Great God! my brother!"

"Your brother! What can you mean?" replied Sherbroke: "there must be some deception in this." And
with that he instantly proceeded into the bedroom, followed by Wynyard. No one to be seen there! They
searched in every part, and convinced themselves that
it was entirely untenanted. Wynyard persisted in declaring that he *had* seen his brother's spirit; but Sherbroke inclined to the belief that they might have been,
in some way or other, deluded, possibly by a trick of a
brother officer.

Nevertheless, both waited with great anxiety for
letters from England; and this anxiety at last became
so apparent on Wynyard's part that his brother officers,
in spite of his resolution to the contrary, finally won
from him the confession of what he had seen. The
story was soon bruited abroad, and produced great
excitement throughout the regiment. When the expected vessel with letters arrived, there were none for
Wynyard, but one for Sherbroke. As soon as that
officer had opened it, he beckoned Wynyard from the
room. Expectation was at its climax, especially as the
two friends remained closeted for an hour. On Sherbroke's return the mystery was solved. It was a letter
from a brother officer, begging Sherbroke to break
to his friend Wynyard the news of the death of his favorite brother, who had expired on the 15th of October,
and at the same hour at which the friends saw the apparition in the block-house.

It remains to be stated that, some years afterward,
Sir John Sherbroke, then returned to England, was
walking in Piccadilly, London, when, on the opposite
side of the street, he saw a gentleman whom he instantly recognized as the counterpart of the mysterious
visitor. Crossing over, he accosted him, apologizing

for his intrusion, and learned that he was a brother (not the *twin* brother, as some accounts have it) of Wynyard.

Such is the story; for the truth of which I have been fortunate enough to obtain vouchers additional to those already given.

Captain Henry Scott, R.N., residing at Blackheath, near London, and with whom I have the pleasure of being acquainted, was, about thirty years ago, when Sir John Sherbroke was Governor of Nova Scotia, under his command as Assistant Surveyor-General of that province; and dining, one day, with Sir John, a guest remarked that an English newspaper, just received, had a most extraordinary ghost-story, in which his (Sir John's) name appeared. Thereupon Sherbroke, with much emotion, quickly replied, "I beg that the subject may not again be mentioned." The impression on the minds of all present was, that he considered the matter too serious to be talked of.

But we are not left to mere inference, suggested by this indirect testimony. I communicated to Captain Scott, in manuscript, the above narrative; and, in returning it, that gentleman wrote to me, with permission to use his name, as follows:—

"About six years ago, dining alone with my dear friend—now gone to his account—General Paul Anderson, C.B., I related to him the story of the Wynyard apparition, in substance exactly as you have it. When I had finished, 'It is extraordinary enough,' said he, 'that you have related that story almost *verbatim* as I had it from Sir John Sherbroke's own lips a short time before his death.'* I asked the general

---

* His death is noticed in Blackwood's Magazine for June, 1830.

whether Sir John had expressed any opinion about the incident.

" 'Yes,' he replied: 'he assured me, in the most solemn manner, that he believed the appearance to have been a ghost or spirit; and added that this belief was shared by his friend Wynyard.'

" General Anderson was a distinguished Peninsular War officer, a major under Sir John Moore, and one of those who assisted to bury that gallant general."*

It will not, I think, be questioned that this evidence is as direct and satisfactory as can well be, short of a record left in writing by one or other of the seers,— which it does not appear is to be found.† Sir John Sherbroke, when forty years had passed by, repeats to a brother officer his unaltered conviction that it *was* the spirit of his friend's brother† that appeared to them in the Canadian block-house, and that that friend was as fully convinced of the fact as himself.

Strongly corroborative, also, is the fact that so deeply imprinted in Sherbroke's memory were the features of the apparition that the recollection called up, after the lapse of years, by the appearance of a stranger casually met in the streets of London, caused him to accost that stranger, who proved to be a brother of the deceased.

In the following we find an example of three persons seeing the same apparition, though at different times :—

---

* Extracted from letter of Captain Henry Scott to me, dated January 26, 1859.

† The brother's name was John Otway Wynyard; and he was at the time of his death on the 15th of October, 1785, Lieutenant in the 3d Regiment of Life-Guards.

APPARITION OF A STRANGER.

In March of the year 1854, the Baron de Gulden-stubbé was residing alone in apartments, at Number 23 Rue St. Lazare, Paris.

On the 16th of that month, returning thither from an evening-party, after midnight, he retired to rest; but, finding himself unable to sleep, he lit a candle and began to read. Very soon his attention was drawn from the book by experiencing first one electric shock, then another, until the sensation was eight or ten times repeated. This greatly surprised him and effectually precluded all disposition to sleep: he rose, donned a warm dressing-gown, and lit a fire in the adjoining saloon.

Returning a few minutes afterward, without a candle, in search of a pocket-handkerchief, to the bedroom, he observed, by light coming through the open door of the saloon, just before the chimney, (which was situated in a corner of the room, at the opposite diagonal from the entrance-door,) what seemed like a dim column of grayish vapor, slightly luminous. It attracted his notice for a moment; but, deeming it merely some effect of reflected light from the lamps in the court-yard, he thought no more of it, and re-entered the parlor.

After a time, as the fire burned badly, he returned to the bedchamber, to procure a fagot. This time the appearance in front of the fireplace arrested his attention. It reached nearly to the ceiling of the apartment, which was fully twelve feet high. Its color had changed from gray to blue,—that shade of blue which shows itself when spirits of wine are burned. It was also more distinctly marked, and somewhat more luminous, than at first. As the baron gazed at it, in some surprise, there gradually grew into sight, within

Z   33

it, the figure of a man. The outlines at first were vague, and the color blue, like the column, only of a darker shade. The baron looked upon it as a hallucination, but continued to examine it steadily from a distance of some thirteen or fourteen feet.

Gradually the outlines of the figure became marked, the features began to assume exact form, and the whole to take the colors of the human flesh and dress. Finally there stood within the column, and reaching about halfway to the top, the figure of a tall, portly old man, with a fresh color, blue eyes, snow-white hair, thin white whiskers, but without beard or moustache; and dressed with some care. He seemed to wear a white cravat and long white waistcoat, high stiff shirt-collar, and a long black frock-coat, thrown back from his chest, as is the wont of corpulent people like him in hot weather. He appeared to lean on a heavy white cane.

After a few minutes, the figure detached itself from the column and advanced, seeming to float slowly through the room, till within about three feet of its wondering occupant. There it stopped, put up its hand, as in form of salutation, and slightly bowed.

The baron's impulse when it first approached had been to ring the bell. So perfectly distinct was the vision, so absolutely material seemed the figure before him, that he could scarcely resist the impression that some stranger (for the features were wholly unknown to him) had invaded his apartment. But the age and friendly demeanor of the intruder arrested his hand. Whether from this world or the other, there seemed nothing hostile or formidable in the appearance that presented itself.

After a time, the figure moved toward the bed, which was to the right of the entrance-door and immediately opposite the fireplace, then, turning to the left, returned to the spot before the fireplace, where it had first appeared, then advanced a second time toward the baron

And this round it continued to make (stopping, however, at intervals) as often as eight or ten times. The baron heard no sound, either of voice or footstep.

The last time it returned to the fireplace, after facing the baron, it remained stationary there. By slow degrees the outlines lost their distinctness; and, as the figure faded, the blue column gradually reformed itself, inclosing it as before. This time, however, it was much more luminous,—the light being sufficient to enable the baron to distinguish small print, as he ascertained by picking up a Bible that lay on his dressing-table and reading from it a verse or two. He showed me the copy: it was in minion type. Very gradually the light faded, seeming to flicker up at intervals, like a lamp dying out.

From the time the figure appeared until it began to fade, mingling with the column, there elapsed about ten minutes: so that the witness of this remarkable apparition had the amplest opportunity fully to examine it. When it turned toward the fireplace, he distinctly saw its back. He experienced little or no alarm, being chiefly occupied during the period of its stay in seeking to ascertain whether it was a mere hallucination or an objective reality. On one or two previous occasions during his life he had seen somewhat similar apparitions,—less distinct, however, and passing away more rapidly; and, as they were of persons whom in life he had known, he had regarded them as subjective only; the offspring, probably, of his imagination, during an abnormal state of the nervous system.

Pondering over this matter, he went to bed, and, after a time, to sleep. In a dream, the same figure he had just seen again appeared to him, dressed exactly as before. It seemed to sit down on the side of the bed; and, as if in reply to the reflections that had been occupying the baron's mind before he retired to rest, he thought he heard it say to him, in substance, " Hitherto you have not believed in the reality of apparitions, considering them only the recallings of memory: now, since you have seen a stranger, you cannot consider it the reproduction of former ideas." The baron assented, in dream, to this reasoning; but the phantom gave him no clew as to what its name or condition in life had been.

The next morning, meeting the wife of the concierge, Madame Matthieu, who had been in the habit of attending to his rooms, he inquired of her who had been their former occupant, adding that his reason for making the inquiry was, that the night before he had seen in his bedroom an apparition. At first the woman seemed much frightened and little disposed to be communicative; but, when pressed on the subject, she admitted that the last person who had resided in the apartments now occupied by the baron was the father of the lady who was the proprietor of the house,—a certain Monsieur Caron, who had formerly filled the office of mayor in the province of Champagne. He had died about two years before, and the rooms had remained vacant from that time until taken by the baron.

Her description of him, not only as to personal appearance, but in each particular of dress, corresponded in the minutest manner to what the baron had seen. A white waistcoat coming down very low, a white cravat, a long black frock-coat: these he habitually wore. His stature was above the middle height; and he was corpulent, his eyes blue, his hair and whiskers white; and he wore neither beard nor moustache. His age was between sixty and seventy. Even the smaller peculiarities were exact, down to the high standing shirt-collar, the habit of throwing back his coat from his chest, and the thick white cane, his constant companion when he went out.

Madame Matthieu further confessed to the baron that he was not the only one to whom the apparition of M. Caron had shown itself. On one occasion a maid-servant had seen it on the stairs. To herself it had appeared several times,—once just in front of the entrance to the saloon, again in a dimly-lighted passage that led past the bedroom to the kitchen beyond, and more than once in the bedroom itself. M. Caron had dropped down in the passage referred to, in an apoplectic fit, had been carried thence into the bedroom, and had died in the bed now occupied by the baron.

She said to him, further, that, as he might have re-marked, she almost always took the opportunity when he was in the saloon to arrange his bedchamber, and that she had several times intended to apologize to him for this, but had refrained, not knowing what excuse to make. The true reason was that she feared again to meet the apparition of the old gentleman.

The matter finally came to the ears of the daughter, the owner of the house. She caused masses to be said for the soul of her father; and it is alleged—how truly I know not—that the apparition has not been seen in any of the apartments since.

This narrative I had from the Baron de Guldenstubbé himself.* That gentleman stated to me that, up to the time when he saw the apparition, he had never heard of M. Caron, and of course had not the slightest idea of his personal appearance or dress; nor, as may be supposed, had it ever been intimated to him that any one had died, two years before, in the room in which he slept.

The story derives much of its value from the calm and dispassionate manner in which the witness appears to have observed the succession of phenomena, and the

---

* In Paris, on the 11th of May, 1859.

exact details which, in consequence, he has been enabled to furnish. It is remarkable, also, as well for the electrical influences which preceded the appearance, as on account of the correspondence between the apparition to the baron in his waking state and that subsequently seen in dream; the first cognizable by one sense only,— that of sight,—the second appealing (though in vision of the night only) to the hearing also.

The coincidences as to personal peculiarities and details of dress are too numerous and minutely exact to be fortuitous, let us adopt what theory, in explanation, we may.

This series of narratives would be incomplete without some examples of those stories of a tragic cast, seeming to intimate that the foul deeds committed in this world may call back the criminal, or the victim, from another.

A very extraordinary sample of such stories is given in the memoirs of Sir Nathaniel Wraxall, a man of some distinction in his day, and from 1780 to 1794 a member of the British Parliament. It was related to Sir Nathaniel, when on a visit to Dresden, by the Count de Felkesheim. Of him Wraxall says, " He was a Livonian gentleman, settled in Saxony; of a very improved understanding, equally superior to credulity as to superstition." The conversation occurred in October, 1778.

After alluding to the celebrated exhibition, by Schrepfer, of the apparition of the Chevalier de Saxe, and expressing his opinion that "though he could not pretend to explain by what process or machinery that business was conducted, yet he had always considered Schrepfer as an artful impostor," the count proceeded to say that he was not so decidedly skeptical as to the possibility of apparitions as to treat them with ridicule or set them down as unphilosophical. Educated in the University of Königsberg, he had attended the lectures on ethics and moral philosophy of a certain professor there, a very superior man, but who, although an ecclesiastic, was suspected of peculiar opinions on religious subjects. In effect, when, during his course, the professor touched on the doctrine of a future state, his language betrayed so visible an embarrassment that the count, his curiosity excited, ventured privately to broach the subject to his teacher, entreating him to say whether he had held back any thing that dwelt on his mind.

The reply of the professor was embodied in the following strange story.

THE IRON STOVE.

"The hesitation which you noticed," said he, "resulted from the conflict which takes place within me when I am attempting to convey my ideas on a subject where my understanding is at variance with the testimony of my senses. I am, equally from reason and reflection, disposed to consider with incredulity and contempt the existence of apparitions. But an appearance which I have witnessed with my own eyes, as far as they or any of the perceptions can be confided in, and which has even received a sort of subsequent confirmation from other circumstances connected with the original facts, leaves me in that state of skepticism and suspense which pervaded my discourse. I will communicate to you its cause.

"Having been brought up to the profession of the Church, I was presented by Frederick William the First, late King of Prussia, to a small benefice, situated in the interior of the country, at a considerable distance south of Königsberg. I repaired thither in order to take possession of my living, and found a neat parsonage-house, where I passed the night in a bed-chamber which had been occupied by my predecessor.

"It was in the longest days of summer; and on the following morning, which was Sunday, while lying awake, the curtains of the bed being undrawn, and it being broad daylight, I beheld the figure of a man, habited in a loose gown, standing at a sort of reading-desk, on which lay a large book, the leaves of which he seemed to turn over at intervals. On each side of him stood a little boy, in whose face he looked earnestly from time to time; and, as he looked, he seemed always to heave a deep sigh. His countenance, pale and disconsolate, indicated some distress of mind. I had the most perfect view of these objects; but, being impressed with too much terror and apprehension to rise or to address myself to the appearances before me, I remained for some minutes a breathless and silent spectator, without uttering a word or altering my position. At length the man closed the book, and then, taking the two children, one in each hand, he led them slowly across the room. My eyes eagerly followed him till the three figures gradually disappeared, or were lost, behind an iron stove which stood at the farthest corner of the apartment.

"However deeply and awfully I was affected by the sight which I had witnessed, and however incapable I was of explaining it to my own satisfaction, yet I recovered sufficiently the possession of my mind to get up; and, having hastily dressed myself, I left the house. The sun was long risen; and, directing my steps to the church, I found that it was open, though the sexton had quitted it. On entering the chancel, my mind and imagination were so strongly impressed by the scene which had recently passed, that I endeavored to dissipate the recollection by considering the objects around me. In almost all Lutheran churches of the Prussian dominions it is the custom to hang up against the walls, or some part of the building, the portraits of the successive pastors or clergymen who have held the living. A number of these paintings, rudely performed, were suspended in one of the aisles. But I had no sooner fixed my eyes on the last in the range, which was the portrait of my immediate predecessor, than they became riveted on the object; for I instantly recognized the same face which I had beheld in my bed-chamber, though not clouded by the same deep impression of melancholy and distress.

"The sexton entered as I was still contemplating this interesting head, and I immediately began a conversation with him on the subject of the persons who had preceded me in the living. He remembered several incumbents, concerning whom, respectively, I made various inquiries, till I concluded by the last, relative to whose history I was particularly inquisitive. 'We considered him,' said the sexton, 'as one of the most learned and amiable men who have ever resided among us. His character and benevolence endeared him to all his parishioners, who will long lament his loss. But he was carried off in the middle of his days by a lingering illness, the cause of which has given rise to many unpleasant reports among us, and which still form matter of conjecture. It is, however, commonly believed that he died of a broken heart.'

"My curiosity being still more warmly excited by the mention of this circumstance, I eagerly pressed him to disclose to me all he knew, or had heard, on the subject. 'Nothing respecting it,' answered he, 'is absolutely known; but scandal has propagated a story of his having formed ·a criminal connection with a young woman of the neighborhood, by whom, it was even asserted, he had two sons. As confirmation of the report, I know that there certainly were two children who have been seen at the parsonage,—boys, of about four or five·years old; but they suddenly disappeared some time before the decease of their supposed father;

though to what place they were sent, or what is become of them, we are wholly ignorant. It is equally certain that the surmises and unfavorable opinions formed respecting this mysterious business, which must necessarily have reached him, precipitated, if they did not produce, the disorder of which our late pastor died: but he is gone to his account, and we are bound to think charitably of the departed.'

"It is unnecessary to say with what emotion I listened to this relation, which recalled to my imagination, and seemed to give proof of the existence of, all that I had seen. Yet, unwilling to suffer my mind to become enslaved by phantoms which might have been the effect of error or deception, I neither communicated to the sexton the circumstances which I had witnessed, nor even permitted myself to quit the chamber where it had taken place. I continued to lodge there, without ever witnessing any similar appearance; and the recollection itself began to wear away as the autumn advanced.

"When the approach of winter made it necessary to light fires throughout the house, I ordered the iron stove which stood in the room, and behind which the figure which I had beheld, together with the two boys, seemed to disappear, to be heated, for the purpose of warming the apartment. Some difficulty was experienced in making the attempt, the stove not only smoking intolerably, but emitting an offensive smell. Having, therefore, sent for a blacksmith to inspect and repair it, he discovered, in the inside, at the farthest extremity, the bones of two small human bodies, corresponding in size with the description given me by the sexton of the two boys who had been seen at the parsonage.

"This last circumstance completed my astonishment, and appeared to confer a sort of reality on an appearance which might otherwise have been considered as a delusion of the senses. I resigned the living, quitted the place, and retired to Königsberg; but it has produced on my mind the deepest impression, and has, in its effect, given rise to that uncertainty and contra diction of sentiment which you remarked in my late discourse."*

Wraxall adds, "Such was Count Felkesheim's story, which, from its singularity, appeared to me deserving of commemoration, in whatever contempt we may hold similar anecdotes."

If this narrative, and the intimations it conveys, may be trusted to, what a glimpse do these display of a species of future punishment speedy and inevitable!—inevitable so long as wickedness inheres in wicked deeds, unless conscience dies with the body. But conscience is an attribute of the immortal spirit, not of the perishable frame. And if, in very truth, from the world beyond it drags down the evil-doer to the earthly scene of his misdeeds, how false is our phrase, when, in speaking of a murderer who has eluded justice, we say he has escaped punishment! His deed dies not. Even if no vengeful arm of an offended Deity requite the wrong, the wrong may requite itself. Even in the case of some hardened criminal, when the soul, dulled to dogged carelessness during its connection with an obtuse and degraded physical organization, remains impervious, while life lasts, to the stings of conscience, death, removing the hard shell, may expose to sensitiveness and to suffering the disengaged spirit.

There are intimations, however, somewhat similar in general character to the above, which seem to teach us that even in the next world repentance, by its regene-

---

* "*Historical Memoirs of my Own Time*," by Sir N. William Wraxall, Bart., London, 1815, pp. 218 to 226.

rating influence, may gradually change the character and the condition of the criminal; and I shall not be deterred from bringing forward an example, in illustration, by the fear of being charged with Roman Catholic leanings. Eclecticism is true philosophy.

The example to which I refer is one adduced and vouched for by Dr. Kerner, and to which, in part, he could testify from personal observation. It is the history of the same apparition, already briefly alluded to,* as one, the appearance of which to Madame Hauffe was uniformly heralded by knockings, or rappings, audible to all. I entitle it

THE CHILD'S BONES FOUND.

The apparition first presented itself to Madame Hauffe during the winter of 1824–25, one morning at nine o'clock, while she was at her devotions. It was that of a swarthy man, of small stature, his head somewhat drooping, his countenance wrinkled as with age, clad in a dark monk's frock. He looked hard at her, in silence. She experienced a shuddering sensation as she returned his gaze, and hastily left the room.

The next day, and almost daily during an entire year, the figure returned, usually appearing at seven o'clock in the evening, which was Madame Hauffe's wonted hour of prayer. On his second appearance he spoke to her, saying he had come to her for comfort and instruction. "Treat me as a child," he said, "and teach me religion." With especial entreaty, he begged of her that she would pray with him. Subsequently he confessed to her that he had the burden of a murder and of other grievous sins on his soul; that he had wandered

---

* See Book III. chap. 2, "*The Seeress of Prevorst.*" The circumstances, as already stated, occurred near Löwenstein, in the kingdom of Wurtemberg. Dr. Kerner and the seeress and her family were Protestants.

restlessly for long years, and had never yet been able to address himself to prayer.

She complied with his request; and from time to time throughout the long period that he continued to appear to her she instructed him in religious matters, and he joined with her in her devotions.

One evening, at the usual hour, there appeared with him the figure of a woman, tall and meager, bearing in her arms a child that seemed to have just died. She kneeled down with him, and prayed also. This female figure had once before appeared to the seeress; and her coming was usually preceded by sounds similar to those obtained from a steel triangle.

Sometimes she saw the man's figure during her walks abroad. It seemed to glide before her. On one occasion she had been on a visit to Gronau with her parents and her brothers and sisters; and ere she reached home the clock struck seven. Of a sudden she began to run; and when they hastened after her to inquire the cause, she exclaimed, "The spirit is gliding before and entreating my prayers." As they passed hastily along, the family distinctly heard a clapping, as of hands, seeming to come from the air before them; sometimes it was a knocking as on the walls of the houses which they happened to pass. When they reached home, a clapping of hands sounded before them as they ascended the stairs. The seeress hastened to her chamber; and there, as if on bended knees, the spirit prayed with her as usual.

The longer she conversed with him, and the oftener he came for prayer, the lighter and more cheerful and friendly did his countenance become. When their devotions were over, he was wont to say, "Now the sun rises!" or, "Now I feel the sun shining within me!"

One day she asked him whether he could hear other persons speak as well as herself. "I can hear them

34

through you," was his reply. "How so?" she inquired. And he answered, "Because when you hear others speak you think of what you hear; and I can read your thoughts."

It was observed that, as often as this spirit appeared, a black terrier that was kept in the house seemed to be sensible of its presence; for no sooner was the figure perceptible to the seeress than the dog ran, as if for protection, to some one present, often howling loudly; and after his first sight of it he would never remain alone of nights.

One night this apparition presented itself to Madame Hauffe and said, "I shall not come to you for a week; for your guardian spirit is occupied elsewhere. Something important is about to happen in your family: you will hear of it next Wednesday."

This was repeated by Madame Hauffe to her family the next morning. Wednesday came, and with it a letter informing them that the seeress's grandfather, of whose illness they had not even been previously informed, was dead. The apparition did not show itself again till the end of the week.

The "guardian spirit" spoken of by the apparition frequently appeared to the seeress, in the form of her grandmother, the deceased wife of him who had just died, and alleged that it *was* her grandmother's spirit, and that it constantly watched over her. When the spirit of the self-confessed murderer reappeared, after the intermission of a week, she asked him why her guardian spirit had deserted her in these last days. To which he replied, "Because she was occupied by the dying-bed of the recently deceased." He added, "I have advanced so far that I saw the spirit of your relative soon after his death enter a beautiful valley. I shall soon be allowed to enter it myself."

Madame Hauffe's mother never saw the apparition,

nor did her sister. But both, at the times when the spirit appeared to the seeress, frequently felt the sensation as of a breeze blowing upon them.

A friend of the family, a certain forest-ranger, named Böheim, would not believe in the apparition, and wished to be present with Madame Hauffe at the usual hour when it came. He and she were alone in the room. When a few minutes had elapsed, they heard the customary rappings, and, shortly after, the sound as of a body falling. They entered, and found Böheim in a swoon on the floor. When he recovered, he told them that, soon after the rappings commenced, there formed itself, in the corner against the wall, a gray cloud; that this cloud gradually approached the seeress and himself; and when it came quite near it assumed human form. It was between him and the door, so as, apparently, to bar egress. He had returned to consciousness when aid arrived, and he was astonished to see persons pass through the figure without seeming to notice it.

At the expiration of about a year from the time of its first appearance,—namely, on the evening of the 5th of January, 1826,—the spirit said to the seeress, "I shall soon leave you altogether." And he thanked her for all the aid and instruction she had given him, and for her prayers. The next day (January 6, the day her child was christened) he appeared to her for the last time. A servant-girl who was with the seeress at the moment saw and heard (to her astonishment) the door open and close; but it was the seeress alone who saw the apparition enter; and she said nothing to the girl about it.

Afterward, at the christening, Madame Hauffe's father distinctly perceived the same figure, looking bright and pleasant. And going presently into an ante-chamber, he also saw the apparition of the tall, thin, melancholy woman, with the child on her arm. After this day neither of the figures ever appeared to the seeress.

But the fact most strikingly corroborative of all remains to be told. At the instigation of the seeress, they dug, at a spot designated by her, in the yard back of the house, near the kitchen, and there, at a considerable depth, *they found the skeleton and other remains of a small child.**

A single narrative is insufficient proof of a novel theory; and by many the theory will be deemed novel which assumes that the hope of improvement dies not with the body, that beyond the tomb, as on this side of it, progress is the great ruling principle, and that not only may we occasionally receive communications from the denizens of another world, but, under certain circumstances, may sometimes impart to them comfort and instruction in return.

I do not find, however, either from analogy, in Scripture, or elsewhere, any presumptive evidence going to disprove such a hypothesis.† The narrative, so far as it goes, sustains it. All that can be said is, that other coinciding proofs are needed before it can be rationally alleged that

---

* *"Die Seherin von Prevorst,"* by Justinus Kerner, 4th edition, Stuttgart and Tübingen, 1846, pp. 367 to 374.

† In a subsequent chapter (on the Change at Death) I shall have occasion to speak of the doctrine—vaguely conceived by the ancients, adopted in somewhat more definite form by the Jews, and universally received by early Christians—of what is commonly called a mediate state after death,—a state where instruction may still be received, where repentance may still do its work, and where the errors of the present life may be corrected in a life to come.

Several of the early Christian Fathers held to the opinion that the gospel was preached, both by Christ and his apostles, to the dead as well as to the living: among them, Origen and Clement of Alexandria. The latter exclaims, "What! do not the Scriptures manifest that the Lord preached the gospel to those who perished in the deluge, or rather to such as had been bound, and to those in prison and in custody? It has been shown to me that the apostles, in imitation of the Lord, preached the gospel to those in Hades."—*Quoted by Sears, " Foregleams of Immortality,"* p. 264.

we have obtained such an aggregation of evidence as may be pronounced conclusive.

It is none the less to be conceded that Kerner's story bears strong marks of authenticity. The good faith of the author has scarcely been questioned even by his opponents. His opportunities for observation were almost without precedent. "I visited Madame Hauffe, as physician," he tells us, "probably three thousand times. I frequently remained by her sick-bed hours at a time; I knew her surroundings better than she did herself; and I took unspeakable pains to follow up every rumor or suggestion of trickery, without ever detecting the slightest trace of any deception."*

It is to be remarked, also, that in this example there are many strongly corroborative circumstances, beyond the perceptions of the seeress,—the knockings and clappings, heard by all; the cool breeze felt by her mother and sister; the terror of the dog; the fulfillment of the prophecy, communicated beforehand to her family, in connection with the grandfather's death. Add to this that the same apparition was seen, at different times, by three persons,—by Madame Hauffe, by her father, and by Herr Böheim. Names, dates, places, every minute incident is given. The narrative was published, on the spot, at the time. Sixteen years afterward, on the issuing of the fourth edition of his work, Dr. Kerner reiterates in the most solemn manner his conviction of its truth.

It is in vain to assert that we ought to pass lightly by such testimony as this.

In the two preceding narratives, the incidents of which seem to indicate the return of the evil-doer's

---

* "Seherin von Prevorst," p. 324. The entire work will well repay a careful perusal.

spirit to the scene of his evil deed, the deed was one of the greatest of earthly crimes,—murder. But we may find examples where the prompting motive of return appears to be a mere short-coming of the most trivial character. Such a one is given by Dr. Binns, in his "Anatomy of Sleep." It was communicated by the Rev. Charles McKay, a Catholic priest, then resident in Scotland, in a letter addressed by him to the Countess of Shrewsbury, dated Perth, October 21, 1842. This letter was communicated by the earl to Dr. Binns, who publishes it entire, adding that "perhaps there is not a better-authenticated case on record." I extract it from the letter, as follows.

THE DEBT OF THREE-AND-TENPENCE.

"In July, 1838, I left Edinburgh, to take charge of the Perthshire missions. On my arrival in Perth, the principal station, I was called upon by a Presbyterian woman, (Anne Simpson by name,) who for more than a week had been in the utmost anxiety to see a priest. On asking her what she wanted with me, she answered, 'Oh, sir, I have been terribly troubled for several nights by a person appearing to me during the night.' 'Are you a Catholic, my good woman?' 'No, sir: I am a Presbyterian.' 'Why, then, do you come to me? I am a Catholic priest.' 'But, sir, *she* (meaning the person that had appeared to her) desired me to go to the priest, and I have been inquiring for a priest during the last week.' 'Why did she wish you to go to the priest?' 'She said she owed a sum of money, and the priest would pay it.' 'What was the sum of money she owed?' 'Three-and-tenpence, sir.' 'To whom did she owe it?' 'I do not know, sir.' 'Are you sure you have not been dreaming?' 'Oh, God forgive you! for she appears to me every night. I can get no rest.' 'Did you know the woman you say appears to you?' 'I was poorly lodged, sir, near the barracks, and I often saw and spoke to her as she went in and out to the barracks; and she called herself Maloy.'

"I made inquiry, and found that a woman of that name had died who had acted as washerwoman and followed the regiment. Following up the inquiry, I found a grocer with whom she had dealt, and, on asking him if a person, a female, named Maloy owed him any thing, he turned up his books, and told me she did owe him *three-and-tenpence*. I paid the sum. The grocer knew nothing of her death, nor, indeed, of her character, but that she was attached to the barracks. Subsequently the Presbyterian woman came to me, saying that she was no more troubled."*

It is not a plausible supposition, in this case, that for so paltry a sum a tradesman should concert with an old woman (she was past seventy years of age) to trump up a story of an apparition and impose on the good nature and credulity of a priest. Had it been such a trick, too, it is scarcely supposable that the woman should not have mentioned the grocer's name, but should have left the reverend gentleman to grope after the creditor as he best might.

If the whole was related in good faith, the indication seems to be that human character may be but little altered by the death-change,—sometimes preserving in another state of existence not only trifling recollections, but trivial cares.

Some narratives appear to favor the supposition that not the criminal only, but the victim of his crime, may, at times, be attracted in spirit to the earthly scene of suffering. The Hydesville story may have been an ex-

---

* *"Anatomy of Sleep,"* by Edward Binns, M.D., pp. 462, 463.

ample of this. While in Paris, in the spring of 1859, I
obtained what appears to be another. The narrative
was communicated to me by a clergyman of the Church
of England, the Rev. Dr. ——, Chaplain to the British
Legation at ——. Having heard from a brother clergyman something of the story, I asked, by letter, to be
favored with it; stating, in general terms, the purpose
of my work. The request was kindly complied with,
and produced an interesting contribution to this branch
of the subject.

THE STAINS OF BLOOD.

"In the year 185- I was staying, with my wife and
children, at the favorite watering-place ——. In order
to attend to some affairs of my own, I determined
to leave my family there for three or four days. Accordingly, on the —th of August, I took the railway,
and arrived that evening, an unexpected guest, at ——
Hall, the residence of a gentleman whose acquaintance
I had recently made, and with whom my sister was
then staying.

"I arrived late, soon afterward went to bed, and
before long fell asleep. Awaking after three or four
hours, I was not surprised to find I could sleep no
more; for I never rest well in a strange bed. After
trying, therefore, in vain again to induce sleep, I began
to arrange my plans for the day.

"I had been engaged some little time in this way,
when I became suddenly sensible that there was a light
in the room. Turning round, I distinctly perceived a
female figure; and what attracted my special attention
was, *that the light by which I saw it emanated from itself.*
I watched the figure attentively. The features were
not perceptible. After moving a little distance, it disappeared as suddenly as it had appeared.

"My first thoughts were that there was some trick.

I immediately got out of bed, struck a light, and found my bedroom-door still locked. I then carefully examined the walls, to ascertain if there were any other concealed means of entrance or exit; but none could I find. I drew the curtains and opened the shutters; but all outside was silent and dark, there being no moonlight.

"After examining the room well in every part, I betook myself to bed and thought calmly over the whole matter. The final impression on my mind was, that I had seen something supernatural, and, if supernatural, that it was in some way connected with my wife. What was the appearance? What did it mean? Would it have appeared to me if I had been asleep instead of awake? These were questions very easy to ask and very difficult to answer.

"Even if my room-door had been unlocked, or if there had been a concealed entrance to the room, a practical joke was out of the question. For, in the first place, I was not on such intimate terms with my host as to warrant such a liberty; and, secondly, even if he had been inclined to sanction so questionable a proceeding, he was too unwell at the time to permit me for a moment to entertain such a supposition.

"In doubt and uncertainty I passed the rest of the night; and in the morning, descending early, I immediately told my sister what had occurred, describing to her accurately every thing connected with the appearance I had witnessed. She seemed much struck with what I told her, and replied, 'It is *very* odd; for you have heard, I dare say, that a lady was, some years ago, murdered in this house; but it was not in the room you slept in.' I answered, that I had never heard any thing of the kind, and was beginning to make further inquiries about the murder, when I was interrupted by the entrance of our host and hostess, and afterward by breakfast.

"After breakfast I left, without having had any opportunity of renewing the conversation. But the whole affair had made upon me an impression which I sought in vain to shake off. The female figure was ever before my mind's eye, and I became fidgety and anxious about my wife. 'Could it in any way be connected with her?' was my constantly recurring thought. So much did this weigh on my mind that, instead of attending to the business for the express purpose of transacting which I had left my family, I returned to them by the first train; and it was only when I saw my wife and children in good health, and every thing safe and well in my household, that I felt satisfied that, whatever the nature of the appearance might have been, it was not connected with any evil to them.

"On the Wednesday following, I received a letter from my sister, in which she informed me that, since I left, she had ascertained that the murder *was* committed in the very room in which I had slept. She added that she purposed visiting us next day, and that she would like me to write out an account of what I had seen, together with a plan of the room, and that on that plan she wished me to mark the place of the appearance, and of the disappearance, of the figure.

"This I immediately did; and the next day, when my sister arrived, she asked me if I had complied with her request. I replied, pointing to the drawing-room table, 'Yes: there is the account and the plan.' As she rose to examine it, I prevented her, saying, 'Do not look at it until you have told me all you have to say, because you might unintentionally color your story by what you may read there.'

"Thereupon she informed me that she had had the carpet taken up in the room I had occupied, and that the marks of blood from the murdered person were there, plainly visible, on a particular part of the floor. At my request she also then drew a plan of the room, and marked upon it the spots which still bore traces of blood.

"The two plans—my sister's and mine—were then compared, and we verified the most remarkable fact *that the places she had marked as the beginning and ending of the traces of blood coincided exactly with the spots marked on my plan as those on which the female figure had appeared and disappeared.*

"I am unable to add any thing to this plain statement of facts. I cannot account, in any way, for what I saw. I am convinced no human being entered my chamber that night; yet I know that, being wide awake and in good health, I *did* distinctly see a female figure in my room. But if, as I must believe, it was a supernatural appearance, then I am unable to suggest any reason why it should have appeared to me. I cannot tell whether, if I had not been in the room, or had been asleep at the time, that figure would equally have been there. As it was, it seemed connected with no warning nor presage. No misfortune of any kind happened then, or since, to me or mine. It is true that the host, at whose house I was staying when this incident occurred, and also one of his children, died a few months afterward; but I cannot pretend to make out any connection between either of these deaths and the appearance I witnessed. The 'cui bono,' therefore, I do not attempt to explain. But what I distinctly saw, that, and that only, I describe."*

---

* Communicated to me, under date April 25, 1859, in a letter from the Rev. Dr. ——, who informs me that the relation is in the very words, so

In this case, the narrative bears testimony to accuracy and dispassionate coolness in the observer. It is one of those examples, also, which give support to the opinion that such phenomena sometimes present themselves without any special purpose so far as we can discover. Moreover, it is evident that sufficient precautions were taken to prevent the possibility of suggestion becoming the cause of the coincidence between the two plans of the room,—that executed by the brother and that afterward drawn by the sister. They were, clearly, made out quite independently of each other. And if so, to what can we ascribe the coincidence they exhibited? Evidently, not to chance.

In the preceding cases, the attraction to earth seems to have been of a painful nature. But a more frequent and influential motive seems to be that great principle of human love, which even in this world, cold though it be, is the most powerful incentive to virtue, and which in another will doubtless assert far more supremely its genial sway. It may be the affection of remote kindred, apparently evinced by some ancestor, or the stronger love of brother to sister, of parent to child, of husband to wife. Of the last an example will be found in the following narrative, for which I am indebted to the kindness of London friends; and though, in accordance with the wishes of the family, some of the names are initialized only, they are all known to myself. Of the good faith of the narrators there cannot be a doubt.

---

far as his memory serves, in which the narrator, his brother, repeated it to him. Though not at liberty to print the reverend gentleman's name, he has permitted me to furnish it privately in any case in which it might serve the cause to advance which these pages have been written.

THE FOURTEENTH OF NOVEMBER.

In the month of September, 1857, Captain G——W——, of the 6th (Inniskilling) Dragoons, went out to India to join his regiment.

His wife remained in England, residing at Cambridge. On the night between the 14th and 15th of November, 1857, toward morning, she dreamed that she saw her husband, looking anxious and ill,—upon which she immediately awoke, much agitated. It was bright moonlight; and, looking up, she perceived the same figure standing by her bedside. He appeared in his uniform, the hands pressed across the breast, the hair disheveled, the face very pale. His large dark eyes were fixed full upon her; their expression was that of great excitement, and there was a peculiar contraction of the mouth, habitual to him when agitated. She saw him, even to each minute particular of his dress, as distinctly as she had ever done in her life; and she remembers to have noticed between his hands the white of the shirt-bosom, unstained, however, with blood. The figure seemed to bend forward, as if in pain, and to make an effort to speak; but there was no sound. It remained visible, the wife thinks, as long as a minute, and then disappeared.

Her first idea was to ascertain if she was actually awake. She rubbed her eyes with the sheet, and felt that the touch was real. Her little nephew was in bed with her: she bent over the sleeping child and listened to its breathing; the sound was distinct; and she became convinced that what she had seen was no dream. It need hardly be added that she did not again go to sleep that night.

Next morning she related all this to her mother, expressing her conviction, though she had noticed no marks of blood on his dress, that Captain W—— was either killed or grievously wounded. So fully impressed

35

was she with the reality of that apparition that she thenceforth refused all invitations. A young friend urged her, soon afterward, to go with her to a fashionable concert, reminding her that she had received from Malta, sent by her husband, a handsome dress-cloak, which she had never yet worn. But she positively declined, declaring that, uncertain as she was whether she was not already a widow, she would never enter a place of amusement until she had letters from her husband (if, indeed, he still lived) of later date than the 14th of November.

It was on a Tuesday in the month of December, 1857, that the telegram regarding the actual fate of Captain W—— was published in London. It was to the effect that he was killed before Lucknow on the *fifteenth* of November.

This news, given in the morning paper, attracted the attention of Mr. Wilkinson, a London solicitor, who had in charge Captain W——'s affairs. When at a later period this gentleman met the widow, she informed him that she had been quite prepared for the melancholy news, but that she felt sure her husband could not have been killed on the 15th of November, inasmuch as it was during the night between the 14th and 15th that he appeared to herself.*

The certificate from the War Office, however, which it became Mr. Wilkinson's duty to obtain, confirmed the date given in the telegram; its tenor being as follows:—

---

* The difference of longitude between London and Lucknow being about five hours, three or four o'clock A.M. in London would be eight or nine o'clock A.M. at Lucknow. But it was in the *afternoon*, not in the morning, as will be seen in the sequel, that Captain W—— was killed. Had he fallen on the 15th, therefore, the apparition to his wife would have appeared several hours before the engagement in which he fell, and while he was yet alive and well.

"No. $\frac{9579}{1}$.   WAR OFFICE,
                                                      30th January, 1858.

"These are to certify that it appears, by the records in this office, that Captain G—— W——, of the 6th Dragoon Guards, was killed in action on the 15th November, 1857.*   (Signed)   B. HAWES."

While Mr. Wilkinson's mind remained in uncertainty as to the exact date, a remarkable incident occurred, which seemed to cast further suspicion on the accuracy of the telegram and of the certificate. That gentleman was visiting a friend, whose lady has all her life had perception of apparitions, while her husband is what is usually called an impressible medium; facts which are known, however, only to their intimate friends. Though personally acquainted with them, I am not at liberty to give their names. Let us call them Mr. and Mrs. N——.

Mr. Wilkinson related to them, as a wonderful circumstance, the vision of the captain's widow in connection with his death, and described the figure as it had appeared to her. Mrs. N——, turning to her husband, instantly said, "That must be the very person I saw, the evening we were talking of India, and you drew an elephant, with a howdah on his back. Mr. Wilkinson has described his exact position and appearance; the uniform of a British officer, his hands pressed across his breast, his form bent forward as if in pain. The figure," she added to Mr. W——, "appeared just behind my husband, and seemed looking over his left shoulder."

"Did you attempt to obtain any communication from him?" Mr. Wilkinson asked.

"Yes: we procured one through the medium of my husband."

"Do you remember its purport?"

---

* Into this certificate, of which I possess the original, an error has crept. Captain G—— W—— was of the 6th (Inniskilling) Dragoons, not of the 6th Dragoon Guards.

"It was to the effect that he had been killed in India that afternoon, by a wound in the breast; and adding, as I distinctly remember, 'That thing I used to go about in is not buried yet.' I particularly marked the expression."

"When did this happen?"

"About nine o'clock in the evening, several weeks ago; but I do not recollect the exact date."

"Can you not call to mind something that might enable you to fix the precise day?"

Mrs. N—— reflected. "I remember nothing," she said, at last, "except that while my husband was drawing, and I was talking to a lady friend who had called to see us, we were interrupted by a servant bringing in a bill for some German vinegar, and that, as I recommended it as being superior to English, we had a bottle brought in for inspection."

"Did you pay the bill at the time?"

"Yes: I sent out the money by the servant."

"Was the bill receipted?"

"I think so; but I have it up-stairs, and can soon ascertain."

Mrs. N—— produced the bill. Its receipt bore date the *fourteenth* of November!

This confirmation of the widow's conviction as to the day of her husband's death produced so much impression on Mr. Wilkinson, that he called at the office of Messrs. Cox & Greenwood, the army agents, to ascertain if there was no mistake in the certificate. But nothing there appeared to confirm any surmise of inaccuracy. Captain W——'s death was mentioned in two separate dispatches of Sir Colin Campbell; and in both the date corresponded with that given in the telegram.

So matters rested, until, in the month of March, 1858, the family of Captain W—— received from Captain G—— C——, then of the Military Train, a letter dated near Lucknow, on the 19th December, 1857. This letter informed them that Captain W—— had been killed before Lucknow, while gallantly leading on the squadron, not on the 15th of November, as reported in Sir Colin Campbell's dispatches, but on the *fourteenth, in the afternoon.* Captain C—— was riding close by his side at the time he saw him fall. He was struck by a fragment of shell in the breast, and never spoke after he was hit. He was buried at the Dilkoosha; and on a wooden cross erected by his friend, Lieutenant R—— of the 9th Lancers, at the head of his grave, are cut the initials G. W. and the date of his death, the 14th of November, 1857.*

The War Office finally made the correction as to the date of death, but not until more than a year after the event occurred. Mr. Wilkinson, having occasion to apply for an additional copy of the certificate in April, 1859, found it in exactly the same words as that which I have given, only that the 14th of November had been substituted for the 15th.†

This extraordinary narrative was obtained by me directly from the parties themselves. The widow of Captain W—— kindly consented to examine and correct the manuscript, and allowed me to inspect a copy of Captain C——'s letter, giving the particulars of her husband's death. To Mr. Wilkinson, also, the manuscript was submitted, and he assented to its accuracy so far as he is concerned. That portion which relates to Mrs. N—— I had from that lady herself. I have neg-

---

* It was not in his own regiment, which was then at Meerut, that Captain W—— was serving at the time of his death. Immediately on arriving from England at Cawnpore, he had offered his services to Colonel Wilson, of the 64th. They were at first declined, but finally accepted; and he joined the Military Train, then starting for Lucknow. It was in their ranks that he fell.

† The originals of both these certificates are in my possession: the first bearing date 30th January, 1858, and certifying, as already shown, to the 15th; the second dated 5th April, 1859, and testifying to the 14th.

lected no precaution, therefore, to obtain for it the warrant of authenticity.

It is, perhaps, the only example on record where the appearance of what is usually termed a ghost proved the means of correcting an erroneous date in the dispatches of a commander-in-chief, and of detecting an inaccuracy in the certificate of a War Office.

It is especially valuable, too, as furnishing an example of a double apparition. Nor can it be alleged (even if the allegation had weight) that the recital of one lady caused the apparition of the same figure to the other. Mrs. W—— was at the time in Cambridge, and Mrs. N—— in London; and it was not till weeks after the occurrence that either knew what the other had seen.

Those who would explain the whole on the principle of chance coincidence have a treble event to take into account: the apparition to Mrs. N——, that to Mrs. W——, and the actual time of Captain W——'s death; each tallying exactly with the other.

Examples of apparitions at the moment of death might be multiplied without number. Many persons—especially in Germany—who believe in no other species of apparition admit this. *Anzeigen* is the German term employed to designate such an intimation from the newly dead.

Compelled by lack of space, I shall here close the list of narratives connected with alleged apparitions of the dead, by giving one—certainly not the least remarkable —a portion of the corroborative proofs of which were sought out and obtained by myself.

THE OLD KENT MANOR-HOUSE.

In October, 1857, and for several months afterward, Mrs. R——,* wife of a field-officer of high rank in the British

---

* The initials of the two names here given are not the actual ones; but I have the pleasure of a personal acquaintance with both these ladies.

army, was residing in Ramhurst Manor-House, near Leigh, in Kent, England. From the time of her first occupying this ancient residence, every inmate of the house had been more or less disturbed at night—*not* usually during the day—by knockings and sounds as of footsteps, but more especially by voices which could not be accounted for. These last were usually heard in some unoccupied adjoining room; sometimes as if talking in a loud tone, sometimes as if reading aloud, occasionally as if screaming. The servants were much alarmed. They never saw any thing; but the cook told Mrs. R—— that on one occasion, in broad daylight, hearing the rustle of a silk dress close behind her, and which seemed to touch her, she turned suddenly round, supposing it to be her mistress, but, to her great surprise and terror, could see nobody. Mrs. R——'s brother, a bold, light-hearted young officer, fond of field-sports, and without the slightest faith in the reality of visitations from another world, was much disturbed and annoyed by these voices, which he declared must be those of his sister and of a lady friend of hers, sitting up together to chat all night. On two occasions, when a voice which he thought to resemble his sister's rose to a scream, as if imploring aid, he rushed from his room, at two or three o'clock in the morning, gun in hand, into his sister's bedroom, there to find her quietly asleep.

On the second Saturday in the above month of October, Mrs. R—— drove over to the railway-station at Tunbridge, to meet her friend Miss S——, whom she had invited to spend some weeks with her. This young lady had been in the habit of seeing apparitions, at times, from early childhood.

When, on their return, at about four o'clock in the afternoon, they drove up to the entrance of the manor-house, Miss S—— perceived on the threshold the appearance of two figures, apparently an elderly couple, habited in the costume of a former age. They appeared as if standing on the ground. She did not hear any voice; and, not wishing to render her friend uneasy, she made at that time no remark to her in connection with this apparition.

She saw the appearance of the same figures, in the same dress, several times within the next ten days, sometimes in one of the rooms of the house, sometimes in one of the passages,—always by daylight. They appeared to her surrounded by an atmosphere nearly of the color usually called neutral tint. On the third occasion they spoke to her, and stated that they had been husband and wife, that in former days they had possessed and occupied that manor-house, and that their name was *Children.* They appeared sad and downcast; and, when Miss S—— inquired the cause of their melancholy, they replied that they had idolized this property of theirs; that their pride and pleasure had centered in its possession; that its improvement had engrossed their thoughts; and that it troubled them to know that it had passed away from their family and to see it now in the hands of careless strangers.

I asked Miss S—— *how* they spoke. She replied that the voice was audible to her as that of a human being's; and that she believed it was heard also by others in an adjoining room. This she inferred from the fact that she was afterward asked with whom she had been conversing.*

After a week or two, Mrs. R——, beginning to suspect that something unusual, connected with the constant disturbances in the house, had occurred to her friend,

---

* Yet this is not conclusive. It might have been Miss S——'s voice only that was heard, not any reply—though heard by her—made by the apparitions. Visible to her, they were invisible to others. Audible to her, they may to others have been inaudible also.

Yet it is certain that the voices at night were heard equally by all.

questioned her closely on the subject; and then Miss S—— related to her what she had seen and heard, describing the appearance and relating the conversation of the figures calling themselves Mr. and Mrs. Children.

Up to that time, Mrs. R——, though her rest had been frequently broken by the noises in the house, and though she too has the occasional perception of apparitions, had seen nothing; nor did any thing appear to her for a month afterward. One day, however, about the end of that time, when she had ceased to expect any apparition to herself, she was hurriedly dressing for a late dinner,—her brother, who had just returned from a day's shooting, having called to her in impatient tones that dinner was served and that he was quite famished. At the moment of completing her toilet, and as she hastily turned to leave her bed-chamber, not dreaming of any thing spiritual, there in the doorway stood the same female figure Miss S—— had described,—identical in appearance and in costume, even to the old point-lace on her brocaded silk dress,—while beside her, on the left, but less distinctly visible, was the figure of her husband. They uttered no sound; but above the figure of the lady, as if written in phosphoric light in the dusk atmosphere that surrounded her, were the words "*Dame Children,*" together with some other words, intimating that, having never aspired beyond the joys and sorrows of this world, she had remained "earth-bound." These last, however, Mrs. R—— scarcely paused to decipher; for a renewed appeal from her brother, as to whether they were to have any dinner that day, urged her forward. The figure, filling up the doorway, remained stationary. There was no time for hesitation: she closed her eyes, rushed through the apparition and into the dining-room, throwing up her hands and exclaiming to Miss S——, " Oh, my dear, I've walked through Mrs. Children !"

2 B

This was the only time during her residence in the old manor-house that Mrs. R—— witnessed the apparition of these figures.

And it is to be remarked that her bed-chamber, at the time, was lighted, not only by candles, but by a cheerful fire, and that there was a lighted lamp in the corridor which communicated thence to the dining-room.

This repetition of the word "Children" caused the ladies to make inquiries among the servants and in the neighborhood whether any family bearing that name had ever occupied the manor-house. Among those whom they thought likely to know something about it was a Mrs. Sophy O——, a nurse in the family, who had spent her life in that vicinity. But all inquiries were fruitless; every one to whom they put the question, the nurse included, declaring that they had never heard of such a name. So they gave up all hopes of being able to unravel the mystery.

It so happened, however, that, about four months afterward, this nurse, going home for a holiday to her family at Riverhead, about a mile from Seven Oaks, and recollecting that one of her sisters-in-law, who lived near her, an old woman of seventy, had fifty years before been housemaid in a family then residing at Ramhurst, inquired of her if she had ever heard any thing of a family named Children. The sister-in-law replied that no such family occupied the manor-house when she was there; but she recollected to have then seen an old man who told her that in his boyhood he had assisted to keep the hounds of the Children family, who were then residing at Ramhurst. This information the nurse communicated to Mrs. R—— on her return; and thus it was that that lady was first informed that a family named Children really had once occupied the manor-house.

All these particulars I received in December, 1858,

directly from the ladies themselves, both being together at the time.

Even up to this point the case, as it presented itself, was certainly a very remarkable one. But I resolved, if possible, to obtain further confirmation in the matter.

I inquired of Miss S—— whether the apparitions had communicated to her any additional particulars connected with the family. She replied that she recollected one which she had then received from them, namely, that the husband's name was *Richard*. At a subsequent period, likewise, she had obtained the date of Richard Children's death, which, as communicated to her, was 1753. She remembered also that on one occasion a third spirit appeared with them, which they stated was their son; but she did not get his name. To my further inquiries as to the costumes in which the (alleged) spirits appeared, Miss S——replied " that they were of the period of Queen Anne or one of the early Georges, she could not be sure which, as the fashions in both were similar." These were her exact words. Neither she nor Mrs. R——, however, had obtained any information tending either to verify or to refute these particulars.

Having an invitation from some friends residing near Seven Oaks, in Kent, to spend with them the Christmas week of 1858, I had a good opportunity of prosecuting my inquiries in the way of verification.

I called, with a friend, Mr. F——, on the nurse, Mrs. Sophy O——. Without alluding to the disturbances, I simply asked her if she knew any thing of an old family of the name of Children. She said she knew very little except what she had heard from her sister-in-law, namely, that they used in former days to live at a manor-house called Ramhurst. I asked her if she had ever been there. "Yes," she said, " about a year ago, as nurse to Mrs. R——." "Did Mrs. R——," I asked her, " know any thing about the Children family?" She replied that her mistress had once made inquiries of her about them, wishing to know if they had ever occupied the manor-house, but at that time she (Mrs. Sophy) had never heard of such a family : so she could give the lady no satisfaction.

"How did it happen," I asked, "that Mrs. R—— supposed such a family might once have occupied the house?"

"Well, sir," she replied, "that is more than I can tell you,—unless, indeed, [and here she hesitated and lowered her voice,] it was through a young lady that was staying with mistress. Did you ever hear, sir," she added, looking around her in a mysterious way, "of what they call *spirit-rappers?*"

I intimated that I had heard the name.

"I'm not afraid of such things," she pursued: "I never thought they would harm me; and I'm not one of your believers in ghosts. But then, to be sure, we *did* have such a time in that old house!"

"Ah! what sort of a time?"

"With knockings, sir, and the noise of footsteps, and people talking of nights. Many a time I've heard the voices when I was going along the passage at two or three o'clock in the morning, carrying the baby to my mistress. I don't believe in ghosts; but you may be sure, sir, it was something serious when mistress's brother got up in the middle of the night and came to his sister's room with his loaded gun in his hand. And then there was another brother: he got out of his bed one night and declared there were robbers in the house."

"Did you see any thing?"

"No, sir, never."

"Nor any of the other servants?"

"I think not, sir; but cook was *so* frightened!"

"What happened to her?"

"Well, sir, no harm happened to her, exactly: only

she was kneeling down making her fire one morning when up she started with a cry like. I heard her, and came in to see what was the matter. 'Oh,' says she, 'nurse, if I didn't hear the rustling of a silk dress all across the kitchen!' 'Well, cook,' says I, 'you know it couldn't be me, being I never wear silk.' 'No,' says she,—and she sort of laughed,—'no, I knew it wasn't you, for I've heard the same three or four times already; and whenever I look round there's nothing there.'"

I thanked the good woman, and then went to see the sister-in-law, who fully confirmed her part of the story.

But as all this afforded no clew either to the Christian name, or the date of occupation, or the year of Mr. Children's death, I visited, in search of these, the church and graveyard at Leigh, the nearest to the Ramhurst property, and the old church at Tunbridge; making inquiries in both places on the subject. But to no purpose. All I could learn was, that a certain George Children left, in the year 1718, a weekly gift of bread to the poor, and that a descendant of the family, also named George, dying some forty years ago, and not residing at Ramhurst, had a marble tablet, in the Tunbridge church, erected to his memory.

Sextons and tombstones having failed me, a friend suggested that I might possibly obtain the information I sought by visiting a neighboring clergyman. I did so, and with the most fortunate result. Simply stating to him that I had taken the liberty to call in search of some particulars touching the early history of a Kentish family of the name of Children, he replied that, singularly enough, he was in possession of a document, coming to him through a private source, and containing, he thought likely, the very details of which I was in search. He kindly intrusted it to me; and I found in it, among numerous particulars regarding another member of the family, not many years since deceased, certain extracts from the "Hasted Papers," preserved in the British Museum; these being contained in a letter addressed by one of the members of the Children family to Mr. Hasted. Of this document, which may be consulted in the Museum library, I here transcribe a portion, as follows:—

"The family of Children were settled for a great many generations at a house called, from their own name, Childrens, situated at a place called Nether Street, otherwise Lower Street, in Hildenborough, in the parish of Tunbridge. George Children of Lower Street, who was High-Sheriff of Kent in 1698, died without issue in 1718, and by will devised the bulk of his estate to *Richard* Children, eldest son of his late uncle, William Children of Hedcorn, and his heirs. This Richard Children, *who settled himself at Ramhurst,* in the parish of Leigh, married Anne, daughter of John Saxby, in the parish of Leeds, by whom he had issue four sons and two daughters," &c.

Thus I ascertained that the first of the Children family who occupied Ramhurst as a residence was named Richard, and that he settled there in the early part of the reign of George I. The year of his death, however, was not given.

This last particular I did not ascertain till several months afterward; when a friend versed in antiquarian lore, to whom I mentioned my desire to obtain it, suggested that the same Hasted, an extract from whose papers I have given, had published, in 1778, a history of Kent, and that, in that work, I might possibly obtain the information I sought. In effect, after considerable search, I there found the following paragraph:—

"In the eastern part of the Parish of Lyghe, (now Leigh,) near the river Medway, stands an ancient mansion called Ramhurst, once reputed a Manor and held of the honor of Gloucester." . . . "It continued in the Culpepper family for several generations." . . . "It passed by sale into that of Saxby, and Mr. William Saxby con-

ADDITIONAL CORROBORATIVE FACTS.

veyed it, by sale, to Children. Richard Children, Esq., resided here, *and died possessed of it in* 1753, aged eighty-three years. He was succeeded in it by his eldest son, John Children, of Tunbridge, Esq., whose son, George Children, of Tunbridge, Esq., is the present possessor."*

Thus I verified the last remaining particular, the date of Richard Children's death. It appears from the above, also, that Richard Children was the *only* representative of the family who lived and died at Ramhurst; his son John being designated not as of Ramhurst, but as of Tunbridge. From the private memoir above referred to I had previously ascertained that the family seat after Richard's time was Ferox Hall, near Tunbridge.

It remains to be added that in 1816, in consequence of events reflecting no discredit on the family, they lost all their property, and were compelled to sell Ramhurst, which has since been occupied, though a somewhat spacious mansion, not as a family residence, but as a farmhouse. I visited it; and the occupant assured me that nothing worse than rats or mice disturbs it now.

I am not sure that I have found on record, among what are usually termed ghost-stories, any narrative better authenticated than the foregoing. It involves, indeed, no startling or romantic particulars, no warning of death, no disclosure of murder, no circumstances of terror or danger; but it is all the more reliable on that account; since those passions which are wont to excite and mislead the imaginations of men were not called into play.

It was communicated to me, about fourteen months only after the events occurred, by both the chief witnesses, and incidentally confirmed, shortly afterward, by a third.

---

* That is, in 1778, when the work was published. See, for the above quotation, Hasted's History of Kent, vol. i. pp. 422 and 423.

The social position and personal character of the two ladies to whom the figures appeared preclude, at the outset, all idea whatever of willful misstatement or deception. The sights and sounds to which they testify *did* present themselves to their senses. Whether their senses played them false is another question. The theory of hallucination remains to be dealt with. Let us inquire whether it be applicable in the present case.

Miss S—— first saw the figures, not in the obscurity of night, not between sleeping and waking, not in some old chamber reputed to be haunted, but in the open air, and as she was descending from a carriage, in broad daylight. Subsequently she not only saw them, but heard them speak; and that always in daylight. There are, however, cases on record in which the senses of hearing and sight are alleged to have been both hallucinated; that of Tasso, for example.* And if the case rested here, such is the interpretation which the physician would put upon it.

But some weeks afterward another lady sees the appearance of the selfsame figures. This complicates the case. For, as elsewhere shown,† it is generally admitted, by medical writers on the subject, that, while cases of collective illusion are common, it is doubtful whether there be on record a single authentic case of collective hallucination: the inference being that if two persons see the same appearance, it is not mere imagination; there is *some* objective foundation for it.

It is true, and should be taken into account, that Miss S—— had described the apparition to her friend, and that for a time the latter had some expectation of witnessing it. And this will suggest to the skeptic, as

---

* *"Essay towards a Theory of Apparitions,"* by John Ferr'ar, M.D., London, 1813, p. 75.

† See Book IV. chap. i.

explanation, the theory of expectant attention. But, in the first place, it has never been proved* that mere expectant attention could produce the appearance of a figure with every detail of costume, to say nothing of the phosphorescent letters appearing above it, which Mrs. R—— certainly did *not* expect; and, secondly, Mrs. R—— expressly stated to me that, as four weeks had elapsed and she had seen nothing, she had ceased to expect it at all. Still less can we imagine that her thoughts would be occupied with the matter at the moment when, hurried by a hungry and impatient brother, she was hastily completing, in a cheerfully-lighted room, her dinner-toilet. It would be difficult to select a moment out of the twenty-four hours when the imagination was less likely to be busy with spiritual fancies, or could be supposed excited to the point necessary to reproduce (if it can ever reproduce) the image of a described apparition.

But conceding these extreme improbabilities, what are we to make of the name Children, communicated to the one lady through the sense of hearing and to the other through that of sight?

The name is a very uncommon one; and both the ladies assured me that they had never even heard it before, to say nothing of their being wholly ignorant whether any family bearing that name had formerly occupied the old house. This latter point they seek to clear up; but neither servants nor neighbors can tell them any thing about it. They remain for four months without any explanation. At the end of that time, one of the servants, going home, accidentally ascertains that about a hundred years ago, or more, a family named Children *did* occupy that very house.

What could imagination or expectation have to do

---

* The contrary appears. See page 354.

with this? The images of the figures may be set down, in the case of both the ladies, as hallucination; but the name remains, a stubborn link, connecting these with the actual world.

If even we were to argue—what no one will believe—that this agreement of family name was but a chance coincidence, there remain yet other coincidences to account for before the whole difficulty is settled. There is the alleged Christian as well as family name,—Richard Children; there is the date indicated by the costume, "the reign of Queen Anne or one of the early Georges;" and, finally, there is the year of Richard Children's death.

These the ladies stated to me, not knowing, when they did so, what the actual facts were. These facts I myself subsequently disinterred; obtaining the evidence of a document preserved in the British Museum in proof that Richard Children *did* inherit the Ramhurst property in the fourth year of the reign of George I., and *did* make the Ramhurst mansion-house his family residence. And he is the only representative of the family who lived and died there. His son John may have resided there for a time; but previous to his decease he had left the place for another seat, near Tunbridge.

Then there is the circumstance that misfortunes compelled the descendants of Richard Children to sell the Ramhurst property, and that their ancestor's family mansion, passing into the hands of strangers, was degraded (as that ancestor would doubtless have considered it) to an ordinary farm-house; all this still tallying with the communications made.

It is perfectly idle, under the circumstances, to talk of fancy or fortuitous coincidence. Something other than imagination or accident, be it what it may, determined the minute specifications obtained from the apparitions in the Old Kent Manor-House.

The lesson taught by this story—if we admit the figures which presented themselves to the two ladies to have been, in verity, the apparitions of the Children family—is, that crime is not necessary to attract the spirits of the departed back to earth; that a frame of mind of an exclusively worldly cast—a character that never bestowed a thought upon any thing beyond this earth, and was troubled only by the cares of possession and the thoughts of gain—may equally draw down the spirit, though freed from the body, to gather cumber and sorrow amid the scenes of its former care. If this be so, how strong the motive not to suffer the present and the temporal, necessary and proper in their places as they are, so completely to engross us as to usurp the place, and wholly to exclude the thoughts, of the future and the spiritual!

I presume not to anticipate the judgment which the reader may pass on the evidence here submitted to him. If his decision be, that there is not, in any of the preceding examples, proof that an objective reality, be its nature what it may, was presented to the senses of the observers, then he would do well to consider whether the rule of evidence according to which he may have reached that decision, if applied to history, sacred and profane, would not sweep off nine-tenths, and more, of all we have been accustomed to trust to as foundation for historical deduction and religious belief.

If, on the other hand, adopting in this investigation the same rules in scanning testimony by which we are governed, day by day, in ordinary life, the reader should decide that something other than hallucination must be conceded, and that the senses of some of these observers *did* receive actual impressions produced by an external reality, the question remains, of what precise character that reality is.

Daniel De Foe has an elaborate work on this subject, illustrated by many examples; of which some, it must be confessed, exhibit more of that inimitable talent which makes Robinson Crusoe one of the most vivid realities of childhood, than of that more prosaic precision which scorns not names and dates and authenticating vouchers.

De Foe's opinion is, "The inquiry is not, as I take it, whether the inhabitants of the invisible spaces do really come hither or no, but who they are who do come?"*

From the "meanness of some of the occasions on which some of these things happen," he argues that it cannot be angels, properly so called, such as appeared to Gideon or to David. "Here," says he, "you have an old woman dead, that has hid a little money in the orchard or garden; and an apparition, it is supposed, comes and discovers it, by leading the person it appears to, to the place, and making some signal that he should dig there for somewhat. Or, a man is dead, and, having left a legacy to such or such, the executor does not pay it, and an apparition comes and haunts this executor till he does justice. Is it likely an angel should be sent from heaven to find out the old woman's earthen dish with thirty or forty shillings in it, or that an angel should be sent to harass this man for a legacy of five or ten pounds? And as to the devil, will any one charge Satan with being solicitous to see justice done? They that know him at all must know him better than to think so hardly of him." (p. 34.)

Nor can it, he argues, be the soul or ghost of the departed person; "for if the soul is happy, is it reason-

---

* "*Universal History of Apparitions*," by Andrew Moreton, Esq., 3d ed., London, 1738, p. 2. De Foe's biographers acknowledge for him the authorship of this work. The first edition appeared in 1727.

able to believe that the felicity of heaven can be interrupted by so trivial a matter and on so slight an occasion? if the soul be unhappy, remember the great gulf fixed : there is no reason to believe these unhappy souls have leisure or liberty to come back upon earth on errands of such a nature."

The idea of Hades, or a mediate state, evidently did not enter into De Foe's mind; and thus he found himself in a dilemma. "There is nothing," says he, "but difficulty in it on every side. Apparitions there are : we see no room to doubt the reality of that part; but what, who, or from whence, is a difficulty which I see no way to extricate ourselves from but by granting that there may be an appointed, deputed sort of stationary Spirits in the invisible world, who come upon these occasions and appear among us; which inhabitants or spirits, (you may call them angels, if you please,—bodies they are not and cannot be, neither had they been ever embodied,) but such as they are, they have a power of conversing among us, and can, by dreams, impulses, and strong aversions, move our thoughts, and give hope, raise doubts, sink our souls to-day, elevate them to-morrow, and in many ways operate on our passions and affections."*

Again he says, "The spirits I speak of must be heaven-born: they do Heaven's work, and are honored by his special commission; they are employed in his immediate business : namely, the common good of his creature, man."†

If there be no mediate state which the spirit enters at death, and whence it may occasionally return, then De Foe's hypothesis may be as good as any other. But if we admit a Sheol or Hades, and thus do away with all difficulty about disturbing the ecstatic felicity of

* "Universal History of Apparitions," p. 35. † Work cited, p. 52.

heaven or escaping across the gulf from the fast-binding chains of hell, why should we turn aside from a plain path, and seek to evade a straightforward inference, that, if God really does permit apparitions, these may be what they allege they are? Why should we gratuitously create, for the nonce, a nondescript species of spirits, not men, though a little lower than the angels; protectors, who simulate; guardians who lie; ministering spirits commissioned by God, who cheat men by assuming false forms,—to one appearing as an aunt, to another as a grandmother, now personating a murderer and imploring prayer, now playing the part of the murdered and soliciting pity? Is this God's work? Are these fitting credentials of heavenly birth, plausible evidences of Divine commission?

The question remains as to the existence of a mediate state, whence human spirits that have suffered the Great Change may be supposed to have the occasional power of returning. Before touching upon it, I pause, to add a few examples of what seem visitings from that unknown sphere; interferences, of which some assume the aspect of retribution, some of guardianship, all being of a peculiarly personal character.

BOOK V.

INDICATIONS OF PERSONAL INTERFERENCES.

CHAPTER I.

RETRIBUTION.

EVER since the days of Orestes, the idea of a spiritual agency, retributive and inevitable, has prevailed, in some shape, throughout the world. If we do not now believe in serpent-haired furies, the ministers of Divine vengeance, pursuing, with their whips of scorpions, the doomed criminal, we speak currently of the judgments of God, as evinced in some swift and sudden punishment overtaking, as if by the direct mandate of Heaven, the impenitent guilty.

On the other hand, Christianity sanctions, in a general way, the idea of spiritual care exerted to guide human steps and preserve from unforeseen danger. Protestantism does not, indeed, admit as sound the doctrine of patron saints, to whom prayers may properly be addressed and from whom aid may reasonably be expected. Yet we must deny not only the authority of St. Paul, but, it would seem, that of his Master also, if we reject the theory of spirits, protective and guardian, guiding the inexperience of infancy and ministering at least to a favored portion of mankind.*

Among modern records of alleged ultramundane influences we come upon indications which favor, to a certain

---

* Matthew xviii. 10; Hebrews i. 14.

extent, both ideas; that of requital for evil done, and that of guardian care exerted for the good of man. The latter is more frequent and more distinctly marked than the former. There is nothing giving color to the idea of permission to inflict serious injury, still less to the notion of implacable vengeance.* The power against the evil-doer seems to be of a very limited nature, reaching no further than annoyance, of petty effect unless conscience give sting to the infliction. On the other hand, the power to guide and protect appears to be not only more common, but more influential; with its limits, however, such as a wise parent might set to the free agency of a child. If warnings are given, it is rather in the form of dim hints or vague reminders than of distinct prophecy. If rules of action are suggested, they are of a general character, not relieving the spiritual ward from the duty of forethought and the task of self-decision, nor yet releasing him from the employment of that reason without the constant exercise of which he would speedily be degraded from his present position at the head of animal nature.

The modern examples to which I have referred are more or less definite in their character.

Among the narratives, for instance, appearing to involve retributive agency, Dr. Binns vouches for one admitting of various interpretation. He records it as "a remarkable instance of retributive justice which occurred very recently in Jamaica." The story is as follows:—

"A young and beautiful quadroon girl, named Duncan, was found murdered in a retired spot, a few paces from the main road. From the evidence given on the coro-

---

* The Grecians themselves do not represent the Furies as implacable. These were held to be open—as their name of Eumenides implies—to benevolent and merciful impulses, and might, by proper means, be propitiated.

ner's inquest, it was satisfactorily established that she had been violated previous to the murder. A large reward was offered for any information that might lead to the apprehension of the murderer; but nearly a year elapsed without any clew whatever being obtained. It happened that, about this period from the discovery of the murder, two black men, named Pendril and Chitty, were confined for separate petty offenses; one in the Kingston penitentiary, on the south, the other in Falmouth gaol, on the north, side of the island. Their imprisonment was unknown to each other, and the distance between their places of incarceration was eighty miles. Each of these men became restless and talkative in his sleep, repeatedly expostulating as if in the presence of the murdered girl, and entreating her to leave him. This happened so frequently that it led to inquiries, which terminated in the conviction of the two men."*

This case may be regarded either as an example of accidentally synchronous dreams, or else of an apparition presenting itself simultaneously, or nearly so, to the sleeping senses of two men at a distance from each other.

The former is a supposable explanation. Conscience may be conceived likely to dog the thoughts of men guilty of such an infamy. But that to both, distant and disconnected from each other, and after a year had passed, its retributive reminders should assume the selfsame shape at the very same time, by mere chance, is a contingency possible, indeed, but of very improbable occurrence.

And why should it be considered unlikely that some agency other than chance was here at work? We know that warnings have been given in dreams: why should dreams not embody requitals also?

* "*Anatomy of Sleep,*" by Edward Binns, M.D., 2d ed., London, 1845, p. 152.

But, since the above case presents two possible phases, let us pass to another, of less equivocal character.

WHAT A FRENCH ACTRESS SUFFERED.

Mademoiselle Claire-Josèphe Clairon was the great French tragedian of the last century. She occupied, in her day, a position similar to that which Rachel has recently filled. Marmontel was one of her warmest eulogists; and her talents were celebrated in the verses of Voltaire.

Her beauty, her grace, and her genius won for her many enthusiastic admirers; some professing friendship, others offering love. Among the latter, in the year 1743, was a young man, Monsieur de S——, son of a merchant of Brittany, whose attachment appears to have been of the most devoted kind.

The circumstances connected with this young man's death, and the events which succeeded it, are of an extraordinary character; but they come to us from first hand, and remarkably well authenticated, being detailed by Mademoiselle Clairon herself, in her autobiography, from which I translate the essential part of the narrative, as follows :—

"The language and manners of Monsieur de S—— gave evidence of an excellent education and of the habit of good society. His reserve, his timidity, which deterred all advances except by little attentions and by the language of the eyes, caused me to distinguish him from others. After having met him frequently in society, I at last permitted him to visit me at my own house, and did not conceal from him the friendship with which he inspired me. Seeing me at liberty, and well inclined toward him, he was content to be patient; hoping that time might create in me a warmer sentiment. I could not tell—who can?—how it would result. But, when he came to reply candidly to the questions which my

reason and curiosity prompted, he himself destroyed the
chance he might have had. Ashamed of being a com-
moner only, he had converted his property into ready
funds, and had come to Paris to spend his money, aping
a rank above his own. This displeased me. He who
blushes for himself causes others to despise him. Besides this, his temperament was melancholy and misanthropic: he knew mankind too well, he said, not to
contemn and to avoid them. His project was to see no
one but myself, and to carry me off where I should see
only him. That, as may be supposed, did not suit me
at all. I was willing to be guided by a flowery band,
but not to be fettered with chains. From that moment,
I saw the necessity of destroying entirely the hopes he
nourished, and of changing his assiduities of every day
to occasional visits, few and far between. This caused
him a severe illness, during which I nursed him with
every possible care. But my constant refusals aggravated the case; and, unfortunately for the poor fellow,
his brother-in-law, to whom he had intrusted the care
of his funds, failed to make remittances, so that he was
fain to accept the scanty supply of spare cash I had, to
furnish him with food and medical assistance." . . .
"Finally he recovered his property, but not his health;
and, desiring for his own sake to keep him at a distance
from me, I steadily refused both his letters and his visits.

"Two years and a half elapsed between the time of
our first acquaintance and his death. He sent, in his
last moments, to beg that I would grant him the happiness of seeing me once more; but my friends hindered
me from doing so. He died, having no one near him
but his servants and an old lady, who for some time
had been his only society. His apartments were then
on the Rempart, near the Chaussée d'Antin; mine, in
the Rue de Bassy, near the monastery of Saint-Germain.

"That evening my mother and several other friends

were supping with me,—among them, the Intendant of the Menus-Plaisirs, whose professional aid I constantly required, that excellent fellow Pipelet, and Rosely, a comrade of mine and a young man of good family, witty and talented. The supper was gay. I had just been singing to them, and they applauding me, when, as eleven o'clock struck, a piercing cry was heard. Its heart-rending tone and the length of time it continued struck every one with astonishment. I fainted, and remained for a quarter of an hour totally unconscious."

. . . "When I recovered, I begged them to remain with me part of the night. We reasoned much in regard to this strange cry; and it was agreed to have spies set in the street, so that, in case of its repetition, we might detect its cause and its author.

"Every succeeding night, always at the same hour, the same cry was repeated, sounding immediately beneath my windows, and appearing to issue from the vacant air. My people, my guests, my neighbors, the police, all heard it alike. I could not doubt that it was intended for me. I seldom supped from home, but when I did, nothing was heard there; and several times, when I returned later than eleven, and inquired of my mother, or the servants, if any thing had been heard of it, suddenly it burst forth in the midst of us.

"One evening the President de B——, with whom I had been supping, escorted me home, and, at the moment he bade me good-night at the door of my apartment, the cry exploded between him and myself. He was quite familiar with the story, for all Paris knew it; yet he was carried to his carriage more dead than alive.

"Another day, I begged my comrade, Rosely, to accompany me, first to the Rue Saint-Honoré, to make some purchases, afterward to visit my friend Mademoiselle de Saint-P——, who resided near the Porte Saint-Denis. Our sole topic of conversation all the way was my ghost, as I used to call it. The young man, witty and unbelieving, begged me to evoke the phantom, promising to believe in it if it replied. Whether from weakness or audacity, I acceded to his request. Thrice, on the instant, the cry sounded, rapid and terrible in its repetition. When we arrived at my friend's house, Rosely and I had to be carried in. We were both found lying senseless in the carriage.

"After this scene, I remained several months without hearing any thing more; and I began to hope that the disturbance had ceased. I was mistaken.

"The theater had been ordered to Versailles, on occasion of the marriage of the Dauphin. We were to remain there three days. We were insufficiently provided with apartments. Madame Grandval had none. We waited half the night in hopes that one would be assigned to her. At three o'clock in the morning I offered her one of the two beds in my room, which was in the Avenue de Saint-Cloud. She accepted it. I occupied the other bed; and as my maid was undressing, to sleep beside me, I said to her, 'Here we are at the end of the world, and with such frightful weather! I think it would puzzle the ghost to find us out here.' The same cry, on the instant! Madame Grandval thought that hell itself was let loose in the room. In her night-dress she rushed down-stairs, from the top to the bottom. Not a soul in the house slept another wink that night. This was, however, the last time I ever heard it.

"Seven or eight days afterward, while chatting with my ordinary circle of friends, the stroke of eleven o'clock was followed by a musket-shot, as if fired at one of my windows. Every one of us heard the report; every one of us saw the flash; but the window had received no injury. We concluded that it was an attempt on my life, that for this time it had failed, but that precautions must be taken for the future. The Intendant hastened to M. de Marville, then Lieutenant of Police, and a personal friend of his. Officers were instantly sent to examine the houses opposite mine. Throughout the following days they were guarded from top to bottom. My own house, also, was thoroughly examined. The street was filled with spies. But, in spite of all these precautions, for three entire months, every evening, at the same hour, the same musket-shot, directed against the same pane of glass, was heard to explode, was seen; and yet no one was ever able to discover whence it proceeded. This fact is attested by its official record on the registers of the police.

"I gradually became in a measure accustomed to my ghost, whom I began to consider a good sort of fellow, since he was content with tricks that produced no serious injury; and, one warm evening, not noticing the hour, the Intendant and myself, having opened the haunted window, were leaning over the balcony. Eleven o'clock struck; the detonation instantly succeeded; and it threw both of us, half-dead, into the middle of the room. When we recovered, and found that neither of us was hurt, we began to compare notes; and each admitted to the other the having received, he on the left cheek and I on the right, a box on the ear, right sharply laid on. We both burst out laughing.

"Next day nothing happened. The day after, having received an invitation from Mademoiselle Dumesnil to attend a nocturnal fête at her house, near the Barrière Blanche, I got into a hackney-coach, with my maid, at eleven o'clock. It was bright moonlight; and our road was along the Boulevards, which were then beginning to be built up. We were looking out at the houses they were building, when my maid said to me, 'Was it not somewhere near here that Monsieur de S—— died?' 'From what they told me,' I replied, 'it must have been in one of these two houses in front of us,'—pointing to them at the same time. At that moment the same musket-shot that had been pursuing me was fired from one of the houses, and passed through our carriage.* The coachman set off at full gallop, thinking he was attacked by robbers; and we, when we arrived at our destination, had scarcely recovered our senses. For my own part, I confess to a degree of terror which it was long before I could shake off. But this exploit was the last of its kind. I never again heard any discharge of fire-arms.

"To these shots succeeded a clapping of hands, given in measured time and repeated at intervals. These sounds, to which the favor of the public had accustomed me, gave me but trifling annoyance, and I took little trouble to trace their origin. My friends did, however. 'We have watched in the most careful manner,' they would say to me: 'it is under your very door that the sounds occur. We hear them; but we see nobody. It is another phase of the same annoyances that have followed you so long.' As these noises had nothing alarming in them, I did not preserve a record of the period of their continuance.

"Nor did I take special note of the melodious sounds by which, after a time, they were succeeded. It seemed as if a celestial voice warbled the prelude to some noble air which it was about to execute. Once the voice commenced at the Carrefour de Bussy, and continued all the way until I reached my own door. In this case, as in all the preceding, my friends watched, followed the sounds, heard them as I did, but could never see any thing.

"Finally all the sounds ceased, after having continued,

---

* Whether a *ball* passed through the carriage does not clearly appear. The expression is, "D'une des maisons partit ce même coup de fusil qui me poursuivait; il traversa notre voiture."

with intermissions, a little more than two years and a half."

Whether the sequel may be regarded as supplying a sufficient explanation or not, it is proper to give it, as furnished by Mademoiselle Clairon.

That lady desiring to change her residence, and the apartments she occupied being advertised to rent, several persons called to see them. Among the rest there was announced a lady advanced in years. She exhibited much emotion, which communicated itself to Mademoiselle Clairon. At last she confessed that it was not to look at the apartments she came, but to converse with their occupant. She had thought of writing, she said, but had feared that her motives might be misinterpreted. Mademoiselle Clairon begged for an explanation; and the conversation which ensued is thus reported by herself.

"'I was, mademoiselle,' said the lady, 'the best friend of Monsieur de S——; indeed, the only one he was willing to see during the last year of his life. The hours, the days, of that year were spent by us in talking of you, sometimes setting you down as an angel, sometimes as a devil. As for me, I urged him constantly to endeavor to forget you, while he protested that he would continue to love you even beyond the tomb. You weep,' she continued, after a pause; 'and perhaps you will allow me to ask you why you made him so unhappy, and why, with your upright and affectionate character, you refused him, in his last moments, the consolation of seeing you once more.'

"'Our affections,' I replied, 'are not within our own control. Monsieur de S—— had many meritorious and estimable qualities; but his character was somber, misanthropic, despotic, so that he caused me to fear alike his society, his friendship, and his love. To make him happy, I should have had to renounce all human intercourse, even the talent I exercise. I was poor and proud. It has been my wish and my hope to accept no favor,—to owe every thing to my own exertions. The friendship I entertained for him caused me to try every means to bring him back to sentiments more calm and reasonable. Failing in this, and convinced that his obstinate resolve was due less to the extremity of his passion than to the violence of his character, I adopted, and adhered to, the resolution to separate from him forever. I refused to see him on his death-bed, because the sight of his distress would have made me miserable, to no good end. Besides, I might have been placed in the dilemma of refusing what he might ask me, with seeming barbarity, or acceding to it with certain prospect of future unhappiness. These, madame, were the motives which actuated me. I trust you will not consider them deserving of censure.'

" 'It would be unjust,' she replied, 'to condemn you. We can be reasonably called upon to make sacrifices only to fulfill our promises or in discharge of our duty to relatives or to benefactors. I know that you owed him no gratitude; he himself felt that all obligation was on his part; but the state of his mind and the passion which ruled him were beyond his control; and your refusal to see him hastened his last moments. He counted the minutes until half-past ten, when his servant returned with the message that most certainly you would not come. After a moment of silence, he took my hand, and, in a state of despair which terrified me, he exclaimed, " *Barbarous creature! But she shall gain nothing by it. I will pursue her as long after my death as she has pursued me during my life.*" . . . I tried to calm him. He was already a corpse.' "*

---

* " *Mémoires de Mademoiselle Clairon, Actrice du Théâtre Français, écrits par elle-même,*" 2d ed., Paris, 1822, pp. 78 to 96. The editors state that

This is the story as Mademoiselle Clairon herself relates it. She adds, " I need not say what effect these last words produced on me. The coincidence between them and the disturbances that had haunted me filled me with terror. . . . I do not know what chance really is; but I am very sure that what we are in the habit of calling so has a vast influence upon human affairs."

In the Memoirs of the Duchesse d'Abrantès, written by herself, and containing so many interesting particulars of the French Revolution and the stirring events which succeeded it, she states that, during the Consulate, when Mademoiselle Clairon was upward of seventy years of age, she (the duchess) made her acquaintance, and heard from her own lips the above story, of which she gives a brief and not very accurate compendium. In regard to the impression which Mademoiselle Clairon's mode of relating it produced on the duchess, that lady remarks,—

"I know not whether in all this there was a little exaggeration; but she who usually spoke in a tone savoring of exaltation, when she came to relate this incident, though she spoke with dignity, laid aside all affectation and every thing which could be construed into speaking for effect. Albert, who believed in magnetism, wished, after having heard Mademoiselle Clairon, to persuade me that the thing was possible. I laughed at him then. Alas! since that time I have myself learned a terrible lesson in credulity."[*]

I know not according to what sound principles of evidence we can refuse credit to a narrative so well authenticated as this. The phenomena were observed,

---

these Memoirs are published " without the change of a single word from the original manuscript."

[*] " *Mémoires de Madame la Duchesse d'Abrantès, écrits par elle-même,*" 2d ed., Paris, 1835, vol. ii. p. 39.

not by Mademoiselle Clairon only, but by numerous other witnesses, including the most sharp-eyed and suspicious of beings,—the police-officers of Paris. The record of them is still to be found in the archives of that police. They were not witnessed once, twice, fifty times only. They were observed throughout more than two entire years. The shot against a certain pane of her window was fired, so Mademoiselle Clairon expressly tells us, every night, at the same hour, for three months,—therefore ninety times in succession. What theory, what explanation, will account for a trick of such a character that could for so long a space of time escape the argus eyes of the French police? Then the cry at the moment when, at Rosely's suggestion, the phantom was evoked; the shot against the carriage from the house where Monsieur de S—— had resided: what imaginable trickery could be at the bottom of these?

The incidents occurred in Mademoiselle Clairon's youth; commencing when she was twenty-two years and a half old and terminating when she was twenty-five. Nearly fifty years afterward, toward the close of her life, in that period of calm reflection which comes with old age, she still preserved that deep conviction of the reality of these marvels which imparted to the tone and manner of her narrative the attesting simplicity of truth.

Finally, the coincidence to which Mademoiselle Clairon alludes is a double one; first as to the incidents themselves, then as to the period of their continuance. Monsieur de S——, with his dying breath, declared that he would haunt her; and this she knew not till the persecution, commencing within half an hour after his decease, was ended. He said, further, that she should be followed by his spirit for as long a period as she had held him enthralled. But from the period of his acquaintance with her till his death was two years and a half, while from this latter event till the close of the disturbances there elapsed, as the sufferer tells us, two years and a half more.

Yet even if we admit in this case the reality of ultra-mundane agency, I do not presume to assert, as a corollary positively proved, that it *was* the spirit of Monsieur de S—— which fulfilled the threat he had made. That is certainly the most natural explanation which suggests itself. And if it be not the true one, chance, at least, is insufficient to account for the exact manner in which the declaration of the dying man tallies with the sufferings of her who was the object of his unfortunate and unavailing love.

If we accept this narrative, it bears with it an additional lesson. Supposing the agency of the disturbances to be spiritual, we cannot regard it as commissioned from God, any more than we do the annoyances which a neighbor, taking unjust offense, may inflict, in this world, on his offending neighbor in retaliation. Mademoiselle Clairon's conduct seems to have been justifiable and prudent; certainly not meriting persecution or punishment.

Why, then, were these annoyances permitted? When we can tell why *earthly* annoyances are often allowed to overtake the innocent, it will be time enough to insist upon an answer to the spiritual question.

Natural phenomena occur under general laws, not by special dispensation. But the disturbances above recorded were doubtless natural phenomena.

We may imagine that every thing in the next world is governed by principles totally different from those which we see in operation here. But why should we imagine this? Does not the same Providence preside on the further as on the hither side of the Dark River?

An example somewhat more closely resembling punish-

ment really merited and expressly sent is the following,
—a narrative which I owe to the kindness of Mrs. S. C.
Hall, the author, and to the truth of which, as will be
seen, she bears personal testimony. But even in this
case can we rationally assert more than that the agency
was permitted, not commissioned?

I give the story in Mrs. Hall's own words. The circumstances occurred in London.

WHAT AN ENGLISH OFFICER SUFFERED.

"All young girls have friendships one with another;
and when I was seventeen my friend, above all others,
was Kate L——. She was a young Irish lady, my senior
by three years,—a gentle, affectionate, pretty creature,
much devoted to her old mother, and exercising constant
forbearance toward a disagreeable brother who would
persist in playing the flute, though he played both out
of time and tune. This brother was my *bête noire;* and
whenever I complained of his bad playing, Kate would
say, 'Ah, wait till Robert comes home; he plays and
sings like an angel, and is *so* handsome!'

"This 'Robert' had been with his regiment for some
years in Canada; and his coming home was to be *the*
happiness of mother and daughter. For three months
before his return nothing else was talked of. If I had
had any talent for falling in love, I should have done
so, in anticipation, with Robert L——; but *that* was
not my weakness; and I was much amused with my
friend's speculations as to whether Robert would fall in
love with me, or I with him, *first.*

"When we met, there was, happily, no danger to either.
He told Kate that her friend was always laughing; and
I thought I had never looked on a face so beautiful in
outline and yet so haggard and painful. His large blue
eyes were deeply set, but always seemed looking for
something they could not find. To look at *him* made

me uncomfortable. But this was not so strange as the change which, after a time, was evident in Kate. She had become, in less than a week, cold and constrained. I was to have spent a day with her; but she made some apology, and, in doing so, burst into tears. Something was evidently wrong, which I felt satisfied time must disclose.

"In about a week more she came to see me by myself, looking ten years older. She closed the door of my room, and then said she desired to tell me something which she felt I could hardly believe, but that, if I was not afraid, I might come and judge for myself.

"After Robert's return, she said, for a week or so they had been delightfully happy. But very soon— she thought about the tenth day, or rather night—they were alarmed by loud raps and knocks in Robert's room. It was the back room on the same floor on which Mrs. L—— and her daughter slept together in a large front bed-chamber. They heard him swearing at the noise, as if it had been at his servant; but the man did not sleep in the house. At last he threw his boots at it; and the more violent he became, the more violent seemed to grow the disturbance.

"At last his mother ventured to knock at his door and ask what was the matter. He told her to come in. She brought a lighted candle and set it on the table. As she entered, her son's favorite pointer rushed out of the room. 'So,' he said, 'the dog's gone! I have not been able to keep a dog in my room at night for years; but under your roof, mother, I fancied, I hoped, I might escape a persecution that I see now pursues me even here. I am sorry for Kate's canary-bird that hung behind the curtain. I heard it fluttering after the first round. Of course it is dead!'

"The old lady got up, all trembling, to look at poor

Kate's bird. It *was* dead, at the bottom of the cage,—all its feathers ruffled.

"'Is there no Bible in the room?' she inquired. 'Yes,'—he drew one from under his pillow: 'that, I think, protects me from blows.' He looked so dreadfully exhausted that his mother wished to leave the room, to get him some wine. 'No: stay here: do not leave me!' he entreated. Hardly had he ceased speaking, when some huge, heavy substance seemed rolling down the chimney and flopped on the hearth; but Mrs. L—— saw nothing. The next moment, as from a strong wind, the light was extinguished, while knocks and raps and a rushing sound passed round the apartment. Robert L—— alternately prayed and swore; and the old lady, usually remarkable for her self-possession, had great difficulty in preventing herself from fainting. The noise continued, sometimes seeming like violent *thumps*, sometimes the sounds appearing to *trickle* around the room.

"At last her other son, roused by the disturbance, came in, and found his mother on her knees, praying.

"That night she slept in her son's room, or rather attempted to do so; for sleep was impossible, though her bed was not touched or shaken. Kate remained outside the open door. It was impossible to see, because, immediately after the first plunge down the chimney, the lights were extinguished.

"The next morning, Robert told his family that for more than ten years he had been the victim of this spirit-persecution. If he lay in his tent, it was there, disturbing his brother officers, who gradually shunned the society of 'the haunted man,' as they called him,—one who 'must have done something to draw down such punishment.' When on leave of absence, he was generally free from the visitation for three or four nights; then it found him out again. He never was suffered to remain in a lodging; being regularly 'warned out' by the house-holders, who would not endure the noise.

"After breakfast, the next-door neighbors sent in to complain of the noises of the preceding night. On the succeeding nights, several friends (two or three of whom I knew) sat up with Mrs. L——, and sought to investi-gate, according to human means, the cause. In vain! They verified the fact; the cause remained hidden in mystery.

"Kate wished me to hear for myself; but I had not courage to do so, nor would my dear mother have per-mitted it.

"No inducement could prevail on the pointer to return to his master's room, by day or night. He was a recent purchase, and, until the first noise in London came, had appreciated Robert's kindness. After that, he evidently disliked his master. 'It is the old story over again,' said Robert. 'I could never keep a dog. I thought I would try again; but I shall never have any thing to love, and nothing will ever be permitted to love me.' The animal soon after got out; and they supposed it ran away, or was stolen.

"The young man, seeing his mother and sister fading away under anxiety and want of rest, told them he could bear his affliction better by himself, and would therefore go to Ireland, his native country, and reside in some detached country cottage, where he could fish and shoot.

"He went. Before his departure I once heard the poor fellow say, 'It is hard to be so punished; but per-haps I have deserved it.'

"I learned, afterward, that there was more than a suspicion that he had abandoned an unfortunate girl who

'Loved not wisely, but too well;'

and that she died in America. Be this as it may, in Ireland, as elsewhere, the visitation followed him unceasingly.

"This spirit never spoke, never answered questions: and the mode of communicating now so general was not then known. If it had been, there might have been a different result.

"As it was, Robert L———'s mode of life in his native country gave his mother great anxiety. I had no clew, however, to his ultimate fate; for his sister would not tell me where in Ireland he had made his miserable home.

"My friend Kate married immediately after her brother left. She was a bride, a mother, and a corpse within a year; and her death really broke her mother's heart: so that in two years the family seemed to have vanished, as if I had never known them. I have sometimes thought, however, that if the dear old lady had not received such a shock from her son's spiritual visitor, she would not have been crushed by the loss of her daughter; but she told me she had nothing left to bind her to this world.

"I have often regretted that I had not watched with my young friend one night; but the facts I have thrown together were known to certainly twenty persons in London."*

One rarely finds a narrative better authenticated, or more strongly indicating the reality of an ultramundane agency, than this. It is attested by the name of a lady well and favorably known to the literary world. It is true that, deterred by her fears, she did not personally witness the disturbances. But if she had, would it have added materially to the weight of her testimony as it stands? Could she doubt the reality of these appalling

---

* Extracted from Mrs. Hall's letter to me, dated London, March 31, 1859

demonstrations? Can we doubt it? The testimony of
the sister and the mother, whose lives this fearful visitation darkened if it did not shorten, to say nothing
of the corroborative evidence furnished by friends who
sat up with them expressly to seek out some explanation,—can we refuse credit to all this? The haggard
and careworn looks of the sufferer, his blighted life,—
could these have been simulated? The confession to his
family, wrung from him by the recurrence, in his mother's
house, of the torment he could no longer conceal,—could
that be a lie? Dumb animals attested the contrary.
The death of the canary-bird, the terror of the dog,—
could fancy cause the one or create the other? Or shall
we resort to the hypothesis of human agency? Ten
years had the avenging sounds pursued the unfortunate
man. In tent or tavern, in country or city, go where
he would, the terrible Intrusion still dogged his steps.
The maternal home was no city of refuge from the pur-
suer. To the wilds of Ireland it followed the culprit
in his retreat. Even if such human vengeance were
conceivable, would not human ingenuity be powerless to
carry it out?

But, if we concede the reality and the spiritual character of the demonstration, are we to admit also the
explanation hypothetically suggested by the narrator?
Was Robert L—— really thus punished, through life,
for one of the worst, because one of the most selfish and
heartless and misery-bringing, in the list of human sins?
He himself seemed to be of that opinion: "Perhaps I
have deserved it" was the verdict of his conscience. It
may be rash, with our present limited knowledge of
ultramundane laws, to assert any thing in the premises; knowing as we do that tens of thousands of
such offenders pass through life unwhipped of justice.*

---

* It does not by any means follow, however, that because many similar
offenders escape unpunished, there was nothing retributive in the incidents

Yet, if we reject that hypothesis, what other, more plausible, remains?

Even if we accept that explanation, however, it is not to be assumed, as of course, that it was the spirit of his poor victim that thus ceaselessly followed her deserter, the betrayer of her trust. Love may be changed, for a time, into vehement dislike: it is difficult to believe that, after the earthly tenement is gone, it should harden into hate eternal and unrelenting. And we can conceive that some other departed spirit, of evil nature, obtaining power over the wretched man by the aid of an impressible temperament wrought upon by a conscience haunted by remorse, might have been permitted (who can tell under what law or for what purpose?) to visit, with such retribution, the evil deed.

But here we enter the regions of conjecture. These events happened long before Spiritualism had become a distinctive name. No attempt was made to communicate with the sounds. No explanation, therefore, trustworthy or apocryphal, was reached. There was no chance, then, given to conciliate; no opportunity afforded for propitiation.

It has been alleged that, in many modern instances of what had assumed the character of spiritual interference, the disturbance ceased when communication, by knockings, was sought and obtained. So it might have been, as Mrs. Hall suggests, in the case of Robert L——. And, if so, the spirit-rap, lightly esteemed by many as it is, might have brought to repentance and saved from hopeless suffering—possibly premature death—a young man with heavy guilt, indeed, upon his soul, yet not a sinner above all men that dwelt in London.

---

here related. In this mysteriously-governed world some criminals escape, while others, less guilty perhaps, are overtaken. "Those eighteen upon whom the tower in Siloam fell, and slew them, think ye that they were sinners above all men that dwelt in Jerusalem?"—Luke xiii. 4.

CHAPTER II.

GUARDIANSHIP.

A PLEASANTER task remains; to speak, namely, of the indications that reach us of ultramundane aid and spiritual protection.

Three stories have come to my knowledge, in each of which the subject of the narrative is alleged to have been saved from death by an apparition seeming to be the counterpart of himself: one related of an English clergyman, traveling, late at night, in a lonely lane, by whose side the figure suddenly appeared, and thus (as the clergyman afterward ascertained) deterred two men, bent on murder and robbery, from attacking him; and both the others—the one occurring to a student in Edinburgh, the other to a fashionable young man in Berlin—being examples in which the seer is said to have been warned from occupying his usual chamber, which had he occupied, he would have perished by the falling in of a portion of the house.

But these anecdotes, though for each there is plausible evidence, do not come within the rule I have laid down to myself of sufficient authentication.

A somewhat similar story is related and vouched for by Jung Stilling, of a certain Professor Böhm, of Marburg, in whose case, however, the warning came by an urgent presentiment only, not by an actual apparition.*

Such a case of presentiment, though the danger was to another, not to the subject of it, came to me, through the kindness of a lady, at first hand, as follows:—

---

* *"Theorie der Geisterkunde."*

HOW SENATOR LINN'S LIFE WAS SAVED.

Those who were familiar with the political history of our country twenty years ago remember well Dr. Linn, of Missouri. Distinguished for talents and professional ability, but yet more for the excellence of his heart, he received, by a distinction as rare as it was honorable, the unanimous vote of the Legislature for the office of Senator of the United States.

In discharge of his Congressional duties, he was residing with his family in Washington, during the spring and summer of 1840, the last year of Mr. Van Buren's administration.

One day during the month of May of that year, Dr. and Mrs. Linn received an invitation to a large and formal dinner-party, given by a public functionary, and to which the most prominent members of the Administration party, including the President himself and our present Chief Magistrate, Mr. Buchanan, were invited guests. Dr. Linn was very anxious to be present; but, when the day came, finding himself suffering from an attack of indigestion, he begged his wife to bear his apology in person, and make one of the dinner-party, leaving him at home. To this she somewhat reluctantly consented. She was accompanied to the door of their host by a friend, General Jones, who promised to return and remain with Dr. Linn during the evening.

At table Mrs. Linn sat next to General Macomb, who had conducted her to dinner; and immediately opposite to her sat Silas Wright, Senator from New York, the most intimate friend of her husband, and a man by whose death, shortly after, the country sustained an irreparable loss.

Even during the early part of the dinner, Mrs. Linn felt very uneasy about her husband. She tried to reason herself out of this, as she knew that his indisposition

was not at all serious; but in vain. She mentioned her
uneasiness to General Macomb; but he reminded her of
what she herself had previously told him,—that General
Jones had promised to remain with Dr. Linn, and that,
in the very unlikely contingency of any sudden illness,
he would be sure to apprize her of it.   Notwithstanding
these representations, as dinner drew toward a close
this unaccountable uneasiness increased to such an uncontrollable impulse to return home, that, as she expressed
it to me, she felt that she *could* not sit there a moment
longer.   Her sudden pallor was noticed by Senator
Wright, and excited his alarm.   "I am sure you are ill,
Mrs. Linn," he said: "what is the matter?"   She replied that she was quite well, but that she *must* return
to her husband.   Mr. Wright sought, as General Macomb
had done, to calm her fears; but she replied to him, "If
you wish to do me a favor for which I shall be grateful
while I live, make some excuse to our host, so that we
can leave the table."   Seeing her so greatly excited, he
complied with her request, though they were then but
serving the dessert; and he and Mrs. Wright accompanied Mrs. Linn home.

As they were taking leave of her at the door of her
lodgings, Senator Wright said, "I shall call to-morrow
morning, and have a good laugh with the doctor and
yourself over your panic apprehensions."

As Mrs. Linn passed hastily up-stairs, she met the
landlady. "How is Dr. Linn?" she anxiously asked.
"Very well, I believe," was the reply: "he took a bath
more than an hour ago, and I dare say is sound asleep
by this time.   General Jones said he was doing extremely
well."

"The general is with him, is he not?"

"I believe not.   I think I saw him pass out about
half an hour ago."

In a measure reassured, Mrs. Linn hastened to her

husband's bed-chamber, the door of which was closed. As she opened it, a dense smoke burst upon her, in such stifling quantity that she staggered and fell on the threshold. Recovering herself after a few seconds, she rushed into the room. The bolster was on fire, and the feathers burned with a bright glow and a suffocating odor. She threw herself upon the bed; but the fire, half smothered till that moment, was fanned by the draught from the opened door, and, kindling into sudden flame, caught her light dress, which was in a blaze on the instant. At the same moment her eye fell on the large bath-tub that had been used by her husband. She sprang into it, extinguishing her burning dress; then, returning to the bed, she caught up the pillow and a sheet that was on fire, scorching her arms in so doing, and plunged both into the water. Finally, exerting her utmost strength, she drew from the bed her insensible husband. It was then only that she called to the people of the house for aid.

Dr. Sewell was instantly summoned. But it was full half an hour before the sufferer gave any signs whatever of returning animation. He did not leave his bed for nearly a week; and it was three months before he entirely recovered from the effects of this accident.

"How fortunate it was," said Dr. Sewell to Mrs. Linn, "that you arrived at the very moment you did! Five minutes more,—nay, three minutes,—and, in all human probability, you would have never seen your husband alive again."

Mr. Wright called, as he promised, the next morning. "Well, Mrs. Linn," said he, smiling, "you have found out by this time how foolish that strange presentiment of yours was."

"Come up-stairs," she replied. And she led him to his friend, scarcely yet able to speak; and then she showed him the remains of the half-consumed bolster and partially-burned bed-linen.

Whether the sight changed his opinion on the subject of presentiments I cannot tell; but he turned pale as a corpse, (Mrs. Linn said,) and did not utter a word.

I had all the above particulars from Mrs. Linn herself,* together with the permission to publish them in illustration of the subject I am treating, attested by date and names.

There is one point in connection with the above narrative which is worthy of special examination. In case we admit that Mrs. Linn's irresistible impulse to leave the dinner-table was a spiritual impression, the question remains, was it a warning of evil then existing, or was it a presentiment of evil that was still to arise? In other words, was it in its character only clairvoyant, or was it in its nature clearly prophetic?

The impression was distinctly produced on Mrs. Linn's mind, as that lady told me, at least half an hour before it became so urgent as to compel her to leave the entertainment. When she did leave, as the carriages were not ordered till eleven o'clock, and no hackney-coach was at hand, she and Mr. and Mrs. Wright, as she further stated to me, returned on foot. The distance being a mile and a half, they were fully half an hour in walking it. It follows that Mrs. Linn was impressed to return more than an hour before she opened the door of the bedroom.

Now, it is highly improbable that the fire should have caught, or that any thing should have happened likely to lead to it, in the bedroom as much as an hour, or even half an hour, before Mrs. Linn's arrival. But if not,—if, at the moment Mrs. Linn was first impressed, no condition of things existed which, to human percep-

* In Washington, on the 4th of July, 1859.

tions, could indicate danger,—then, unless we refer the whole to chance coincidence, the case is one involving not only a warning presentiment, but a prophetic instinct.

More distinct still, as an example of what seems protective agency, is the following from a recent work by the Rev. Dr. Bushnell.

HELP AMID THE SNOW-DRIFTS.

"As I sat by the fire, one stormy November night, in a hotel-parlor, in the Napa Valley of California, there came in a most venerable and benignant-looking person, with his wife, taking their seats in the circle. The stranger, as I afterward learned, was Captain Yount, a man who came over into California, as a trapper, more than forty years ago. Here he has lived, apart from the great world and its questions, acquiring an immense landed estate, and becoming a kind of acknowledged patriarch in the country. His tall, manly person, and his gracious, paternal look, as totally unsophisticated in the expression as if he had never heard of a philosophic doubt or question in his life, marked him as the true patriarch. The conversation turned, I know not how, on spiritism and the modern necromancy; and he discovered a degree of inclination to believe in the reported mysteries. His wife, a much younger and apparently Christian person, intimated that probably he was predisposed to this kind of faith by a very peculiar experience of his own, and evidently desired that he might be drawn out by some intelligent discussion of his queries.

"At my request, he gave me his story. About six or seven years previous, in a mid-winter's night, he had a dream in which he saw what appeared to be a company of emigrants arrested by the snows of the mountains and perishing rapidly by cold and hunger. He noted the very cast of the scenery, marked by a huge perpendicular front of white rock cliff; he saw the men cutting off what appeared to be tree-tops rising out of deep gulfs of snow; he distinguished the very features of the persons and the look of their particular distress. He woke profoundly impressed with the distinctness and apparent reality of his dream. At length he fell asleep and dreamed exactly the same dream again. In the morning he could not expel it from his mind. Falling in, shortly, with an old hunter comrade, he told him the story, and was only the more deeply impressed by his recognizing, without hesitation, the scenery of the dream. This comrade had come over the Sierra by the Carson Valley Pass, and declared that a spot in the pass answered exactly to his description. By this the unsophisticated patriarch was decided. He immediately collected a company of men with mules and blankets and all necessary provisions. The neighbors were laughing, meantime, at his credulity. 'No matter,' said he: 'I am able to do this, and I will; for I verily believe that the fact is according to my dream.' The men were sent into the mountains, one hundred and fifty miles distant, directly to the Carson Valley Pass. And there they found the company in exactly the condition of the dream, and brought in the remnant alive."*

Dr. Bushnell adds, that a gentleman present said to him, "You need have no doubt of this; for we Californians all know the facts and the names of the families brought in, who now look upon our venerable friend as a kind of Savior." These names he gave, together with the residences of each; and Dr. Bushnell avers that he found the Californians everywhere ready to second the old man's testimony. "Nothing could be more natural,"

---

* "Nature and the Supernatural," by Horace Bushnell, New York, 1858, pp. 475. 476. George C. Yount was the trapper's name.

continues the doctor, "than for the good-hearted patriarch himself to add that the brightest thing in his life,
and that which gave him the greatest joy, was his simple
faith in that dream."

Here is a fact known and acknowledged by a whole
community. That it actually occurred is beyond cavil.
But how could it occur by chance? In the illimitable
wintry wilderness, with its hundred passes and its thousand emigrants, how can a purely accidental fancy be
supposed, without ultramundane interference, to shape
into the semblance of reality a scene actually existing
a hundred and fifty miles off, though wholly unknown
to the dreamer,—not the landscape only, with its white
cliffs and its snow-buried trees, but the starving travelers cutting the tree-tops in a vain effort to avert cold
and famine? He who credits this believes a marvel far
greater than the hypothesis of spiritual guardianship.

In support of that hypothesis, however, there are
well-attested narratives, indicating, more directly than
this story of the Californian trapper, loving care on the
part of the departed. One of these will be found in a
work on the supernatural by the Rev. Dr. Edwards. He
communicates it in the shape of an "extract of a letter
from an enlightened and learned divine in the north of
Germany." The incident occurred, he tells us, at Levin,
a village belonging to the Duchy of Mecklenburg, not
far from Demmin, in Prussian Pomerania, on the Sunday before Michaelmas, in the year 1759. The extract
referred to (the title only added by me) is as follows:—

UNEXPECTED CONSOLATION.

"I will now, in conclusion, mention to you a very
edifying story of an apparition, for the truth of which
I can vouch, with all that is dear to me. My late
mother, a pattern of true piety, and a woman who

was regular in prayer, lost, quite unexpectedly
after a short illness, arising from a sore throat, my
younger sister, a girl of about fourteen years of age.
Now, as during her illness she had not spoken much
with her on spiritual subjects, by no means supposing
her end so near, (although my father had done so,) she
reproached and grieved herself most profoundly, not
only on this account, but also for not having sufficiently
nursed and attended upon her, or for having neglected
something that might have brought on her death. This
feeling took so much hold of her, that she not only
altered much in her appearance, from loss of appetite,
but became so monosyllabic in speaking that she never
expressed herself except on being interrogated. She
still, however, continued to pray diligently in her chamber. Being already grown up at the time, I spoke with
my father respecting her, and asked him what was to
be done, and how my good mother might be comforted.
He shrugged his shoulders, and gave me to understand
that, unless God interposed, he feared the worst.

Now, it happened, some days after, when we were all,
one Sunday morning, at church, with the exception of
my mother, who remained at home, that on rising up
from prayer, in her closet, she heard a noise as though
some one was with her in the room. On looking about
to ascertain whence the noise proceeded, something
took hold of her invisibly and pressed her firmly to it,
as if she had been embraced by some one, and the same
moment she heard,—without seeing any thing whatever,
—very distinctly, the voice of her departed daughter,
saying quite plainly to her, '*Mamma! mamma! I am
so happy! I am so happy!*' Immediately after these
words, the pressure subsided, and my mother felt and
heard nothing more. But what a wished-for change
did we all perceive in our dear mother on coming home!
She had regained her speech and former cheerfulness;

she ate and drank, and rejoiced with us at the mercy which the Lord had bestowed upon her; nor during her whole life did she even notice again, with grief, the great loss which she had suffered by the decease of this excellent daughter."*

That this was a case of hallucination of two senses, hearing and feeling, can be considered probable only if no unequivocal examples of similar agency can be found. And if, to some persons, speech by an inhabitant of another world, audible upon earth, seem an impossible phenomenon, let them read the following, communicated to me by a gentleman to whose lady, as our readers have seen, I am already indebted for one of the most striking narratives in connection with personal interferences.

GASPAR.

"At Worcester, a few weeks since, I accidentally met, at the house of a banker in that city, a lady whom I had not previously known; and from her lips I heard a story of a character so extraordinary that no commonplace voucher for the veracity of the narrator would suffice, in the eyes of most people, to establish its authenticity.

"Nor was it an ordinary testimonial which, on applying to our host, he furnished to me. He had known the lady, he said, for more than thirty years. 'So great is her truth,' he added, 'so easily proved is her uprightness, that I cannot entertain a doubt that she herself believes whatever she says.' Blameless in her walk and conversation, he regarded it as an incredibility that she should *seek* to deceive. Of strong mind, and intelligent upon all subjects, it seemed almost as difficult for him to

* *"The Doctrine of the Supernatural Established,"* by Henry Edwards, D.D., LL.D., F.A.S., F.G.S., &c., London, 1845, pp. 226 to 228.

imagine that in the narrative he had himself frequently heard from her lips—clear and circumstantial as it was— she should have been a self-deceiver. And thus he was in a dilemma. For the facts were of a character which he was extremely reluctant to admit; while the evidence was of a stamp which it seemed impossible to question.

"My own observation of the lady, stranger as she was to me, confirmed every thing which her friend the banker had told me in her favor. There was in her face and manner, even in the tones of her voice, that nameless something, rarely deceptive, which carries conviction of truth. As she repeated the story, I could not choose but trust to her sincerity; and this the rather because she spoke with evident reluctance. 'It was rarely,' the banker said, 'that she could be prevailed on to relate the circumstances,—her hearers being usually skeptics, more disposed to laugh than to sympathize with her.'

"Add to this, that neither the lady nor the banker were believers in Spiritualism,—having heard, as they told me, 'next to nothing' on the subject.

"I commit no breach of confidence in the following communication. 'If you speak of this matter,' said the lady to me, 'I will ask you to suppress the name of the place in France where the occurrences took place.' This I have accordingly done. I may add that the incidents here related had been the frequent subject of conversation and comment between the lady and her friends.

"Thus premising, I proceed to give the narrative as nearly as I can in the lady's words.

"'About the year 1820,' she said, 'we were residing at the seaport town of ——, in France, having removed thither from our residence in Suffolk. Our family consisted of my father, mother, sister, a young brother about the age of twelve, and myself, together with an English servant. Our house was in a lonely spot, on the outskirts of the town, with a broad, open beach around it, and with no other dwelling, nor any outbuildings, in its vicinity.

"'One evening my father saw, seated on a fragment of rock only a few yards from his own door, a figure enveloped in a large cloak. Approaching him, my father bid him "good-evening;" but, receiving no reply, he turned to enter the house. Before doing so, however, he looked back, and, to his very great surprise, could see no one. His astonishment reached its height when, on returning to the rock where the figure had seemed seated, and searching all round it, he could discover no trace whatever of the appearance, although there was not the slightest shelter near where any one could have sought concealment.

"'On entering the sitting-room, he said, "Children, I have seen a ghost!"—at which, as may be supposed, we all heartily laughed.

"'That night, however, and for several succeeding nights, we heard strange noises in various parts of the house,—sometimes resembling moans underneath our window, sometimes sounding like scratches against the window-frames, while at other times it seemed as if a number of persons were scrambling over the roof. We opened our window again and again, calling out to know if any one were there, but received no answer.

"'After some days, the noises made their way into our bedroom, where my sister and myself (she twenty and I eighteen years of age) slept together. We alarmed the house, but received only reproaches, our parents believing that we were affected by silly fancies. The noises in our room were usually knocks,—sometimes repeated twenty or thirty times in a minute, sometimes with the space perhaps of a minute between each.

"'At length our parents also heard both the knockings in our room and the noises outside, and were fain to admit that it was no imagination. Then the incident of the ghost was revived. But none of us were seriously alarmed. We became accustomed to the disturbances.

"'One night, during the usual knockings, it occurred to me to say, aloud, "If you are a spirit, knock six times." Immediately I heard six knocks, very distinctly given, and no more.

"'As time passed on, the noises became so familiar as to lose all terrifying, even all disagreeable, effect; and so matters passed for several weeks.

"'But the most remarkable part of my story remains to be told. I should hesitate to repeat it to you, were not all the members of my family witnesses of its truth. My brother—then, it is true, a boy only, now a man in years, and high in his profession—will confirm every particular.

"'Besides the knockings in our bedroom, we began to hear—usually in the parlor—what seemed a human voice. The first time this startling phenomenon occurred, the voice was heard to join in one of the domestic songs of the family while my sister was at the piano. You may imagine our astonishment. But we were not long left in doubt as to whether, in this instance, our imaginations had deceived us. After a time, the voice began to speak to us clearly and intelligibly, joining from time to time in the conversation. The tones were low, slow, and solemn, but quite distinct: the language was uniformly French.

"'The spirit—for such we called it—gave his name as GASPAR, but remained silent whenever we made inquiry touching his history and condition in life. Nor did he ever assign any motive for his communications with us. We received the impression that he was a Spaniard; but I cannot recall any certain reason, even, for such belief. He always called the family by their Christian names. Occasionally he would repeat to us lines of poetry. He never spoke on subjects of a religious nature or tendency, but constantly inculcated Christian morality, seeming desirous to impress upon us the wisdom of virtue and the beauty of harmony at home. Once, when my sister and myself had some slight dispute, we heard the voice saying, "M—— is wrong; S—— is right." From the time he first declared himself he was continually giving us advice, *and always for good.**

"'On one occasion my father was extremely desirous to recover some valuable papers which he feared might have been lost. Gaspar told him exactly where they were, in our old house in Suffolk; and there, sure enough, in the very place he designated, they were found.

"'The matter went on in this manner *for more than three years*. Every member of the family, including the servants, had heard the voice. The presence of the spirit—for we could not help regarding him as present—was always a pleasure to us all. We came to regard him as our companion and protector. One day he said, "I shall not be with you again for some months." And, accordingly, for several months his visits intermitted. When, one evening at the end of that time, we again heard the well-known voice, "I am with you again!" we hailed his return with joy.

"'At the times the voice was heard, we never saw any appearance; but one evening my brother said, "Gaspar, I should like to see you;" to which the voice replied, "You shall see me. I will meet you if you go to the farthest side of the square." He went, and returned presently, saying, "I have seen Gaspar. He was in a large cloak, with a broad-brimmed hat. I looked under the hat, and he smiled upon me." "Yes," said the voice, joining in, "that was I."

"'But the manner of his final departure was more

* The italics are in the original manuscript.

2 E

touching, even, than his kindness while he stayed. We returned to Suffolk; and there, as in France, for several weeks after our arrival, Gaspar continued to converse with us, as usual. One day, however, he said, "I am about to leave you altogether. Harm would come to you if I were to be with you here in this country, where your communications with me would be misunderstood and misinterpreted."

"'From that time,' concluded the lady, in that tone of sadness with which one speaks of a dear friend removed by death,—'from that time to this, we never heard the voice of Gaspar again!'

"These are the facts as I had them. They made me think; and they may make your readers think. Explanation or opinion I pretend not to add, further than this: that of the perfect good faith of the narrator I entertain no doubt whatever. In attestation of the story as she related it, I affix my name.

"S. C. HALL.

"LONDON, June 25, 1859."

What are we to think of a narrative coming to us so directly from the original source, and told in so straightforward a manner, as this? What hypothesis, be it of trickery, self-delusion, or hallucination, will serve us to set it aside? One, two, a dozen, incidents, running through a week or two, might, at utmost need, be explained away, as the result, perhaps, of some mystification,—possibly of some mistake of the senses. But a series of phenomena extending throughout three years, witnessed, long before the era of Spiritualism, in the quiet of domestic privacy, by every member of an enlightened family, observed, too, without the slightest terror to mislead, or excitement to disqualify as witness, making, day after day, on all the witnesses, the same impression,—upon what rational plea, short of suspicion of willful deception, can we set aside, as untrustworthy, such observations as these?

I seek in vain any middle ground. Either an oral communication, apparently from an ultramundane source, is possible; or else a cultivated and intelligent family, of high standing and unimpeached honor, combined to palm upon their friends a stark lie. Not the narrator alone: her father, mother, brother, sister, must all have been parties to a gross and motiveless falsehood, persisted in through a lifetime; nay, a falsehood not motiveless only, but of certain and evident injury in a worldly sense. For such a story, as every one knows, cannot, in the present prejudiced state of public opinion, be told (let the narrator be ever so highly respected) without risk of painful comment and injurious surmise.

On the other hand, that a disembodied spirit should speak to mortal ears, is one of those ultramundane phenomena, alleged in several of the preceding narratives, which the reader may have found it the most difficult to credit or conceive.

But my task as a compiler draws near its termination. I must set a limit to the number of my narrative-proofs, or else depart from the rule I have laid down to myself, to study brevity, and to place these proofs, so far as I may, within the reach of all, by restricting this treatise to the limits of a single duodecimo volume. With one additional narrative, therefore, out of a multitude that remain on my hands, I here, for the present, close the list.

THE REJECTED SUITOR.

In a beautiful country residence, at no great distance from London, in one of the prettiest portions of England, live a gentleman and his wife, whom I shall designate as Mr. and Mrs. W. They have been married sixteen years, but have no children.

Four or five years ago, there came to reside with them a friend of the family, an aged gentleman who had already passed his eightieth year, and whose declining strength and increasing infirmities gradually demanded more and more constant care. Mrs. W. tended him with the anxious affection of a daughter; and when, after some four years, he died, she mourned him as if she had indeed lost a father. Her sorrow for his loss was the deeper because of that beautiful characteristic of her sex, which causes a true-hearted woman to lament most the feeble child, or the aged sufferer, whose helplessness has seemed to cast them upon her as a constant burden, but whom that very dependence has so endeared to her, that, when death takes from her the object of her care, she feels rather a blank in her existence than a release from daily toil or nightly watch.

In such a frame of mind as this, and feeling more than usually depressed, Mrs. W. went one morning, not long after her old friend's death, into her garden, in search of some distraction from the grief that oppressed her. She had been there but a few minutes, when she felt a strong impulse to return to the house and write.

It ought here to be stated that Mrs. W. is not, nor ever has been, what, in modern phrase, is called a Spiritualist. Indeed, what she had heard of Spiritualism years before had caused her to regard it as a mischievous delusion; and though, later, she had begun somewhat to doubt how far she might have been unjustly prejudiced, she had never sat at a table, nor otherwise evoked Spiritual phenomena; it cannot be regarded as such that on one or two occasions she had sat down, out of curiosity, to see if her hand would write automatically; a few unintelligible figures or unimportant words having been the only result.

On the present occasion, however, the impulse to write, gradually increasing, and attended with a nervous

yo one doreening a any

without hope Cael thy churdom

your God and lewill help thee

R G D

and uneasy sensation in the right arm, became so strong that she yielded to it; and, returning to the house and picking up a sheet of note-paper and a small portfolio, she sat down on the steps of the front door, put the portfolio on her knee, with the sheet of note-paper across it, and placed her hand, with a pencil, at the upper left-hand corner, as one usually begins to write. After a time the hand was gradually drawn to the lower right-hand corner, and began to write *backward;* completing the first line near the left-hand edge of the sheet, then commencing a second line, and finally a third, both on the right, and completing the writing near to where she had first put down her pencil. Not only was the last letter in the sentence written first, and so on until the commencing letter was written last, but each separate letter was written backward, or inversely; the pencil going over the lines which composed each letter from right to left.

Mrs. W. stated to me that (as may well be conceived) she had not the slightest perception of what her hand was writing; no idea passing through her mind at the time. When her hand stopped, she read the sentence as she would have read what any other person had written for her. The handwriting was cramped and awkward, but, as the fac-simile will show,* legible enough. The sentence read thus:—

"*Ye are sorrowing as one without hope. Cast thy burden upon God, and he will help thee.*"

---

* See Plate I. It would seem that it ought to have read, "*Thou art sorrowing,*" &c. If I am asked whence this error in the grammatical construction of the sentence, I reply that I can no more account for it than I can for the writing itself. No one could write more correctly or grammatically than does Mrs. W. It was not through her, therefore, as in the case of an illiterate scribe we might have imagined it, that the error occurred. Its occurrence is additional proof that her mind had no agency in the matter; though it would probably be stretching conjecture too far to imagine that it was so intended.

Mrs. W. afterward said to me that if an angel from heaven had suddenly appeared to her and pronounced these words, her astonishment could scarcely have exceeded that with which she first read them. She felt awe-stricken, as if in the presence of some superior power. She sat long in silent contemplation. Then she perused, again and again, the sentence before her, half doubting, the while, the evidence of her own senses. After a time she again took pencil in hand, and tried to write something backward. But the simplest word, of three or four letters, was too much for her. She puzzled over it without being able to trace it backward, so as to be legible when done.

Then the question arose in her mind, "Whence is this? Who caused me to write that sentence?"

Her thoughts involuntarily reverted to the aged friend whom she had just lost. Could his spirit, from its home in another world, have dictated those words of consolation? Could he have been permitted to guide her hand so that she might thus receive assurance that he sympathized with her sorrow and took thought how he might relieve it?

That was the conclusion to which she finally inclined. Yet, desiring further assurance, she silently prayed that the spirit which had written this sentence through her hand might also be allowed, through the same medium, to subscribe its name. And then she placed her pencil at the foot of the paper, confidently expecting that the name of the friend whom she had lost would be written there.

The event, however, wholly belied her expectation. The pencil, again drawn nearly to the right-hand edge of the paper, wrote, backward as before, not the expected name, but the initials R. G. D.

Mrs. W., as she read them, felt herself shudder and turn pale. The grave seemed giving forth its dead

The initials were those of a young man who, eighteen years before, had sought her in marriage, but whom, though she had long known and highly esteemed him, she had rejected,—not experiencing for him any sentiment warmer than friendship, and perhaps having other preferences. He had received her refusal without complaint or expostulation. "You never gave me reason to expect," he said, gently, "that I should be accepted. But I was resolved to know my fate; for I could endure suspense no longer. I thank you for having dealt so candidly with me. I see now that you can never be my wife; but no one else ever shall be. So much, at least, is within my power."

And with that he had left her. Twelve years afterward he died, a bachelor. When Mrs. W. had first heard of his death, she had felt a momentary pang, as the thought arose that she perhaps, in crossing his life's path, had darkened and made solitary his existence. But, as she had nothing with which to reproach herself in the matter, and as she had never felt for him more than for any other deserving friend, she soon ceased to think of him; and she solemnly assured me that she could not call to mind that his name, even, had recurred to her remembrance, for several years, until the moment when it was thus suddenly and unexpectedly called up.

This occurred on the afternoon of Tuesday, March 1, 1859. A little more than a month afterward, to wit, on Monday, April 4, about four o'clock in the afternoon, while Mrs. W. was sitting in her parlor, reading, she suddenly heard, apparently coming from a small side-table near her, three distinct raps. She listened; and again there came the same sounds. Still uncertain whether it might not be some accidental knocking, she said, "If it be a spirit who announces himself, will he repeat the sound?" Whereupon the sounds were instantly and still more distinctly repeated; and Mrs.

W. became assured that they proceeded from the side-table.

She then said, "If I take pencil and paper, can I be informed who it is?" Immediately there were three raps, as of assent; and when she sat down to write, her hand, writing backward, formed the same initials as before,—R. G. D.

Then she questioned, "For what purpose were these sounds?" To which the reply, again written backward, was, "*To show you that we are thinking and working for you.*"*

Nor was this all. Ten days after the last incident, namely, on Thursday afternoon, April 14, Mrs. W., happening to call to mind that R. G. D. had once presented to her a beautiful black Newfoundland dog, thought within herself, "How much I should like to have just such an animal now!" And, one of her servants happening to be near at the time, she said to her, "I wish I had a fine large Newfoundland for a walking-companion."

The next morning, after breakfast, a gentleman was announced. He proved to be an entire stranger, whom Mrs. W. did not remember to have ever seen before. He was a surveyor, from a neighboring town, and led with him a noble black Newfoundland, as high as the table. After apologizing for his intrusion, he said he had taken the liberty to call, in order to ask Mrs. W.'s acceptance of the dog he had brought with him. "You could not have offered me a more acceptable gift," said Mrs. W.; "but will you allow me to ask what induced you to think of bringing him to me?" "I brought him," he said, "because I do not intend, for the future, to keep dogs, and because I felt assured that in you he would find a kind mistress."

Mrs. W. informed me that she had ascertained, to

* For fac-simile, see Plate II.

Plate 2

R G D

to show you that we

are thinking and working for you

an absolute certainty, that the girl to whom she had spoken on the matter had not mentioned to any one her wish to have a dog, and, indeed, that the casual remark had passed from the girl's mind and she had never thought of it again. A few hours only, it will be observed, intervened between the expression of the wish and the offer of the animal.

Those who are as well acquainted with Mrs. W. as I am know that uprightness and conscientiousness are marked traits in her character, and that the above incidents may be confidently relied on as the exact truth. I had them direct from Mrs. W. herself, a few days after they occurred; and that lady kindly ceded to me the original manuscript of the two communications.

The circumstances, taken in connection, are, of their kind, among the most extraordinary with which I am acquainted. And to the candid reader it will not be matter of surprise to learn that Mrs. W., until then a skeptic in the reality of any direct agencies from another world, should have confessed to me that her doubts were removed, that she felt comforted and tranquilized, and that she accepted the indications thus vouchsafed to her, unsought, unlooked for, as sufficient assurance that she was, in a measure, under spiritual protection,—thought of, cared for, even from beyond the tomb.

Before we decide that a faith so consolatory is unfounded, we shall do well to review the facts of this case.

Whence the sudden impulse in the garden? People are not in the habit of imagining that they desire to write, unless they have something to say. Mrs. W. was not a Spiritualist, nor residing among Spiritualists: so that no epidemic agency can be urged in explanation, even if such a suggestion have weight. The phenomenon which presented itself was strictly spontaneous.

40*

Whence, again, the writing backward? In that the will had no agency. As little had expectation. Mrs. W., in her normal state, had not the power so to write. By diligent practice she might, doubtless, have acquired it. But she *had* no such practice. She had *not* acquired it. And, not having acquired it, it was as much a physical impossibility for her, of herself, so to write, as for a man, picking up a violin for the first time, to execute thereon, at sight, some elaborate passage from Handel or Beethoven.

Again, whence the intention to write after so unexampled and impracticable a manner? Where there is an intention there must be an intelligence. It was not Mrs. W. who intended; for the result struck her with awe,—almost with consternation. It was not her intelligence, therefore, that acted. What intelligence was it?

Nor can we reasonably doubt what the intention was. Had Mrs. W.'s hand written forward, she would, in all probability, have remained in uncertainty whether, half unconsciously perhaps, the words were not of her own dictation. The expedient of the backward writing precluded any such supposition; for she could not of herself do unconsciously a thing which she could not do at all. And this expedient seems to have been ingeniously devised to cut off any supposition of the kind. Then here we have the invention of an expedient, the display of ingenuity. But who is the inventor? Who displays the ingenuity? I confess my inability to answer these questions.

The incident of the dog, if it stood alone, would be less remarkable. A thing may happen when there are ten thousand chances to one against it. A lady might to-day express a wish for a Newfoundland dog, and a perfect stranger, who knew nothing of that wish, might to-morrow offer her one. And all this might occur, as we usually say, by chance. But in the case before us there are the attendant circumstances to be taken into account. R. G. D. had, in former days, given Mrs. W. just such a dog. She had been thinking of him and of his gift. She had been told, ten days before, through some agency which she had found it impossible to interpret as mundane, that he was thinking and working for her. Was she superstitious when she said to me, as she did, that "nothing could convince her that a spirit did not influence the owner of the dog to bring it to her"?

I think her conclusion, under the circumstances, was a natural one. I believe that few having the same personal experience as had Mrs. W. would have resisted it. Was it reasonable, as well as natural? It is difficult to say why it was not, unless we assume it beyond question as a thing impossible that a departed spirit should communicate with a living person, should read a living person's thoughts, should influence a living person's actions.

But it is clearly a waste of time to examine a question at all which we have resolved in advance to decide in the negative.

And, if we have not so resolved, shall we not do well fairly to meet the questions which this and the preceding narratives suggest? If outside of this material existence there be occasionally exercised a guardian thought for the welfare of men; if, sometimes, comfort may reach us, and agencies may work for us, coming over from that world to which we are all fast hastening; if there be an earthly love that is stronger than death; are these influences, if actual influences they be, so undesirable in themselves, fraught with so little of consolation, so incapable of cheering a drooping soul, so powerless to sustain a sinking spirit, so impotent to vivify the faith in a Hereafter, that we may properly repulse them, at the threshold, as graceless aberrations, or put them aside, unscrutinized, as unholy or incredible?

BOOK VI.

THE SUGGESTED RESULTS.

CHAPTER I.

THE CHANGE AT DEATH.

"Natura non fecit saltum."—LINNÆUS.

IT suffices not that a theory be supported by a strong array of proofs. To merit grave notice or challenge rational belief, it must not involve results in themselves absurd.

But how stands the case in regard to the theory for which, in the preceding pages, I have been adducing evidence?—the hypothesis, namely, that when the spirit of man, disengaged from the body, passes to another state of existence, its thoughts and affections may still revert to earth; and that, in point of fact, it does occasionally make itself perceptible to the living, whether in dream or in the light of day,—sometimes to the sense of sight, sometimes to that of hearing or of touch, sometimes by an impression which we detect in its effect but cannot trace to its origin; these various spiritual agencies wearing in this instance a frivolous, in that a solemn, aspect, now assuming the form of petty annoyance, now of grave retribution, but more frequently brightening into indications of gentle ministry and loving guardianship.

If these things cannot be admitted without giving entrance in their train to inferences clearly absurd, it avails little how great a weight of evidence may have been brought to bear in their favor: the decision must be against them at last.

So thought De Foe.* A disciple of Luther, and sharing his aversions, he rejected, with that sturdy reformer, not only the Purgatory of Romish theology, but the idea of *any* future state mediate between heaven and hell. Therefore, he argued, the dead cannot return. From heaven they cannot: who can imagine the beatitude of the eternally blessed rudely violated for purpose so trivial? And for the damned in hell, how shall we suppose for them leisure or permission to leave, on earthly errand, a prison-house of which the gates are closed on them forever?

The premises conceded, these conclusions fairly follow. The dead cannot reasonably be imagined to return either from heaven or from hell. Then, if there be no mediate state after death, the theory of spiritual appearance or agency upon earth, by those who have gone before us, is inadmissible.

This must be conceded the rather because the occasions of alleged return are sometimes of very slight moment. A servant-girl is attracted to earth by the letters and the portrait of her lover. The proprietors of an old house return to lament over its decay and grieve for its change of ownership. A father appears to his son to prevent him from unnecessarily disbursing a few pounds. A poor-camp follower, at death, has left unsatisfied a debt scantly reaching a dollar, and to effect the repayment of that pittance her spirit forsakes, night after night, its eternal abode!

Here we come upon another necessary inference. If these stories be true, the recently-departed spirit must retain, for a longer or shorter period, not only

---

* See page 428.

its general habits of thought and motives of action, but even its petty peculiarities and favorite predilections. There must be no sudden change of individuality at the moment of death, either for the better or for the worse. Men will awake in another life, the body indeed left behind, and, with it, its corporeal instincts, its physical infirmities; yet each will awake the same individual, morally, socially, intellectually, as when on his earthly death-bed he lay down to rest.

In all this there is nothing tending to affect, either affirmatively or negatively, the doctrine of a final Day of Judgment. My argument but regards the state of the soul at the time of its emancipation by death, and for a certain period thereafter.

But so far it evidently does go. It is idle to deny it. The theory that departed friends may revisit us, and watch over us here, clearly involves two postulates:—

First, that, when death prostrates the body, the spirit remains not, slumbering in the grave, beside moldering flesh and bone, but enters at once upon a new and active phase of life; not a state of ineffable bliss, nor yet of hopeless misery, but a condition in which cares may affect, and duties may engage, and sympathies may enlist, its feelings and its thoughts.

Secondly, that the death-change reaches the body only, not the heart or the mind; discarding the one, not transforming the others.

In other words, Death destroys not, in any sense, either the life or the identity of man. Nor does it permit the spirit, an angel suddenly become immaculate, to aspire at once to heaven. Far less does it condemn that spirit, a demon instantly debased, to sink incontinently to hell.

All this may sound heterodox. The more important inquiry is, whether it be irrational. Nor was it heterodox, but most strictly. canonical, until many centuries had intervened between the teachings of Christ and the creeds of his followers. If we adopt it now, we may be running counter to the preponderating sentiment of modern Protestantism, but we are returning to the faith, universally confessed, of primitive Christianity.* I do not state this as an argument for its truth, but only as a reminder of its lineage.

Luther was a man to be praised and admired,— courageous, free-thoughted, iron-willed,—a man for his time and his task. But Luther, like other men, had his sins and his errors to answer for. Every thing about him was strong, his prejudices included. When his will reacted against deep-rooted opposition, the power of its stubborn spring sometimes carried him beyond truth and reason. He always plied his reforming besom with gigantic effect, not always with deliberate consideration. He found Purgatory an abuse; and, to make radical work, he swept out Hades along with it.†

---

* " Thus the matter stands historically. In the last quarter of the second century, when the Christian churches emerge clearly into the light, we find them universally in possession of the idea of a mediate place of souls,—one which was neither heaven nor hell, but preliminary to either. It was not an idea broached by heretics here and there. It was the belief of the Church universal, which nobody called in question."—"*Foregleams of Immortality,*" by Edward H. Sears, 4th edition, Boston, published by the American Unitarian Association, 1858, p. 268.

Unable, for lack of space, to enter on the historical evidences for the above, I refer the reader to Mr. Sears's work, where he will find these succinctly set forth. Also to " *The Belief of the First Three Centuries concerning Christ's Mission to the Under-World,*" by Frederick Huidekoper, where he may read the following passage, with numerous quotations from the Fathers in attestation :—" It can scarcely be that, at the opening of the second century, or the close of the first, the doctrine of Christ's under-world mission, so far, at least, as regards the preaching to, and liberation of, the departed, was not a widely-spread and deeply-seated opinion among Christians." . . . " On the essential features of this doctrine the Catholics and heretics were of one mind. It was a point too settled to admit dispute."—p. 135, quoted by Sears, p. 262.

† A more scrupulous man would have been arrested by the consideration

It is a question of infinite importance whether, in outrooting the faith of preceding ages,* he committed not only a grave error in fact, but also a grievous mischief in practice.

When the great Reformer denied a mediate state after death, the denial involved a hypothesis of an extraordi-

---

that Peter, who must have known his Master's views on the subject, speaks of the gospel being communicated to the dead, and of Christ himself preaching even to the spirits of those who perished in the Deluge. (1 Peter iii. 19, 20; and iv. 6.) But where, except in Hades, could this have happened?

If it be objected that the word *Hades* does not even occur in the New Testament, the reply is, that Luther—whom our English translators followed—unceremoniously shut it out. He caused the two words *Gehenna* and *Hades* to be equally rendered *Hell*. "Yet," (I quote from Sears,) " as Dr. Campbell has shown conclusively in his admirable and luminous essay, those two words have not the same meaning; and only the former answers to the modern and Christian idea of hell. The word Hades, occurring eleven times in the New Testament, *never answers to that idea, and never ought to have been so rendered.*"— *Work cited*, p. 277.

If it be further argued that, at least, there is in Scripture no deliberate expounding of this doctrine of Hades, the reply is, that an item of faith universally admitted as beyond question by Jew as well as Christian was not likely to be unnecessarily elaborated, but only incidentally adverted to.

* The Greeks had their Hades; though, with a Chinese reverence for the rites of sepulture, they conceived it to be filled chiefly by the restless and wandering shades of those whose bones lay exposed, neglected and forgotten: and if at last funeral honors were paid to appease the soul, its reward was not heaven, but eternal rest. Nor do they appear to have had the idea of spiritual guardianship, except as exerted by the gods. The Trojan hero does not anticipate any return from Pluto's realm to watch over the spouse he loved, but rather an eternal separation :—

> "Thy Hector, wrapped in everlasting sleep,
>   Shall neither hear thee sigh nor see thee weep."

The *Sheol* of the Jews—at least, according to the later Rabbins—had three regions: an upper sphere, of comparative happiness, where were the patriarchs, prophets, and others worthy to be their associates; a second, lower region, dull and dark, the temporary abode of the wicked; and, lowest of all, Gehenna, untenanted now, and to remain empty until the Day of Judgment shall have sent the condemned to occupy it.

nary character. Since without Hades there can be neither hope nor reform nor preparation beyond the grave, we are compelled to suppose, in the case of man, what Linnæus says is not to be found in the entire economy of Nature,—a sudden leap, as it were, across a great chasm,—a transforming change as instantaneous as it is complete. We are compelled to imagine that this change is preceded by no gradual progress nor effected by any human exertion.

According to the varying notions of the believers in this abrupt metamorphosis, it may occur at the moment of dissolution, or else at some epoch indefinitely distant. A portion of Luther's followers, embarrassed to dispose of the human soul in the interval between its separation from the body and its summons at some remote period by the last trump, partially adopt, in their difficulty, the Grecian doctrine of peaceful rest. According to them, the soul, overcome by Death, like any mortal thing, steeped in unconsciousness, suffers a virtual sepulture, a suspension of sentient existence, a species of temporary annihilation, to endure, He alone knows how long who has fixed the Day of Judgment. Other Lutherans, however, shocked at this approach to the dictum of revolutionary philosophy promulgated in France's Days of Terror,—"Death is an eternal sleep,"—seek to evade the dilemma by supposing that there *is* no great, universal, far-off Day of Judgment at all, but that the day of death is to each one of us the day of retribution also; that the soul, at the moment of emancipation, ascends to the tribunal of God, there instantly to be preferred to heaven or consigned to hell.

Under either hypothesis, the conception of a sudden revolution of all thought and feeling is clearly involved. Man, bright though his virtues be, and dark his sins, is, while he remains here, neither seraph nor demon. Among all our associates, be they valued friends or

2 F   41

mere distant acquaintances, how many, even of the very best, are suited to enter heaven? How many, even of the very worst, are fit only for hell? What an over-whelming majority are far too imperfect for the one, yet, with some redeeming virtue, much too good for the other! With exceptions, if any, altogether too rare to invalidate the general rule, man does not attain, upon earth, either the perfection of virtue or the extremity of degradation.

But what future may we reasonably expect for a being so constituted, at the hands of a God throughout whose works no principle shines out more luminously than that of universal adaptation? A final doom, or a further novitiate?—which?

The latter, evidently, unless we assume that the adaptation is to be precipitated, as by unexampled miracle; unless, in the twinkling of an eye, the comparatively good man is to be relieved, without effort of his, of all frailty that were unworthy of celestial membership, while the comparatively wicked man is to be shorn, equally by an agency which he controls not, of every latent spark or lingering scruple that rates, if ever so little, above the infernal.

Let us say nothing of the injustice apparently involved in such a theory. But where do we find, in a single page of that Great Book which has been spread open since the creation of the world to all God's rational creatures, one indication, even the most trifling, that sustains by the probabilities of analogy the theory itself?

We find every portion of God's handiwork instinct with the principle of progression. The seed, the plant, the blossom, the fruit,—these are the types of Nature's gradual workings. All change is a harmonious, connected succession.

Gradual, above all, are the influences through which,

under God's visible economy, man's character is formed. The constant dropping of circumstance, the slow hardening of habit, the unfolding, by imperceptible swell, of the affections, the enlistment, one by one, of governing motives, the tardy expansion, stretching from infancy to ripe manhood, of the intellectual powers,—these are the means at work, acting so silently, modifying by degrees so microscopically minute, that, like the motion of the hour-hand over the dial of a small watch, the advance escapes our perception. We detect, when months or years have elapsed, a certain space passed over. We know that the unbroken chain of influences has stretched on, though its links are invisible to mortal eyes.

Such is the mode, so strictly gradual, so constantly operating through the intervention of slow-working agencies, under which alone, here upon earth, man's character is influenced. And this could not have been otherwise unless man had been created, not the progressive free agent he is, but some creature essentially different.

Nor in the development of the human being, such as he is, do we find that God ever permits Himself (if one may so speak) to depart from the law inherent in the organization and attributes of the creature He has made. Progressively and mediately, by the intervention of motive presented, by the agency of will, by the influence of surroundings physical and social,—thus, and not otherwise, does God suffer man gradually to become what circumstance, daily acting on a constitution like his, determines that he shall be. Thus, and not otherwise, so far as we can follow him, is man taught and guided.

At last this progressive being reaches a point at which the body, that during its earlier vigor seconded in a measure the promptings of its immortal associate, faints and fails.   It has served its purpose, like an aged, decaying tree.   That which was erewhile felt as a comfort and an aid becomes a burden and an incumbrance. The Immortal has outgrown its perishable envelope. The larva drops off.   The unmasked spirit is gone, beyond our ken.

In following—as in thought we may—its invisible progress, since the ablest theologians differ in their interpretation of authority, what earthly guide can we follow more trustworthy than analogy?   Where but in the rule of the Past can we find reliable indication touching the probable rule in the Future?

The conclusion is evident.   He who conducts the soul to the brink of the Dark River deserts it not on the hither side.   Nor is that river the boundary of His realm.   His laws operate beyond.   But these laws, so far as we know them, exhibit no variableness nor shadow of turning.   And I see neither reason nor likelihood in the supposition that in any portion of creation they are suspended or reversed.   I see neither reason nor likelihood in the theory that, in any portion of creation, progress and exertion will fail to precede improvement, or that man will ever be degraded by agency other than his own.

I find nothing absurd or irrational, therefore, in the postulates which the theory of spiritual interference involves.   On the contrary, it seems to me probable enough that the attention of men may have been especially called, in our modern day, to this very theory, in order to correct an important error, and thus to put an end to the mischief which that error may have occasioned.

If it be true that Hades exists, the truth is an important one.   But in proportion to the importance of a truth denied are the evil consequences likely to result from the denial.

Does this apply in the instance under consideration? Do grave and serious evils result from rejecting the doctrine of a mediate state after death?

Man is so constituted that remote inducements act upon him with feeble force. Experience proves that the power of reward, as an incentive, is in the inverse ratio of the distance at which it is set. And no maxim in jurisprudence is better established than this: that punishment, to be effectual, should tread close on the heels of the offense.

If, then, we assume—as mental philosophers are wont to do—that a belief in future rewards and punishments is a chief incentive to truth and virtue, it is essential that their effect should not be enfeebled by remoteness.

But this is precisely what Luther did in his eager desire to be rid of Purgatory. He postponed to a Day of Judgment, that may not arrive for untold ages, the reward and the punishment of earthly deeds. It avails little to add that the interval was to be passed in unconscious slumber, and to be told, as we sometimes are, that a thousand years of dreamless sleep are to the sleeper but as a moment of time: so subtle a distinction does not reach the feelings nor convince the common mind.

What wonder, then, that the murderer is deterred by the fear of earthly punishment, uncertain as it is, in a thousand cases in which the dread of a Day of Judgment, scarcely discerned in the illimitable distance, exerts an influence too feeble to arrest his arm?

What wonder that the self-indulgent man of the world, like a spoiled child whom one vainly seeks to tempt from some injurious pleasure of to-day by the promise of a greater pleasure laid up for to-morrow, recklessly snatches at every sensual enjoyment now, undeterred by the risk of losing celestial happiness commencing he knows not when?

What wonder that the pulpit ceaselessly declaims against man's blindness and folly in preferring the fleeting joys of a moment to the bliss of life everlasting, and that the declamation so often falls on dull ears and closed hearts?

When the philosopher places a magnet beyond the sphere of its usual action, he wonders not that he can no longer detect its manifestations. The theologian, less reasonable, removes to a distance, rendered endless by the dilating effect of uncertainty, all that attracts of future reward, all that repels of future punishment, and still expects that the magnetic agency of a Hereafter will retain its force and win over its converts.

My argument, it may be objected, does not apply to those who believe that God sits in perpetual judgment, and that each moment, as it surrenders its victim, witnesses also his doom.

To a limited extent the objection is valid, but to a limited extent only. A separation may be effected by other means almost as completely as by distance. In the parable, the gulf between Dives and Lazarus is not represented as of vast width: sight across it is possible, question is put and answer received; yet it is spoken of as impassable.

But have we not, in breaking down the old doctrine of Hades,—the spiritual bridge connecting the Here with the Hereafter,—left open a great gulf, if not impassable, yet hard for mortal conceptions to pass? To human feelings, have we not separated, almost as effectually as if limitless time intervened, the existence of man on earth from his future life in heaven?

The question of identity—that theme of ancient sophists—is a difficult one. In a physical sense, a man is not, strictly speaking, the identical individual to-day that he was yesterday or that he will be to-morrow. Nevertheless, the change from one day to another is usually so imperceptible that we instinctively conceive of the individual as the same.

But if the changes now running through twenty years were condensed into a single night; if an infant, such as he appears to us when twelve months only have elapsed since his birth, put to sleep to-night, were to awake to-morrow morning exactly the same, in mind and body, as he will be when he shall have attained his majority, he would be for us not the same individual, but another. The case, in modified form, actually occurs. We part with an infant two or three years old, to see him again a man of twenty-five. Theoretically, we regard him as the same person; practically, he is a new acquaintance, whom we never met before.

There is this difference, however, between the two cases. In the latter, the absent individual has retained, in his own feelings, his identity, though we have lost all perception of it. In the former, in which we have supposed the transformation effected in a night, the identity would be lost as surely to the person transformed as to us, the witnesses of the transformation.

But we cannot suppose that the change from infancy to manhood, great as it is, can for a moment be compared in its thoroughness to that radical transformation which alone could fit the best of us to join the seraphic hosts, or make an erring brother or a frail sister the proper associate of the devils in Luther's hell.

Still less can we imagine that the God of a world like this, disclosing, at every step we take in it, adaptations infinite in number and in character marvelous beyond all human conception, should consign any one of his creatures to an abode for which he was not strictly adapted.

But if the change instantly succeeding the momentary sleep of death be far greater than that we have imagined in a creature lying down at night an infant and awaking next morning a full-grown man, and if, in this latter case, identity would be lost, how much more in the former!

The body is gone: what continuous links of identity remain? The mind, the feelings. Transform these, and *every* link is severed connecting, FOR US, a Here with a Hereafter.

It is not WE, in any practical sense, who survive, but others. A human being dies on earth; a seraph, or a demon, appears in heaven or in hell.*

It is idle to say that this is a fine-drawn theoretical distinction, the mere sophism of a logician. It is precisely because of its practical character that I am induced here to put it forward.

I do not affirm that men confess to themselves their unbelief that they, the same individuals who now think and feel, will exist in a future state. That is not the form which the evil assumes.

Professing Christians are wont to declare that they will live again, as glorified angels, in heaven. And, in a certain theoretical sense, they believe it. They would be shocked if one were to suggest that they have not faith in an after-life for themselves. So far as a human

---

* A similar idea has been elsewhere expressed :—"An instantaneous change, either from good to evil or from evil to good, if effected in a sovereign manner by a foreign power, and effected irrespectively of an economy of motives, would rather be the annihilation of one being and the creation of another, than the changing of the character of the same being; for it is of the very nature of a change of character that there be an internal process, a concurrence of the will, and yielding of the rational faculties to rational inducements, and also the giving way of one species of desires and one class of habits to another."—"*Physical Theory of Another Life*," London, 1839, chap. xiii. p. 181.

being can identify himself with another creature essen-tially different, they do believe that they, now living, and the glorified angels, hereafter to live, are the self-same persons.

But the very expressions they currently employ betray the imperfect character of this belief. "We shall live *again*," they say. The expression implies a hiatus. And they actually feel as they express themselves. Their faith does not call up the idea of continuous life. Death, for them, is not a herald, but a destroyer,—the fell exterminator, not the welcome deliverer.* The drooping willow, the dark cypress, are his emblems; not the myrtle and the laurel.

Their conception is that of two lives, with a dreary gulf between. The descent to that gulf is fitly accompanied, they think, by lamentation. The mourners go about the streets. It is not a worthless, obscuring incumbrance thrown off and left behind in its kindred earth, while a freed spirit rejoices in its emancipation: it is WE who go down to the gloomy tomb, where there is neither work, nor device, nor knowledge, nor wisdom; nay, where hope itself is extinct.

> "In the cold grave, to which we haste,
> There are no acts of pardon past;
> But fixed the doom of all remains,
> And everlasting silence reigns."

Can such conceptions as these obtain among us, yet interpose between man and his celestial home no distorting medium, no obscuring vail?

---

* If I had the superintendence of a picturesque cemetery, the lines over its entrance-gate should be from Mrs. Hemans:—

> "Why should not he whose touch dissolves our chain
> Put on his robes of beauty, when he comes
> As a deliverer?"

But there is another important view to be taken of this matter.

Veneration is one of the most influential sentiments of our nature,—universal, or nearly so, in its prevalence; and no legislator, with a just knowledge of human kind, ignores or overlooks its influence. But when veneration engrosses the human character, when, as in the case of ancient anchorite or ascetic monk, human life is wholly spent in adoration and in rapt contemplation of God and celestial things, not only is the character dwarfed and injured, but the feelings become morbid and sound judgment disappears. Here upon earth, no one sentiment can be suffered exclusively to occupy a man, without producing an abnormal condition of mind, greatly prejudicial alike to his improvement and to his usefulness.

If the sudden transformation of character which Luther's system presupposes does actually take place immediately after death, or immediately before a Day of Judgment, then all this may be changed; then man, being no longer the creature we find him here, may at once become adapted to a state of being in which prayer and praise are the sole and everlasting avocations. In the mean time, however, on this side the grave, man is *not* so changed. While human beings remain here upon earth, therefore, they are not, nor ever can be, prepared for heaven, in the common acceptation of that word.

But, according to another law of our nature, we sympathize little with that for which we are not prepared. If we set about endeavoring to imagine how we should feel if we were entirely different from what we are, the result is a dull and chill perception, that never reaches the feelings or warms the heart. Can the bold, active, unlettered youth, whose enjoyment centers in the sports of the field, realize, by any mental effort, the happiness of the artist, haunted by visions of beauty, or the deep satisfaction of the student, surrounded by his books and reveling in the vast realms of thought which these disclose? He hears of such delights, perhaps, and denies not their existence; but the cold assent he gives never attains the grade of a governing motive, nor suffices to influence his life.

To human beings, therefore, such as they are upon earth, the eternal life of the "rapt seraph who adores and burns" has no living charm. Men may reason themselves, and sometimes they do, into an artificial rapture of enthusiasm, pending the influence of which they experience an actual longing to join the angelic hosts and share in their changeless occupation. But unless they have become, more or less, secluded from the duties of active life, or have abandoned themselves, in some closed retreat, to a constant routine of exclusively devotional and contemplative exercises, it is, for the most part, the reason that frigidly argues, not the genial impulse of the feelings that adopts and assents. In Protestant Christendom the heart of the millions is not reached by the prospect commonly presented to them of eternal life.

Here is no assertion that heaven, as it has been depicted to us, will not, at some future epoch, be a state adapted to the human race. We know not whither ultramundane progress may lead. We cannot tell what man may become when, in another stage of existence, he has run another career of improvement. It will be time enough to speculate upon this when that future career shall have commenced. But we *do* know what manner of creature man now is; and we *do* know that, while here, he must be governed by the laws of his being. He must appreciate before he is fitted to enjoy. And if that which he is not fitted to enjoy be promised to him on certain conditions, the anticipation of it will,

as a general rule, call forth no strenuous exertion,—
because it will awaken no vivid desire.

Nor let it be said that it is to the man of low desires
or groveling instincts alone that heaven, shorn of a preliminary Hades, is too distant in time, or too remote in
feeling, to be appreciated or longed for. How numerous
and distinct are the virtuous emotions that now move
the heart of man! The promptings to acts of benevolence and deeds of mercy, the stirrings of magnanimity,
the efforts of self-denial; fortitude, courage, energy,
perseverance, resignation; the devotion of love, and the
yearnings of compassion :—what a varied list is here!
And in that man who confesses the practical short-
comings of his life, who feels how far better was his
nature than have been its manifestations, who knows
how often in this world noble impulse has been re-
pressed, how many generous aspirings have here
scarcely been called into action,—in the heart of such
a man must not the hope be strong, that the life which
now is may have a sequel and a complement in that
which is to come? He who has labored long and
patiently to control and discipline a wayward nature,—
he who has striven in this world, with earnest and
patient effort, after self-culture, moral and intellectual,—
may he not properly desire and rationally expect that
he will be allowed to prosecute the task, here so imperfectly commenced, there, where there is no flesh to
be weak if the spirit be willing? Shall the philanthropist, whose life has been one long series of benefactions
to his race, be blamed if he cannot surrender at death,
without regret, the godlike impulse that bids him succor
the afflicted and heal the broken heart? Even he whose
days have been spent in exploring the secrets of nature,
can he be expected, unmoved, to relinquish with his
earthly body the pursuit of that science to which his

heart was wedded?* But, far more, shall a loving and compassionate nature anticipate with complacency the period when the soul, all consecrated to worship or filled with its own supreme felicity, shall no longer select, among its fellow-creatures, its objects either of pity or of love?

In a word, is it the depraved only who are likely to look with coldness on a prospective state that offers scarce any theater for the exercise of the qualities we have been wont to admire, and of the sympathies that have hitherto bound us to our kind? Is it the vicious alone who may find little to attract in a future where one universal sentiment, how holy soever, is to replace all others?—where one virtue, one duty, is instantly to supersede, in the character and the career of man, the varied virtues, the thousand duties, which, here below, his Creator has required at his hands?

Men may take their fellows to task for the indifference with which so many regard a heaven which as yet they are neither prepared to appreciate nor fitted to enjoy; God, who has made man's heart the multiform and richly-dowered thing it is, never will.

I anticipate the objection which may here be made Our conceptions may not rise to the height of that transcendent heaven which has been described to us;

---

* If it be doubted whether such regrets ever haunt the death-bed of a scientific man, let the following vouch for the fact:—"Berzelius then became aware that his last hour had come, and that he must bid adieu to that science he had loved so well. Summoning to his bedside one of his devoted friends, who approached him weeping, Berzelius also burst into tears; and then, when the first emotion was over, he exclaimed, 'Do not wonder that I weep. You will not believe me a weak man, nor think I am alarmed by what the doctor has to announce to me. I am prepared for all. But I have to bid farewell to science; and you ought not to wonder that it costs me dear.' . . . "This was Berzelius's leave-taking of science; in truth, a touching farewell."—"*Siljeström's Minnesfest öfver Berzelius*," Stockholm, 1849, pp. 79, 80.

our feelings may not warm under the description of it; but, if we know nothing of a mediate state of existence except that *it is*,—if we have scarcely a glimpse disclosing its character, or indicating its privileges, or revealing its enjoyments,—how much better or happier shall we be for a belief so vague and shapeless? Rather a Heaven whose beatific glories dazzle without attracting, than a Paradise of which the very outlines are indistinguishable. How can we vividly desire an unknown life, or be comforted or influenced by anticipation of a state so dim and shadowy?

If those who put forth this objection assumed only facts that must be admitted, the objection would be fatal. What they *do* assume is, that we can know nothing of a Hades in the future. Are they right in this?

Beyond the scanty and (be it admitted) insufficient indications to be gleaned from Scripture, I perceive but two sources whence such knowledge can be derived: first, analogy; and, secondly, such revelings as may come to us through narratives similar in character to those I have brought together in this volume, or otherwise from ultramundane source.

We study our instincts too little. We listen to their lessons too carelessly. Instincts are from God.

None of the instincts which we observe among animal races other than our own are useless, or ill adapted, or incomplete. The impulse induces an action strictly corresponding to future contingencies which actually arise. In one sense, these instincts are of a prophetic character. When the bee, before a flower has been rifled of its sweets, prepares the waxen cells, when a bird, in advance of incubation, constructs its downy nest, the adaptation is as perfect as if every coming incident had been expressly foretold.

Man has reason *and* instincts. Sometimes he forgets this. It is his right and duty, in the exercise of his reason, to judge his instincts; yet reverently, as that in which there may be a hidden wisdom. Men, sometimes from a religious error, more frequently from a worldly one, are wont to fall into the thought that it is expedient to discard or to repress them.

There is a strange mystery pervading human society. It is the apparent anomaly presented by man's character taken in connection with his position here.

Let us speak of the better portion of mankind,—the true and worthy type of the race. What, in a word, is the history of their lives? A bright vision and a disenchantment. A struggle between two influences: one, native, inherent; the other, foreign, extraneous, earthly; a warring between the man's nature and his situation.

Not that the world he enters can be said to be unadapted to receive him. For in it there is knowledge to impart, experience to bestow, effort to make, progress to attain; there are trials to test courage and firmness; there are fellow-creatures to love; there are helpless creatures to aid; there are suffering creatures to pity. There is much to interest, and not a little to improve. The present is, doubtless, an appropriate and necessary stage in the journey of life. None the less is it a world the influences of which never fully develop the character of its noblest inhabitant. It is a world of which the most fortunate combinations, the highest enjoyments, leave disappointed and unsatisfied some of the most elevated instincts of man. All religions, more or less distinctly, admit this.

We speak of our *better* nature, as though there were two. There is but one,—one and the same in childhood, in youth, in manhood, till death.

The same, for the Immortal perishes not; never obliterated, but how often, in the course of this earth-life, dulled, dimmed, obscured! How the fleshly envelope weighs upon it! And what a training, as it runs the gauntlet of society, it has! Warm, impulsive, it meets with cold calculation; generous, it encounters maxims of selfishness; guileless, it is schooled to deceit; believing, it is overwhelmed with doubts, it is cheated with lies. And for the images of its worship,—how are they broken and despoiled! It had set them up on earthly pedestal, and had clothed them, all unworthy, in the robes of its own rich conception. Its creative promptings had assumed, perhaps, their highest and holiest phase,—the phase of love; and then it had embodied, in a material existence, that which was but an ethereal portion of itself; investing—alas, how often!—some leaden idol with the trappings of a hero or the vestments of a god. Bitter the awakening! Dearly rued the self-deception! Yet the garment was of heaven, though the shattered idol was of earth.

Thus, for one encouragement to its holier aspirations, it receives twenty sordid lessons from the children of this world, grown wise in their generation; so wise that, in their conceit, they despise and take to task a child of light. They deride his disinterestedness; they mock at his enthusiasm. Assuming the tone of mentors, they read him prudent warnings against the folly of philanthropy and the imbecility of romance.*

And thus, in ten thousand instances, God's instincts fall, like seed by the wayside, on hard and stony ground. They thrive not. Their growth is stunted. Happy if the divine germ penetrate the crusted surface at all!

Either this is an example of a failure in adaptation, or we are looking at a portion only of a great whole.

Shall we suppose it a failure? Shall we imagine that He who, in the lower, cared for it that the innate impulse should exactly correspond to the future occasion, failed to exert similar care in the higher?—that the instincts

---

* A word of excellent etymology, if of indifferent reputation,—derived from the Welsh *rhamanta*, to rise over, to soar, to reach to a distance.

of the bee and the bird are to find theaters of action perfectly suited to their exercise, while those of a crea ture far above them are to be dwarfed in development and disappointed in fruition?

We outrage all analogy in adopting such a hypo-thesis. We must accept this anomaly, if we accept it at all, as an exception—the only one known to us through-out the entire economy of God—to a rule co-extensive with the universe.

But if, unable to credit the existence of so striking an anomaly, we fall back on the remaining hypothesis, —that here we are but looking on a fraction of human life,—then from that fraction we may obtain some idea of the remainder. Then we may predicate in a general way, and with strong probabilities, something of the character and occupations of Hades.

There are favored moments,—at least, in every good man's life,—moments when the hard and the selfish and the worldly are held in abeyance,—moments when the soul springs forth, like a durance-freed bird, equal to every effort, capable of every sacrifice; when nothing seems too high to reach, nothing too distant to compass, —moments in which the exultant spirit recognizes its like welling up in some other heart's holy confession, or flashing out through true poetry like this :—

> " Past the high clouds floating round,
>   Where the eagle is not found,
>   Past the million-starry choir, . . .
>   Through the midst of foul opinions,
>   Flaming passions, sensual mire,
>   To the Mind's serene dominions,
>   I aspire !"*

These are the moments when the still, small voice—the Immortal one—asserts its supremacy. These are the

---

* The lines are Barry Cornwall's.

moments when man feels that if life were but made up
of such, he would need no other heaven.

And these are the moments when the spirit of man,
Sibyl-like, may be questioned of the future; for the
divine rage is upon her, and her foreboding instincts are
the earnest of what is to be.

This argument from analogy, it will occur to the
reader, is similar to that which has so often been made
in proof of the soul's immortality. A universal desire
must have an ultimate correspondence. But, if we look
closely at it, the argument will be seen to prove much
more than continued existence. The desire has a certain
definiteness. In its purest type, it is not a vague, coward
dread of annihilation; it is not a mere selfish longing
to be. The instinct is of far nobler aim and wider scope
than this: it is the voice of the IDEAL in man; and it
teaches not one lesson, but many. It calls up before
him a thousand varied images of the Grand, and the
Good, and the Beautiful, and tells him, "These are
for thee." It appeals to the divinity within him, and
declares, "This thou mayest be." But as it is *to* man,
so it is *of* man, that it speaks,—of man's capabilities,
of man's career, of the excellence that *he* may attain,—
he, the human creature, and not another. The desires
it awakens are of corresponding character.

But, if we are to take a present desire for proof of a
future condition, let us make clear to ourselves what
that desire demands. Does it crave, at this stage of its
progress, another nature or sublimer dreams? No; but
only that this nature might maintain the elevation which
its aspirations have sometimes reached,—only that its
dream-glimpses of moments might have reality and
endurance in a purer atmosphere and under a brighter
sky.

It is a stage for the unchecked exercise of *earthly*

virtues, toward which, as yet, the heart's magnet points. The good which we would, yet did not, that we would still do. The human virtues which we have loved more than practiced, these we would still cherish and exemplify. The human affections which have suffered shipwreck and pined for some quiet haven, they, too, still hope for exercise, still yearn for satisfaction. Our devotional impulses, also, are rife and aspirant, imploring better knowledge and a clearer light. Yet they constitute but one emotion out of many. They interest deeply, they elevate; but they do not engross.

The prophetic voice, then,—the divine foreboding,—speaks not of one life completed and another to commence. It indicates not, as the next phase of existence, a Day of Judgment on which hope must die, and then (but for the blessed alone) a heaven too immaculate for progress, too holy for human avocation or human endeavor. Its presentiments are of a better world, but of a *world* still,—the abode of emancipated spirits, but of *human* spirits,—a world where there is work to do, a race to run, a goal to reach,—a world where we shall find, transplanted from earth to a more genial land, energy, courage, perseverance, high resolves, benevolent actions, Hope to encourage, Mercy to plead, and Love—the earth-clog shaken off that dimmed her purity—still selecting her chosen ones, but to be separated from them no more.

Such are the utterings of the presaging voice. A state, then, suddenly reached, in which one class only of our emotional impulses should find scope for development or opportunity for action, would leave man's instinct, except in a single phase, unanswered and unsatisfied. There would be an initiative, and no correspondence; a promise, and no fulfillment; a preparation, and no result Our earth-life would, indeed, be succeeded by

another; yet in itself it would forever remain frag-
mentary and incomplete.

If, then, we have accepted man's universal desire for
immortality as proof that his spirit *is* immortal, let us
accept also the trendings of that desire as foreshadow-
ings of the Paradise to which that spirit is bound.

Thus, by the light of analogy alone, we find every
probability in favor of the conclusion that, in the next
phase of his existence, man does not cease to be the
human creature he is, and that the virtues, the occupations, and the enjoyments that await him in Hades are
as many and various as those which surround him here,
—better, indeed, brighter, of nobler type and more extended range, but still supplemental only, as appertaining to a second stage of progression,—to a theater fairer
than this, yet not wholly disconnected from it,—to a land
not yet divine, but in which may be realized the holiest
aspirations of earth.

A step beyond this it is still, perhaps, permitted to go.
If there be footfalls on the boundary of another world,
let us listen to their echoes and take note of the indications these may afford.

I do not pretend that there is to be found in the examples adduced in this volume sufficient to mark fully
and distinctly the character of our next phase of life;
and I will not at the present go beyond these. Yet, few
in number as are the indications, they touch on master-
influences.

Eminent among these is one clearly to be derived from
many of the preceding narratives,*—an earnest of social
progress in the future, which we may hail with joy and

* As in the case of Mary Goffe, and of Mrs. E——, (see "*The Dying
Mother and her Babe;*") also in that of Mr. Wynyard, of Captain G——,
(see "*The Fourteenth of November,*") and, indeed, in all cases in which the
spirit is alleged to have appeared soon after death to some beloved survivor.

should accept with gratitude. If any reliance can be placed on some of the best-authenticated incidents recorded in the foregoing pages, they not only prove (what, indeed, we might rationally assume) that it is the body only which imposes the shackles of distance, but they afford evidence also that the released spirit instinctively seeks its selected ones, and attains in a moment the spot where cluster its affections.

But if, beyond a sound body, a clear conscience, and an absence of the fear of want, we look around us, in this world, in search of that one circumstance which above all others stamps our lot in life as fortunate or the reverse, where shall we find it? When we picture to ourselves some happy prospect in the future, some tranquil retreat whence care shall be excluded and where contentment will dwell, what is the essential to that earthly paradise? Who that deserves such blessing but has the answer on his lips?

In the deepest regrets of the Past, how legibly is that answer written! We meet, among our fellow-creatures, with some, as to whom we feel how mighty for good, upon our minds and hearts, is their power; we have glimpses of others, whose very atmosphere sheds over us a glow of happiness. The stream sweeps us apart, and we find the same influence on earth no more.

But if, hereafter, the principle of insulation that prevails throughout this earthly pilgrimage is to give place to the spirit of communion unchecked by space; if, in another phase of life, desire is to correspond to locomotion; if, there, to long for association is to obtain it, if to love is to mingle in the society of the loved; what an element, not of passive feeling but of active organization, is Sympathy destined to become! And how much that would render this world too blessed to leave is in store for us in another!

If we sit down, in our calmest and most dispassionate

moments, to consider how much of our highest and
least selfish pleasures, moral, social, intellectual, has
been due to a daily interchange of thought and feeling
between kindred minds and hearts, and if we reflect
that all the other losses and crosses of life have been as
nothing when compared with those which, by distance
and by death, our severed sympathies and affections
have suffered, we may be led to conclude that the single
change above indicated as appertaining to our next
phase of life will suffice there to assure a happy existence to pure minds and genial hearts; to those who in
this world, erring and frail as they may have been, have
not wholly quenched the spirit of light; with whom
the voice within has still been more potent than the
din without; who have cherished, if often in silence
and secret, God's holy instincts, the flowers that are
still to bloom; and who may hope in that Hereafter,
where like will attract its like, to find a home where
never shall enter the Summoning Angel to announce
the separation of its inmates,—a home of unsundered
affections among the just and good.

I might proceed to touch on other indications scarcely
less important or less encouraging than the preceding,
but which, in the examples furnished in this work,* are
less palpably marked; as that when, at death, the earth-
mask drops, the mind and the heart are unvailed, and
thoughts are discerned without the intervention of
words; so that, in the spirit-land, we "shall know even
as we are known." It will, then, be a land of TRUTH,
where deceit will find no lurking-place, and where the

* The prayer offered by Mrs. W. (see narrative entitled " *The Rejected
Suitor*") was a silent one; and those who have obtained similar communications know well that a mental question usually suffices to procure a pertinent answer. This phenomenon of thought-reading I have myself verified
again and again.

word "falsehood" will designate no possible sin. Can we imagine an influence more salutary, more nobly regenerating, more satisfying to the heart, than this?

But I pause, and check the impulse to amplify the picture. Hereafter, it may be, in possession of more copious materials, I may be enabled better to carry out such a task.

Meanwhile, in pursuit of my immediate object, there needs not, perhaps, further elaboration. I may have adduced sufficient argument in proof that the hypothesis of spirit-visitation involves no absurd postulate. I may also, perhaps, have proved to the satisfaction of a portion of my readers, that the common conceptions of death are false,—that death is not, as Plato argued and as millions believe, the opposite of life, but only the agency whereby life changes its phase.

Yet I know how fast-rooted are long-cherished opinions. Even while I have been writing, I have occasionally been fain to tolerate current phrases of faulty import. Although in the preceding pages, for the sake of being intelligible, I have employed the expressions "on this side the grave," "beyond the tomb," and the like, these, as applied to human beings, are, strictly speaking, inaccurate. WE have nothing to do with the grave. WE do not descend to the tomb. It is a cast-off garment, encoffined, to which are paid the rites of sepulture.

CHAPTER II.

CONCLUSION.

"In completing this design, I am ignorant neither of the greatness of the work, nor of my own incapacity. My hope, however, is, that if the love of my subject carry me too far, I may, at least, obtain the excuse of affection. It is not granted to man to love and be wise."—BACON.

BEFORE I part from the reader, he may desire to ask me whether I conceive the reality of occasional spiritual interference to be here conclusively made out.

I prefer that he should take the answer from his own deliberate judgment. In one respect, he is, probably, better qualified to judge than I. It is not in human nature to ponder long and deeply any theory,—to spend years in search of its proofs and in examination of its probabilities,—yet maintain that nice equanimity which accepts or rejects without one extraneous bias. He who simply inspects may discriminate more justly than he whose feelings have been enlisted in collecting and collating.

Yet I will not withhold the admission that, after putting the strictest guard on the favoritism of parentage, I am unable to explain much of what my reason tells me I must here receive as true, on any other hypothesis than the ultramundane.

Where there are clear, palpable evidences of thought, of intention, of foresight, I see not how one can do otherwise than refer these to a thinker, an intender, a foreseer. Such reference appears to me not rational only, but necessary. If I refuse to accept such manifestations of intelligence as indicating the workings of a

504

rational mind,—if I begin to doubt whether some mechanical or chemical combination of physical elements may not put on the semblance of reason and counterfeit the expression of thought,—then I no longer perceive the basis of my own right to assume that the human forms which surround me have minds to think or hearts to feel. If our perceptions of the forest, and the ocean, and the plain, are to be accepted as proofs that there really is a material world around us, shall we refuse to receive our perceptions of thoughts and feelings other than our own, as evidence that some being, other than ourselves, exists, whence these emanate?* And if that being belong not to the visible world, are we not justified in concluding that it has existence in the invisible?

That the rational being of which we thus detect the agency *is* invisible, invalidates not at all the evidence we receive. It is but a child's logic which infers that, where nothing is seen, nothing exists.

As to the mode and place of existence of these invisible beings, Taylor's conjecture may be the correct one, when he supposes,—

"That within the field occupied by the visible and ponderable universe, and on all sides of us, there is existing and moving another element, fraught with another

---

* Thus argues an elegant and logical mind:—"On the table before us a needle, nicely balanced, trembles, and turns, as with the constancy of love, towards a certain spot in the arctic regions; but a mass of iron, placed near it, disturbs this tendency and gives it a new direction. We assume, then, the presence of an element universally diffused, of which we have no direct perception whatever. Now, let it be imagined that the sheets of a manuscript, scattered confusedly over the table and the floor, are seen to be slowly adjusting themselves according to the order of the pages, and that at last every leaf and every loose fragment has come into its due place and is ready for the compositor. In such a case we should, without any scruple, assume the presence of an invisible rational agent, just as in the case of the oscillations of the needle we had assumed the presence of an invisible elementary power."—TAYLOR's "*Physical Theory of Another Life,*" London, 1839, p. 244.

species of life, corporeal, indeed, and various in its orders, but not open to the cognizance of those who are confined to the conditions of animal organization,—not to be seen, not to be heard, not to be felt, by man.* We here," he continues, "assume the abstract probability that our five modes of perception are partial, not universal, means of knowing what may be around us, and that, as the physical sciences furnish evidence of the presence and agency of certain powers which entirely elude the senses, except in some of their remote effects, so are we denied the right of concluding that we are conscious of all real existences within our sphere."† Or, as he elsewhere expresses it, "Within any given boundary there may be corporeally present the human crowd and the extra-human crowd, and the latter as naturally and simply present as the former."‡

To these beings, usually invisible and inaudible to us, we also may be usually invisible and inaudible.§ It would seem that there are certain conditions, occasionally existing, which cause exceptions on both sides to this general rule. Whether human beings ought simply to await these conditions, or to seek to create them, is an inquiry which does not enter into the plan of this work.

As to the proofs of the agency upon earth of these Invisibles, I rest them not on any one class of observations set forth in this volume, not specially on the phenomena of dreaming, or of unexplained disturbances, or of apparitions whether of the living or the dead, or

---

* Not *usually* open, not *usually* to be seen, &c., would here have been the correct expression.

† *"Physical Theory of Another Life,"* pp. 232, 233.

‡ Work cited, p. 274.

§ See Oberlin's opinion on this subject, at page 364; see, also, a curious intimation suggested by an alleged observation of Madame Hauffe, at pages 397, 398.

of what seem examples of ultramundane retribution or indications of spiritual guardianship, but upon the aggregate and concurrent evidence of all these. It is strong confirmation of any theory that proofs converging from many and varying classes of phenomena unite in establishing it.

These proofs are spread all over society. The attention of the civilized public has been attracted to them in our day as it has not been for centuries, at least, before. If the narrative illustrations here published, scanty and imperfect as they are, obtain, as perhaps they may, a wide circulation, they will provoke further inquiry; they will call forth, in support or in denial, additional facts; and, in any event, truth must be the gainer at last.

If it should finally prove that through the phenomena referred to we may reach some knowledge of our next phase of life, it will be impossible longer to deny the practical importance of studying them. Yet perhaps, as the result of that study, we ought to expect rather outlines, discerned as through a glass darkly, than any distinct filling up of the picture of our future home. We may reasonably imagine that it would injuriously interfere in the affairs of this world if too much or too certain information came to us from another. The duties of the present might be neglected in the rapt contemplation of the future. The feeling within us that to die is gain might assume the ascendency, might disgust us with this checkered earth-life, and even tempt us rashly to anticipate the appointed summons; thus, perhaps, prematurely cutting short the years of a novitiate, of which God, not man, can designate the appropriate term.

Yet enough may be disclosed to produce, on human conduct, a most salutary influence, and to cheer the darkest days of our pilgrimage here by the confident assurance that not an aspiration after good that fades, nor a dream of the beautiful that vanishes, during the earth-phase of life, but will find noble field and fair realization when the pilgrim has cast off his burden and reached his journey's end.

Meanwhile, what motive to exertion in self-culture can be proposed to man more powerful than the assurance, that not an effort to train our hearts or store our minds made here, in time, but has its result and its reward, hereafter, in eternity? We are the architects of our own destiny: we inflict our own punishments; we select our own rewards. Our righteousness is a meed to be patiently earned, not miraculously bestowed or mysteriously imputed. Our wickedness, too, and the inherent doom it entails, are self imposed. We choose: and our Choice assumes place as inexorable judge. It ascends the tribunal, and passes sentence upon us; and its jurisdiction is not limited to earth. The operation of its decrees, whether penal or beneficient, extends as surely to another phase of existence as to this. When death calls, he neither deprives us of the virtues, nor relieves us of the vices, of which he finds us possessed. Both must go with us. Those qualities, moral, social, intellectual, which may have distinguished us in this world will be ours also in another, there constituting our identity and determining our position. And as the good, so the evil. That dark vestment of sin with which, in a man's progress through life, he may have become gradually endued, will cling to him, close as the tunic of Nessus, through the death-change. He, too, still remains the being he was. He retains his evil identity and decides his degraded rank. He awakes amid the torment of the same base thoughts and brutal passions that controlled him here, and that will attract to him, in the associates of his new life, thoughts as base and passions as brutal. Is there in the anticipation of a material Hell, begirt with flames, stronger influence to deter from vice, than in the terrible looming up of an inevitable fate like that?

Inevitable, but not eternal. While there is life, there is hope; and there is life beyond the vail.

But I should be commencing another volume, instead of terminating the present, were I to enlarge on the benefits that may accrue from spiritual agency. The task I set to myself was to treat of an antecedent inquiry; an inquiry into the reality, not into the advantages, of ultramundane intervention. With a single additional observation, then, touching the bearings of that inquiry on the credence of the Christian world, I here close my task.

It is not possible to rise from the perusal of the Scriptures, Old or New, without feeling that the verity of communication with the Invisible World is the groundwork of all we have read. This is not a matter left to inference or construction,—nothing like a case of chronological or narrational variance, which commentators may reconcile or philologists may explain away. It is a question essential, inherent, fundamental. Admit much to be allegory, make allowance for the phraseology of Oriental tongues, for the language of parable and the license of poetry, there yet remains, vast, calm, and not to be mistaken, the firm faith of that Old World in the reality, and the occasional influence directly exerted, of the world of spirits. That faith undermined, the foundations are sapped of the entire Biblical superstructure.

I speak of a great fact declared, not of minute details supplied. The pneumatology of the Bible is general, not specific, in its character. It enters not upon the mode, or the conditions, under which the denizens of another sphere may become agents to modify the character or influence the destiny of mankind. It leaves man to find his way along that interesting path by the

43*

light of analogy,—perhaps by the aid of such disclosures as this work records. The light may be imperfect, the disclosures insufficient to appease an eager curiosity. In the dimness of the present, our longings for enlightenment may never attain satisfaction. We may be destined to wait. That which human wit and industry cannot compass in this twilight world, may be a discovery postponed only till we are admitted, beyond the boundary, into the morning sunshine of another.

ADDENDA

TO THE TENTH THOUSAND.

SINCE the preceding volume was published, doubts have arisen as to the accuracy of one of the narratives originally published, and, in consequence, (see footnote on page 345,) I have now omitted it, substituting another in its place.

On the other hand, I have been fortunate in obtaining for two narratives additional vouchers, which have been inserted in the English reprint of this work, recently issued. The narratives which have been thus corroborated are the "Wynyard Apparition," (page 381,) and "Gaspar," (page 461.)

In regard to the former, it happens, singularly enough, after the lapse of seventy-five years, that an original document has recently come to light in an article published in that useful London periodical, *"Notes and Queries."*

The article in question contains a certified copy of a letter written, thirty-eight years after the date of the incident, by one who may be said to have been an actor in the scene.

From this letter we learn that, soon after the figure had appeared to Sherbroke and Wynyard, and while these two officers were engaged, in the inner room, seeking some explanation of this intrusion, a brother officer, Lieutenant Ralph Gore, coming in, joined in the search. At his suggestion, also, next day, Sherbroke made a memorandum of the date.

From this letter we also learn the exact locality where the incident occurred,—namely, at Sydney, in the island of Cape Breton, off Nova Scotia, and in a room in the new barracks which had been erected there in the summer of 1784,—and that the regiment to which these officers belonged was the thirty-third, at that time commanded by Lieutenant-Colonel Yorke.

By the article referred to, it further appears that the Lieutenant Gore above mentioned had in the year 1823 attained the grade of lieutenant-colonel, and was then stationed in garrison at Quebec. On the 3d of October of that year, a discussion in regard to the Wynyard apparition having arisen during a party then assembled

511

at the house of the late Chief-Justice Sewell, who resided on the esplanade in Quebec, Sir John Harvey, Adjutant-General of the forces in Canada, despatched in writing to Colonel Gore certain queries on the subject. That officer replied, also in writing, on the same day; and his statements corroborate all the particulars above given, so far as he is concerned. He adds that "letters from England brought the account of John Wynyard's death on the very night his brother and Sherbroke saw the apparition." The questions addressed to Colonel Gore, and his replies, in full, are given in "Notes and Queries," for July 2, 1859, No. 183, p. 14. The colonel is there betrayed into a trifling inaccuracy in speaking of Lieutenant Wynyard, in 1785, as captain. The Army Register for that year shows that Sherbroke then held the grade of captain, but Wynyard that of lieutenant only.

In regard to the second narrative, entitled "Gaspar," which, it will be recollected, was narrated by Mr. S. C. Hall, as obtained by him in Worcester, England, from the mouth of one of the principal witnesses, the supplementary testimony was obtained in this wise:—

The narrative was copied, in June, 1860, into the columns of the "Worcester Herald;" and that paper, in reproducing it, expressed the opinion that it was a hoax played off by Mr. Hall on myself. A few days afterward, however, the editor, with commendable frankness, retracted that opinion in these words:—"We owe Mr. Hall an apology. The banker at whose house the parties met in Worcester—to wit, Mr. Hall and the lady who related her experiences of Gaspar, the familiar spirit—assures us that Mr. Hall has given the story most faithfully and exactly as she told it; and that the accessories—the account of the lady's character and bearing, the impression created on the mind by her truthful manner and apparent earnestness of conviction—are also most faithfully rendered. We trust Mr. Carter Hall will excuse us for suspecting him of playing on a friend's credulity. We know of no man more gifted in the grand and peculiar art of Defoe, of imparting to fiction the reality of fact."

I esteem myself fortunate in thus obtaining an additional voucher for one of the most extraordinary narratives in this volume.

APPENDIX.

NOTE A.

CIRCULAR OF A SOCIETY, INSTITUTED BY MEMBERS OF THE UNIVERSITY OF CAMBRIDGE, ENGLAND, FOR THE PURPOSE OF INVESTIGATING PHENOMENA POPULARLY CALLED SUPERNATURAL.

THE interest and importance of a serious and earnest inquiry into the nature of the phenomena which are vaguely called "supernatural" will scarcely be questioned. Many persons believe that all such apparently mysterious occurrences are due either to purely natural causes, or to delusions of the mind or senses, or to willful deception. But there are many others who believe it possible that the beings of the unseen world may manifest themselves to us in extraordinary ways, and also are unable otherwise to explain many facts, the evidence for which cannot be impeached. Both parties have obviously a common interest in wishing cases of supposed "supernatural" agency to be thoroughly sifted. If the belief of the latter class should be ultimately confirmed, the limits which human knowledge respecting the spirit-world has hitherto reached might be ascertained with some degree of accuracy. But in any case, even if it should appear that morbid or irregular workings of the mind or senses will satisfactorily account for every such marvel, still, some progress would be made toward ascertaining the laws which regulate our being, and thus adding to our scanty knowledge of an obscure but important province of science The main impediment to investigations of this kind is the difficulty of obtaining a sufficient number of clear and well-attested cases. Many of the stories current in tradition, or scattered up and down in books, may be exactly true; others must be purely fictitious; others, again,—probably the greater number,—consist of a mixture of truth and falsehood. But it is idle to examine the significance of an alleged fact of this nature until the trustworthiness, and also the extent, of the evidence for it are ascertained. Impressed with this conviction, some members of the University of Cambridge are anxious, if possible, to form an extensive collection of authenticated cases of supposed "supernatural" agency. When the inquiry is once commenced, it will evidently be needful to seek for information beyond the limits of their own immediate circle. From all those, then, who may be inclined to aid them, they request written communications, with full details of persons, times, and places; but it will not be required that names should be inserted without special permission, unless they have already become public property: it is, however, indispensable that the person making any communication should be acquainted with the names, and should pledge himself for the truth of the narrative from his own knowledge or conviction.

The first object, then, will be the accumulation of an available body of facts: the use to be made of them must be a subject for future consideration; but, in any case, the mere collection of trustworthy information will be of value. And it is manifest that great help in the inquiry may be derived from accounts of circumstances which have been at any time considered "supernatural," and afterward proved to be due to delusions of the mind or senses, or to natural causes; (such, for instance, as the operation of those strange and subtle forces which have been discovered and imperfectly investigated in recent times;) and, in fact, generally, from any particulars which may throw light indirectly, by analogy or otherwise, on the subjects with which the present investigation is more expressly concerned.

The following temporary classification of the phenomena about which information is sought may serve to show the extent and character of the inquiry proposed.

1 Appearances of angels.
    (1.) Good.
    (2.) Evil.

II Spectral appearances of
    (1.) The beholder himself, (*e.g.* "Fetches" or "Doubles.")
    (2.) Other men, recognized or not.
        (i.) Before their death, (*e.g.* "Second-Sight.")
            (*a.*) To one person.
            (*b.*) To several persons.
        (ii.) At the moment of their death.
            (*a.*) To one person.
            (*b.*) To several persons.
                1. In the same place.
                2. In several places.
                    i. Simultaneously.
                    ii. Successively.
        (iii.) After their death.   In connection with
            (*a.*) Particular places, remarkable for
                1. Good deeds.
                2. Evil deeds.
            (*b.*) Particular times, (*e.g.* on the anniversary of any event, or at fixed seasons.)
            (*c.*) Particular events, (*e.g.* before calamity or death.)
            (*d.*) Particular persons, (*e.g.* haunted murderers.)

III. "Shapes" falling under neither of the former classes.
    (1.) Recurrent.   In connection with
        (i.) Particular families, (*e.g.* the "Banshee.")
        (ii.) Particular places, (*e.g.* the "Mawth Dog.")
    (2.) Occasional.
        (i.) Visions signifying events, past, present, or future.
            (*a.*) By actual representation, (*e.g.* "Second-Sight.")
            (*b.*) By symbol.
        (ii.) Visions of a fantastical nature.

IV. Dreams remarkable for coincidences
    (1.) In their occurrence.
        (i.) To the same person several times.
        (ii.) In the same form to several persons.
            (*a.*) Simultaneously.
            (*b.*) Successively.

(2.) With facts
    (i.) Past.
        (*a.*) Previously unknown.
        (*b.*) Formerly known, but forgotten.
    (ii.) Present, but unknown.
    (iii.) Future.

V. Feelings.   A definite consciousness of a fact
    (1.) Past,—an impression that an event has happened.
    (2.) Present,—sympathy with a person suffering or acting at a distance.
    (3.) Future,—presentiment.

VI. Physical effects.
    (1.) Sounds,
        (i.) With the use of ordinary means, (*e.g.* ringing of bells.)
        (ii.) Without the use of any apparent means, (*e.g.* voices.)
    (2.) Impressions of touch, (*e.g.* breathings on the person.)

Every narrative of "supernatural" agency which may be communicated will be rendered far more instructive if accompanied by any particulars as to the observer's natural temperament, (*e.g.* sanguine, nervous, &c.,) constitution, (*e.g.* subject to fever, somnambulism, &c.,) and state at the time, (*e.g.* excited in mind or body, &c.)

Communications may be addressed to
    Rev. B. F. Westcott, *Harrow, Middlesex,*
or to

(Postscript.)

NOTE B.

TESTIMONY:

VIEW TAKEN OF IT BY TWO OPPOSING SCHOOLS.

SINCE the foregoing pages were in type, I have received, and perused with much pleasure, a pamphlet, just published in London and Edinburgh, entitled *"Testimony: its Posture in the Scientific World,"* by ROBERT CHAMBERS, F.R.S.E., F.A.S., &c., being the first of a series of "Edinburgh papers," to be issued by that vigorous thinker,—a man who has contributed as much, perhaps, as any other now living, to the dissemination of useful information among the masses throughout the civilized world. Not the least valuable contribution is this very pamphlet.

Mr. Chambers reviews the posture of two schools of philosophy in regard to the force of testimony: the physicists, of whom Mr. Faraday is the type; and the mental and moral philosophers, represented by Abercrombie and Chalmers.

The first, he reminds us, taking into view "the extreme fallaciousness of the human senses," will admit no evidence of any extraordinary natural fact which is not "absolutely incapable of being explained away." If the physicist can presume any error in the statement, he is bound to reject it. "Practically," (Chambers adds,) "all such facts *are* rejected; for there is, of course, no extraordinary fact resting upon testimony alone, of which it is not possible to presume some error in the observation or reporting, if we set about finding one." (p. 2.)

Thus, Mr. Faraday, "defending the skepticism of his class," argues that "there is no trusting our senses, unless the judgment has been largely cultivated for their guidance." He speaks as if there were a bare possibility that a man not regularly trained to scientific observation should see facts truly at all.

44   517

Not so Abercrombie or Chalmers. The great Scottish theologian "professes to walk by the Baconian philosophy. He acknowledges that knowledge can only be founded on observation, and that we learn 'by descending to the sober work of seeing and feeling and experimenting.' He prefers what has been 'seen by one pair of eyes' to all reasoning and guessing. . . . He does not propose that we only receive the marvelous facts of Scripture if we cannot explain them away. . . . He does not ask us to start with a clear understanding of what is possible or impossible. . . . What *he* requires of us 'on entering into any department of inquiry,' as the best preparation, is a very different thing: namely, '*that docility of mind which is founded on a sense of our total ignorance of the subject.*' "*

"No contrast," Chambers continues, "could well be more complete. In the one case, testimony regarding assumedly natural, though novel, facts and occurrences, is treated with a rigor which *would enable us to battle off any thing whatever that we did not wish to receive,* if it could not be readily subjected to experiment, or immediately shown in a fresh instance,—and perhaps even then. In the other, the power and inclination of men to observe correctly any palpable fact, and report it truly, is asserted without exception or reserve. . . . It is plain that one or other of these two views of testimony must be wholly, or in a great degree, erroneous, as they are quite at issue with each other. It becomes of importance, both with a regard to our progress in philosophy and our code of religious beliefs, to ascertain which it is that involves the greatest amount of truth." (p. 6.)

As to the effect, in every-day life, of adopting the scientific view of testimony, he says, "Just suppose, for a moment, that every fact reported to us by others were viewed in the light of the skeptical system, as to the fallaciousness of the senses and the tendency to self-deception. Should we not from that moment be at a stand-still in all the principal movements of our lives? Could a banker ever discount a bill? Could a merchant believe in a market-report? Could the politician put any trust in the genealogy of the monarch? Could we rest with assurance upon any legal deed or document heretofore thought essential to the maintenance of property? Could evidence for the condemnation of the most audacious and dangerous criminal be obtained? Each geologist distrusting his neighbor as to the actuality of the find of fossils in certain strata, what would be the progress of that science? Could we, with any face, ask the young

* Pamphlet cited, p. 6. The italics, throughout, are as Chambers has them.

to believe in a single fact of history, or geography, or any science concerned in education ? What could be more seriously inconvenient to mortals, short of the withdrawal of the sun from the firmament, than the abstraction of this simple principle from the apparatus of social life, that we can all tolerably well apprehend the nature of an event or fact presented to our senses, and give a fair representation of it in words afterward ?

"I must also make bold to say that the skeptical view appears to me out of harmony with the inductive philosophy. Bacon gives us many warnings against preconceived opinions and prejudices; but he does not bid us despair of ascertaining facts from our own senses and from testimony. He laments that there is an impediment in the acquisition of knowledge from the sense of sight being unable to penetrate 'the spiritual operation in tangible bodies;'* but he nowhere tells us that sight is so fallacious that we require a corrective power to assure us that we have really seen any thing." (p. 8.)

Adverting to Faraday's axiom, that we must set out with clear ideas of the possible and impossible, Chambers shrewdly remarks, "This skeptical method consists very much in vicious circles. You cannot know whether a fact be a fact till you have ascertained the laws of nature in the case; and you cannot know the laws of nature till you have ascertained facts. You must not profess to have learned any thing till you have ascertained if it be possible; and this you cannot ascertain till you have learned every thing." (p. 9.)

The whole pamphlet is singularly logical, as well as practical in tendency, and will well repay a perusal. Unable, for lack of space, much further to extend my extracts from it, I must not omit to quote entire the concluding paragraph, strictly bearing, as it does, on the respect which should be shown, and the credit which may properly be accorded, to those classes of facts which it is the object of this work to place before the public. Chambers says,

"If I have here given a true view of human testimony, it will follow that, among the vast multitude of alleged things often heard of and habitually rejected, there are many entitled to more respect than they ordinarily receive. It is a strange thought, but possibly some truths may have been knocking at the door of human faith for thousands of years, and are not destined to be taken in for many yet to come,—or, at the utmost, may long receive but an unhonoring sanction from the vulgar and obscure, all owing to this principle of skepticism, that facts are value-

---

* *Novum Organum*, Book I. aphorism 50.

less without an obvious relation to ascertained law. Should the contrary and (as I think) more inductive principle be ever adopted, that facts rightly testified to are worthy of a hearing, with a view to the ascertaining of some law under which they may be classed, a liberal retrospect along the history of knowledge will probably show to us that even among what have been considered as the superstitions of mankind there are some valuable realities. Wherever there is a perseverance and uniformity of report on almost any subject, however heterodox it may have appeared, there may we look with some hopefulness that a principle or law will be found, if duly sought for. There is a whole class of alleged phenomena, of a mystically psychical character, mixing with the chronicles of false religions and of hagiology, in which it seems not unlikely that we might discover some golden grains. Perhaps, nay, probably, some mystic law, centering deep in our nature, and touching far-distant spheres of 'untried being,' runs through these undefined phenomena,—which, if it ever be ascertained, will throw not a little light upon the past beliefs and actions of mankind,—perhaps add to our assurance that there is an immaterial and immortal part within us, and a world of relation beyond that now pressing upon our senses."*

* Pamphlet cited, p. 24.

INDEX.

THE END.

Printed in the United States
90091LV00005B/57/A

9 780766 187252